Hearts for Him Through Time: Creation to Christ

A Learning Program for Ages 9-11

(with extensions for older students)

Written by Carrie Austin, M.Ed.

Editor:

Julie Grosz, M.Ed.

Cover Designer:

Merlin DeBoer

Heart of Dakota Publishing
www.heartofdakota.com

Special Thanks to:

Our Lord and Savior, Jesus Christ, for giving us the desire to train up our children in the Lord. May He be glorified through this work.

My parents, Ken and Marlene Mellema, for their faithful example of living for Christ and their steadfast commitment to family that has lasted a lifetime. I am so blessed by their unwavering support. They have lovingly encouraged me to pursue the Lord's will for my life and have watched over my children as I've written this book. I can only hope to live up to their example one day.

Julie Grosz for her countless hours of editing, her teaching expertise and knowledge, her listening ear, and her eye for detail. I am so thankful for her steadfast support and encouragement and her enthusiasm for using our programs with her own children. God blessed me with Julie.

Dave and Cindy Madden for forging a new path by homeschooling their seven precious children. We are so thankful that they have gone before us and are a living example of how to live our lives for Christ. I am blessed to call Cindy my sister and my friend.

Mike Austin for his unending support and love, his patient encouragement, and consistent hard work without complaint. I am blessed by his faithful commitment to prayer. He is the love of my life and a cherished father to our four boys. Without him, there would be no Heart of Dakota Publishing.

Cole, Shaw, Greyson, and Beau Austin, my sons, who are the motivation for my writing and my teaching. They are truly an inspiration to me and are wonderful blessings from our Father in heaven.

Copyright 2009, 2016, 2019, 2023 by Carrie Austin
Heart of Dakota Publishing, Inc.
1004 Westview Drive
Dell Rapids, SD 57022

Website: www.heartofdakota.com
Phone (605) 428-4068

ISBN 978-1-61584-560-6

Table of Contents

Introduction

Complete Plans

Hearts for Him Through Time: Creation to Christ features 35 units with complete daily plans. Each unit lasts 4 days, which gives you the 5th day of each week to use as you wish. The 4-day plan can be stretched to cover 5 days if needed. This guide is meant to save you time planning, so you can instead spend your time teaching and enjoying your children. Activities are rotated daily, so you can cover many areas that might often be neglected, without lengthening your school day. These plans are designed to provide an academic, well-balanced approach to learning.

Easy to Use

Simple daily plans are provided on each two-page spread. The subjects can be done in any order. Each day of plans is divided into the following 2 parts: "Learning Through History" and "Learning the Basics". Each segment of plans is further designated as "Teacher Directed = T", "Semi-Independent = S", or "Independent = I". Dividing the plans in this manner is meant to help you move your children toward more independent work. Easy to follow daily plans are divided into 10 boxes, which can be spaced throughout the day as time allows.

Learning Through History

The "Learning Through History" part of the program is told in story form and provides a deeper look at the ancient time period from Creation to Christ. This year of study is meant to provide students with a Biblical overview of ancient history, as students journey through time toward the birth of Christ the promised Savior. Within the readings, students will learn about the Sumerians, the Hebrews, the Egyptians, the Phoenicians, the Assyrians, the Babylonians, the Persians, the Greeks, and the Romans. Biblical history will be shown to be authoritative, as the history of ancient civilizations weaves in and out of Old Testament stories at the proper places in the narrative. An exciting overview of ancient Greece, ancient Rome, and of Christ's life comes next, and the year concludes with the readings of the gospels of Luke, John, and Acts.

The following areas are linked with the history readings: a prophecy fulfillment chart, guided written narrations, timeline entries, copywork, research questions, history projects, Bible passage memory work, sketching, history notebooking, oral narrations, mapping, Bible quiet time, read-alouds, and an audio overview of history.

Learning the Basics

The "Learning the Basics" part of the program focuses on language arts, math, Bible, geography, and science. It includes dictation practice and passages, a choice of scheduled grammar texts, a creative writing program, reading choices, painting and memorization of the poetry of Robert Frost, oral narrations, a choice of math texts, a Bible study of the roots of the ancient church, geography of the Bible lands, and scheduled science readings with lessons.

Quick Activities

Creation to Christ was written with the busy homeschool teacher in mind. It provides a way to do enriching activities without all of the usual planning and preparation. Quick and easy activities require little or no preparation and use materials you're likely to have on hand.

Fun Ideas

Engaging daily lessons take approximately 4 to 4½ hours to complete. More time will be needed if you linger on activities or draw out discussions. The activities are filled with ideas that get kids thinking, exploring, and learning in a meaningful way.

Balanced

Each day's lessons are carefully planned to provide a balance of oral, written, and hands-on work. In this way, oral narration is practiced daily, but in a variety of subject areas. Written work is required daily, but care is taken to balance it with other forms of assessment. Hands-on experiences are provided in each day's plans, but they do not require overwhelming amounts of time.

Flexible

Lesson plans are written to allow you to customize the program to suit your child's needs. A choice of resources is provided. An Extension Pack Schedule in the Appendix extends the area of history to include more advanced reading material. This allows your older students to learn along with your younger students.

Resources

All of the resources noted in *Creation to Christ* are available from Heart of Dakota Publishing. Resources may be ordered online at www.heartofdakota.com, by mail using the printable online order form, or by telephone at (605) 428-4068. Resource titles are listed below.

History Resources (Required)

The Story of the Ancient World by Christine Miller – A Revised and Expanded Edition of 'The Story of the Chosen People' by H.A. Guerber (Nothing New Press, 2006, Second Edition 2015)

Streams of History: Ancient Greece by Ellwood W. Kemp (Yesterday's Classics, 2008)

Streams of History: Ancient Rome by Ellwood W. Kemp (Yesterday's Classics, 2008)

The Radical Book for Kids by Champ Thornton (New Growth Press, 2016)

A Child's Geography Vol. II – Explore the Holy Land by Ann Voskamp and Tonia Peckover (Second Edition 2008, MasterBooks Edition, 2020)

What in the World? Vol. 1: Ancient Civilizations and the Bible by Diana Waring (Diana Waring, 2012) Note: This audio CD set is available in several versions. The 2012 Diana Waring version matches with the track numbers in this guide and includes the audio material needed for this study.

Draw and Write Through History: Greece and Rome by Carylee Gressman and illustrated by Peggy Dick (CPR Publishing, 2007)

Creation to Christ Student Notebook designed by Merlin DeBoer (Heart of Dakota Publishing, 2009)

Science Resources (Required, unless you have your own science)
Exploring Creation with Zoology 3: Land Animals of the Sixth Day by Jeannie K. Fulbright (Apologia Educational Ministries, 2008)
Birds of the Air by Arabella B. Buckley (Yesterday's Classics, 2008)
Plant Life in Field and Garden by Arabella B. Buckley (Yesterday's Classics, 2008)
Exploring the History of Medicine by John Hudson Tiner (Master Books, 2006, 2022)
Galen and the Gateway to Medicine by Jeanne Bendick (Bethlehem Books, 2002)
An Illustrated Adventure in Human Anatomy by Kate Sweeney (Lippincott Williams & Wilkins, 2002)

Resource Choices (Considered to be necessary choices)
*Choose one of the following reading options to use with this program:
    1. *Drawn into the Heart of Reading: Level 4/5* or *Level 6/7/8* by Carrie Austin (Heart of Dakota Publishing, 2000)
    2. Your own program
*Choose one of the following English options to use with this program:
    1. *Building with Diligence: English 4* by Rod and Staff Publishers (Rod and Staff Publishers, 1992)
    2. *Following the Plan: English 5* by Rod and Staff Publishers (Rod and Staff Publishers, 1993)
    3. Your own program
*Choose one of the following writing options to use with this program:
    1. *Writing & Rhetoric Book 1: Fable* and *Book 2: Narrative I* by Paul Kortepeter (Classical Academic Press, 2013)
    2. Your own program
*Choose one of the following math options to use with this program:
    1. *Singapore Primary Mathematics 4A/4B* or *5A/5B: U.S. Edition* by Singapore Ministry of Education (Times New Media, 2003)
    2. *Apologia Math Level 4* or *5* by Kathryn Gomes (Apologia Educational Ministries, Inc. 2021, 2022)
    3. *Math With Confidence Level 4* or *5* by Kate Snow (Well-Trained Mind Press, Projected dates: 2024, 2025)
    4. Your own program
*Choose one of the following Bible options to use with this program:
    1. *The Illustrated Family Bible* by Dorling Kindersley (DK Publishing, 2016)
    2. Your own Bible
*Choose the following CD to aid in memorizing Philippians 2 (scheduled in guide):
    1. *The Bible Study in Stereo: Philippians 2 CD* composed by Martha Minter (Marianne Greer, 2003)

Note: Resources sometimes go out of print or undergo changes. Brief schedule changes between new guide editions will be available under the "Updates" portion of our website at www.heartofdakota.com. Lengthier replacement schedules will be sent along with your purchase of the corresponding guide or book from Heart of Dakota.

"Learning Through History" Components

Reading About History

The "Learning Through History" part of the program is told in story form and provides a deeper look at the ancient time period from Creation to Christ. This year of study is meant to provide students with a Biblical overview of ancient history, as students journey through time toward the birth of Christ the promised Savior.

History stories are scheduled for the students to read independently each day using the following resources: *The Story of the Ancient World* by Christine Miller, *Streams of History: Ancient Greece* by Ellwood W. Kemp, *Streams of History: Ancient Rome* by Ellwood W. Kemp, and a Bible of your choice. These stories provide the focus for this part of the plans. The areas that follow are linked to the daily stories:

Day 1: Research questions are provided for students to answer on a topic inspired by the history study. Students use an index or a search engine to skim to find answers, and to formulate information from the answers they've gathered.
One or more comprehensive history encyclopedias (in print form or on the internet) is recommended for use with the lessons. A Bible dictionary or encyclopedia would also be helpful.
Day 2: A portion of the history reading is selected by the student to copy in the *Student Notebook*. Students are instructed to select a memorable passage that is worthy of being reread.
Day 3: To understand the flow of history, students keep a timeline within their *Student Notebook* of the major events studied throughout the year.
Day 4: Instruction is provided to guide students in writing narrations. The level of guidance gradually decreases throughout the year, until students are writing narrations independently.

Independent History Study

Daily independent history assignments that correspond with the historical time period are scheduled using these resources: *What in the World? Vol. 1* by Diana Waring, *Draw and Write Through History: Greece and Rome* by Carylee Gressman and illustrated by Peggy Dick, and *Creation to Christ Student Notebook* designed by Merlin DeBoer. Audio presentations, copywork of quotes and verses, notebook entries, sketching, and the completion of a prophecy chart are all part of the independent history study part of the plans.

Accuracy and attention to authentic detail are encouraged. Entries are meant to be factual and to provide a finished product that gives an overview of the history topics studied throughout the year. Reminders are given when work is to be done in cursive. Notebook entries are done within the *Student Notebook*. A 3-ring binder with a place to insert a cover page is needed for storing the *Student Notebook* pages.

"Learning Through History" Components
(continued)

The books in the "Reading About History" part of the plans and the resources listed in the "Independent History Study" part of the plans are sold as a set in the **Economy Package**, or individually, at www.heartofdakota.com.

History Project

Three days in each unit are devoted to a meaningful, hands-on project that is designed to bring the history stories to life. Each project is scheduled to be easily completed by the student semi-independently in three short stages. Projects require little or no preparation and use materials you are likely to have on hand. Projects correlate closely with the history stories and provide an important creative outlet for students to express what they've learned.

Projects range from creating an ancient Phoenician board game, to carving a cylinder seal like the ones used by ancient kings; from painting gemstones for the High Priest's breastplate, to folding an origami prayer box; from constructing a working catapult, to holding Olympic Game Trials; from designing your own Philistine headgear, to baking Egyptian Palace Bread; from making a wordless book for sharing the gospel of Jesus, to etching a cross, and much more!

Bible Quiet Time

Each day includes the following Bible study activities: Bible reading from *The Illustrated Family Bible* or your own Bible, a Scripture focus, a prayer focus, Scripture memory work, and music. As often as possible, Bible readings correspond with the history readings. Within each unit the prayer focus rotates through the 4 parts of prayer: adoration, confession, thanksgiving, and supplication. The Scripture focus sets the tone for the prayer for that day. Students memorize all of Philippians 2 through repetition, copywork, and music. Musical selections from *The Bible Study in Stereo: Philippians 2* correspond with the Bible memory verses in the program. At the end of each unit, students copy the Scripture memory selection in a *Common Place Book*. A *Common Place Book* is often a bound composition book with lined pages. It provides a common place to copy anything that is timeless, memorable, or worthy of rereading.

Storytime

There are 3 book set options for Storytime: History Interest Set, Boy Interest Set, or Girl Interest Set. If you desire to read aloud books that coordinate with the historical time period being studied, you will want to choose the History Interest Set. In keeping with the ancient time period, the History Interest Set does contain some violent content. If you wish to avoid this, choose the Boy Interest or Girl Interest Set instead; these sets do not match the history, but were instead selected to provide excellent read-alouds from 9 different genres. Sixth and seventh graders should either listen to the History Interest Set read aloud, or read the Extension Package books (as scheduled in the Appendix), or do both of these options in order to extend their learning. If you are a family that enjoys reading aloud, you may choose to read aloud more than one set of books from the Basic Package.

"Learning Through History" Components
(continued)

These scheduled read-alouds are highly recommended, unless you need to economize. Complete listings and book descriptions for these books can be found in the Appendix. These books are sold as a set as **Basic Package Option 1, 2**, or **3**, or sold individually, at www.heartofdakota.com.

Each unit includes the following activities in coordination with the "Storytime" read-aloud assignments:

Day 1: give a detailed oral narration
Day 2: rotate through the following 4 narration activities: an outline sketch, a short skit, a question and answer session, and an advertisement speech for the book
Day 3: give a summary narration
Day 4: make connections between the story and Proverbs

Independent History Study for Older Students

An Extension Package Schedule in the Appendix extends the area of history to include more advanced independent reading material. This allows your older students to learn along with your younger students. Due to the more mature content of the books within the ancient time period – both in the violence that was prevalent in this period and the depravity of worship of pagan gods – this extension package is best suited for mature 6th and 7th graders who are strong, independent readers.

A schedule of daily independent readings for these books is provided in the Appendix of *Hearts for Him Through Time: Creation to Christ*. Books are at a mid-sixth to upper seventh grade reading level. For very sensitive sixth or seventh graders, or for those who are not yet strong readers, we recommend the Basic Package Option 1 – History Set for the parent to read aloud instead. Complete listings and book descriptions for these books can be found in the Appendix. These books are sold as a set in the **Extension Package**, or individually, at www.heartofdakota.com. This package is an optional part of *Hearts for Him Through Time: Creation to Christ*.

"Learning the Basics" Components

Geography

Geography is studied using *A Child's Geography Vol. II: Explore the Holy Land*. Two days in each unit focus on the geography of the Holy Land. Students will explore six Middle Eastern countries with vivid scenes through the engaging text of a "living book". Activities include narration prompts, notebooking and mapping activities, as well as "Bringing It Home" suggestions that focus on each country's art, music, poetry, and food. A Prayer Walk for each country is also included. This book is scheduled for the parent and student to read and discuss together.

Bible Study

Two days in each unit take an explorer's approach to the Bible, church history, and life using *The Radical Book for Kids*. This interactive book communicates big truths about the Bible and life. *The Radical Book for Kids* takes children on a journey into the ancient church, deep into the ancient roots and Biblical theology of the Christian faith. Kids learn about ancient weapons, discover ancient languages, use secret codes, locate stars, tell time using the sun, play a board game that's 3,000 years old, and more. They'll also learn about the radical men and women who have gone before them and trusted Jesus in the face of great odds. This book is scheduled for the parent and student to read and discuss together.

Poetry and Painting

Poetry is scheduled daily using *Paint Like a Poet*, with a different classic poem written by Robert Frost introduced each unit. *Paint Like a Poet* combines poetry and painting for a one-of-a-kind approach to watercolor painting. Designed to accompany the "Poetry" plans, *Paint Like a Poet* provides a host of easy-to-follow watercolor tutorials inspired by the scenic poetry of Robert Frost. Each painting lesson introduces a new poem with highlighted text to show which lines to use for copywork. Each poem was chosen for its scenic quality and its ability to withstand the test of time. Each unit includes the following poetry study activities:

Day 1: read and appreciate the poetry of Robert Frost; neatly copy a portion of the poem to be included in the painting project

Day 2: use painting techniques to illustrate poetry

Day 3: explore poetry moods with painting lessons

Day 4: share the poetry of Robert Frost and learn about his life
*Each 9 week term: memorize a previously studied Robert Frost poem

Paint Colors:

The following paint colors will either need to be purchased or mixed from other paint colors to complete the lessons. If you are buying paints within a set, use the general color list below. If you prefer to purchase individual colors, some suggestions for specific shades are listed behind each color; however these specific shades are **not** required.

Note: Heart of Dakota sells a Painting Supplies Kit for *Paint Like a Poet* that includes all necessary materials for the painting lessons.

Yellow (Lemon Yellow or Cadmium Yellow Light)
Red (Alizarin Crimson or Cadmium Red Medium)
Blue (Cobalt Blue or Ultramarine Blue)
Light Blue (Cerulean Blue or Sky Blue)
Dark Blue (Phthalo Blue)
Green (Emerald Green or Viridian)
Dark Green (Hooker's Green)
Orange (Cadmium Orange)
Pink or Rose (Permanent Rose)
Purple (Ultramarine Violet)
Brown (Burnt Sienna or Burnt Umber)
Grey (Payne's Gray)
White (Titanium White)
Black (Lamp Black)
Tan or Peach (Yellow Ochre or Flesh Tint)

Basic Painting Supplies:
*Water container (for rinsing brushes)
*White plastic palette (with wells for paint and areas for mixing)
*9" x 12" Watercolor paper (27-30 sheets 140 lb. cold press paper is recommended)
*Large flat brush (1" flat sable brush recommended, however you may use a
  different brush or type)
*Small flat brush (1/2" flat sable brush recommended, but you may use a
  different brush or type)
*Small round brush (#6 or #8 red sable brushes recommended, but you may
  use a different brush or type)

Other Painting Materials:
*Paper Towels
*Toothpicks
*Water dropper
*Pencil
*Masking Tape
*Plastic Wrap
*Table Salt
*Coin
*Two leaves (optional – can make your own leaf patterns to trace)
*Painting sponge (optional – can use wadded paper towel instead)

Helpful Painting Tips: (go over with students)
There are many ways to paint! For the lessons in *Paint Like a Poet,* you can use
either watercolor tube paints or most cakes/pans. We recommend tube paints if at
all possible. If finances allow, artist grade paints are better, but student grade
paints are acceptable.

If you are using most cakes/pans, you will need two water containers. Use one water container for mixing washes and one for clear water to rinse brushes. Before painting, first wet the brush to prepare it for the color. Next, load the brush with paint moving it back and forth across the surface of the paint in the pan. Do not dig into the paint. Use either the plastic lid of the paints or the mixing surface on the palette to mix the paint. Then, apply it to watercolor paper. If the paints in the wells get muddy colored, dip the brush into clean water and dip the brush tip in the paint well to lift out the muddy part of the color. Or, use a pointed bit of paper towel to lift out the muddy color.

Do not stand brushes on their tips or store them in water overnight. Clean brushes in cool water, gently tapping or flicking off the excess water. Then, dry with a soft cloth or paper towel. Store brushes bristle side up if possible, or in a brush box.

Grammar, Mechanics, Usage, and Writing

Grammar lessons are scheduled twice in each unit and focus on grammar, mechanics, and usage for the purpose of improving writing. Choose **either** *Building with Diligence: English 4* **or** *Following the Plan: English 5*. Half of the grammar text will be covered this year, with the other half to be completed in the guide that follows. Systematic lessons focus on one rule or concept per lesson. In order to keep the lessons short, you may want to do most of the lesson orally or on a white board, requiring only one set of practice exercises to be written by the student each day. The Teacher's Manual is considered to be necessary at this level. See the "Table of Contents" in either *Building with Diligence: English 4* or *Following the Plan: English 5* for a scope and sequence. Students need a lined composition book or notebook for their written work.

Writing lessons are scheduled twice in each unit using *Writing & Rhetoric Book 1* and *Book 2*. This series provides students with forms and models of excellent writing to imitate on their path to becoming a better writer. *Book 1: Fable* teaches close reading and comprehension, summarizing a story, amplifying with description and dialogue, and incorporating point of view. *Book 2: Narrative I* focuses on writing beginning/middle/end, narration, main idea, conflict, dialogue and description, topic writing and more! As students read excellent, whole-story examples of literature, they will learn key writing principles. With the step-by-step lessons in *Writing & Rhetoric,* students will grow their writing skills by using imitation.

Dictation

Studied dictation to practice spelling skills is scheduled three days in each unit. Three different levels of dictation passages are provided in the Appendix. The dictation passages are for use with students who have mastered basic spelling words. Special instructions for the dictation passages are included in the Appendix.

The Charlotte Mason method of studied dictation is used. In this method, students study the passage prior to having it dictated. This is an important step in learning to visualize the correct spelling of words. All items in the passage must be written correctly, including punctuation marks, before going on to the next passage. Studied dictation focuses on the goal of using correct spelling within the context of writing.

Permission is granted for you to make copies of the "Dictation Passages Key" to log your children's progress in dictation. A lined composition book is needed for dictation.

Handwriting/Copywork

Daily practice of cursive handwriting is scheduled from a variety of copywork sources. By copying from a correctly written model, students gain practice in handwriting, spelling, grammar, capitalization, punctuation, and vocabulary. Copywork also prepares students to write their own compositions. Work should be required to be done neatly and correctly. It is more important for students to produce careful, quality work, than to produce a large quantity of work that is carelessly done. If your student has had no formal instruction in cursive handwriting, you may want to use one of the recommended cursive handwriting options from *Bigger Hearts for His Glory*.

Reading

Three days in each unit recommend using *Drawn into the Heart of Reading* for literature study. This reading program is multi-level and is designed to use with any books you choose. It is available for students in levels 2-8. It is divided into nine literature units, which can be used in any order.

Drawn into the Heart of Reading is based on instructions and activities that work with any literature. It can be used with one or more students of multiple ages at the same time because it is structured around daily plans that are divided into three levels of instruction. *Drawn into the Heart of Reading* is intended for use year after year as you move students through the various levels of instruction. It is designed to teach students to evaluate characters using a Christian standard that is based on Godly traits.

In order to use *Drawn into the Heart of Reading* with your independent reader, you need the *Drawn into the Heart of Reading* Teacher's Guide and the *Level 4/5* or *Level 6/7/8 Student Book*. You may also choose whether to purchase these optional resources: *Level 4/5 Girl Interest Book Pack, Level 4/5 Boy Interest Book Pack,* or the *Sample Book Ideas List*. Packages for *Drawn into the Heart of Reading* are available at www.heartofdakota.com. Descriptions of books within each pack can be viewed online.

"Learning the Basics" Components
(continued)

Math Exploration

A math instruction reminder is listed in the plans daily. *Creation to Christ* offers a choice of *Singapore Primary Mathematics, Apologia Math,* or *Math with Confidence.* Both *Apologia Math* and *Math with Confidence* come with their own 4-day a week plan for math within their respective Teacher's Guides. Either *Level 4* or *5* is recommended for use with *Creation to Christ.* Schedules for *Singapore Math 4A/4B* and *5A/5B* are located in the Appendix of *Creation to Christ.* Both an "A" and a "B" set are needed for a full year of Singapore math instruction. For placement, go to www.singaporemath.com and click "placement" for a free math placement test. Choose the U.S. version of the test. Or, if you have a different math program that you are already comfortable using, feel free to substitute it for the math portion of the plans.

Independent Science Exploration

Daily independent science readings are scheduled using books contained in the Science Add-On Package. Reading material is meant for students to read independently. These books are sold as a set in the **Economy Package: Science Add-On,** or individually, at www.heartofdakota.com. This package includes these 6 engaging resources:

- *Land Animals of the Sixth Day* by Jeannie K. Fulbright
- *Birds of the Air* by Arabella B. Buckley
- *Plant Life in Field and Garden* by Arabella B. Buckley
- *Exploring the History of Medicine* by John Hudson Tiner
- *Galen and the Gateway to Medicine* by Jeannne Bendick
- *An Illustrated Adventure in Human Anatomy* by Kate Sweeney

These books provide the focus for this part of the plans. The area of life science is emphasized. "Science Exploration" topics correspond whenever possible with the general history topics being studied in the "Learning Through History" part of the plans.

While students read about God creating the world in history, they learn about God's vast animal kingdom in science. While studying God's plan for human life in ancient history, they study God's plan for bird and plant life in nature. While learning about the history of Rome, they learn about Galen, a doctor of the Roman Empire. While studying ancient people's advances in peace, law, and order they biographically study people's advances in medicine. Studying science in this manner allows for natural connections to be made between the two areas.

Each unit includes the following science activities in coordination with the read-aloud assignments:
Day 1: create a science notebook entry
Day 2: practice oral narration by retelling the science reading

"Learning The Basics" Components
(continued)

Day 3: write answers to five provided questions based on the science reading – including scientific terms and Biblical application

Day 4: conduct an experiment related to the reading and log it in a science notebook or on a copy of the "Science Lab Sheet" found in the Appendix

The students need a place to store their notebook entries, written answers, and science experiment results. Use either a 3-ring binder with plastic page protectors, or a bound sketchbook with unlined pages for the notebook assignments and science experiment results. An optional "Science Lab Sheet" is provided in the Appendix and may be reproduced for students to log their science experiment results. Use lined paper for the written answers on Day 3.

Please note that students will be making a book of animal tracks, bird sketches, and plant sketches as part of their notebook assignments. As directed in the plans, students may either make 3 separate booklets, or use a hardbound nature journal for this purpose.

Lesson Plans

Learning through History
Focus: The Beginning of History and of Sin

Unit 1 - Day 1

Reading about History [I]

Read about history in the following resource:

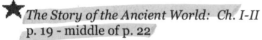

★ *The Story of the Ancient World: Ch. I-II p. 19 - middle of p. 22*

When God created man He placed him in a garden in Eden. Where could you look to research more about the **Garden of Eden**? Read the Bible passage Genesis 2:8-15 for the most accurate resource on the Garden of Eden.

Answer one or more of the following questions from your research: *Where was the Garden of Eden located? What grew in the garden? Why was man placed in the Garden of Eden? Name the 4 rivers that flowed from the river in Eden. Find the Tigris and Euphrates Rivers in Iraq on a globe. How would a worldwide flood make it hard to know where the Garden of Eden was once located?*

<u>Key Idea</u>: God gave man an eternal spirit.

History Project [S]

In this unit you will make a flapbook of the ten generations from Adam to Noah. Fold a white 8 ½ x 11 sheet of paper in half the long way. Next, use a ruler and a pencil to divide the front of the folded paper into eleven 1" strips. Use a dark marker to write, *Generations* on the top strip. Below that write the following ordinal numbers in order from top to bottom, one per strip: *1st, 2nd, 3rd, 4th, 5th, 6th, 7th, 8th, 9th, 10th*. Last, use colored pencils or crayons to lightly draw a scene on the front showing the Garden of Eden. Save your flapbook for Day 2.

<u>Key Idea</u>: Man is made in God's image.

Storytime [T]

Choose one of the following read aloud options:

★ *Dinosaurs of Eden* p. 3-11

★ Read at least one biography for the next 16 days of plans (see Appendix for suggestions).

After the reading, students will give a detailed oral narration. Select one paragraph from the story to read out loud to the students. This will be the starting point for the narration. Set a timer for 3-5 minutes. When the timer rings the narration is over, even if it isn't complete. A detailed, descriptive narration is the goal. See *Narration Tips* in the Appendix as needed.

<u>Key Idea</u>: Use oral narration to retell the story.

Bible Quiet Time [I]

Bible Reading: Choose one option below.

★ *The Illustrated Family Bible* p. 22-25

★ Your own Bible: Genesis chapters 1-2

Scripture Focus: Highlight Genesis 1:26-27.

Prayer Focus: Pray a prayer of adoration to worship and honor God. Begin by reading the highlighted verses out loud as a prayer. End by praying, *I worship you Lord for making me in your image. I admire you for...*

Scripture Memory: Recite Philippians 2:1.
Music: *Philippians 2* CD: Track 1 (verse 1)

<u>Key Idea</u>: God completed the work of creation in six days. He rested on the seventh day and made it holy. We are part of His creation.

Independent History Study [I]

★ Listen to *What in the World?* Disc 1, Tracks 1-2: "Welcome to World History" and "Creation". Note for parents: If you are not of the young earth philosophy, you may wish for your student to omit track 2.

<u>Key Idea</u>: Since no one but God was present at creation, the Bible gives the only clear picture of creation.

Learning the Basics
Focus: Language Arts, Math, Geography, Bible, and Science

Bible Study [T]

Read aloud and discuss with the students the following pages:

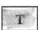 *The Radical Book for Kids* – "A Word of Explanation for Adults" and p. 1-4

Note: Parents should read "A Word of Explanation for Adults" on their own to understand the design of the book.

Key Idea: Study the meanings of the word *radical*. Notice connections in the Bible's big story and message from beginning to end. The Bible's big story is of Jesus and why He came.

Language Arts [S]

Have students complete the first studied dictation exercise (see Appendix for directions and passages).

Help students complete one lesson from the following reading program:

 *Drawn into the Heart of Reading*

Work with the students to complete **one** of the English options listed below:

 Building with Diligence: Lesson 1

 Following the Plan: Lesson 1

 Your own grammar program

Key Idea: Practice language arts skills.

Poetry [I]

Open *Paint Like a Poet* to Lesson 1. Read aloud the poem *"A Late Walk"*. On a 3 x 5 index card, neatly copy in black ink or in pencil the following highlighted lines from the poem:

A tree beside the wall stands bare,
But a leaf that lingered brown,
Disturbed, I doubt not, by my thought,
Comes softly rattling down.
                    -Robert Frost

Check your work to make sure it is correctly copied. Then, cut around your copywork. You may choose to outline the edge of the cut-out with a green marker. Save it for Day 3.

Key Idea: Read and appreciate a variety of classic poetry.

Math Exploration [S]

Choose **one** of the math options listed below.

 Singapore Primary Mathematics 4A/4B or *5A/5B* (see Appendix for schedules), or *Math with Confidence*, or *Apologia Math*

 Your own math program

Key Idea: Use a step-by-step math program.

Science Exploration [I]

 Day 1 of each unit includes a science notebook assignment. Store completed notebook entries in a 3-ring binder with plastic page protectors or a bound sketchbook with unlined pages. To get an overview of how animals are classified, have your parent help you view or print p. **17-19** of the "**Zoology 1 Sample**" from *Elementary Apologia: Zoology 1* at www.apologia.com. Find this sample by clicking on the Zoology 1 textbook image and scrolling down to "See Preview Samples." Then, read p. 17-19 of the sample on your own. Next, at the top of your first notebooking page, copy Genesis 2:19 in cursive. Beneath the verse, cut out and glue in the "Animal Classification Chart" from p. 19 of the pages you printed. If you do not have access to the internet, you may omit this assignment.

Key Idea: Zoologists are scientists who study animals. Taxonomy is used to group animals. All animals belong to the animal kingdom. Then, animals are grouped into phylums and after that into classes.

Reading about History 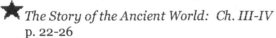 I

Read about history in the following resource:

★ *The Story of the Ancient World: Ch. III-IV* p. 22-26

You will be choosing a portion from today's reading that you found memorable or worthy of being reread to copy. Open your *Student Notebook* to Unit 1. In Box 3, carefully copy in cursive the portion from today's reading that you selected. Then, compare your written work to the original. Last, draw a small colorful picture in Box 3 to illustrate your sentences.

Key Idea: Adam and Eve dwelled in a garden in Eden filled with beautiful trees and animals. Adam was commanded by God not to eat the fruit from the tree of knowledge.

History Project S

Get the flapbook that you saved from Day 1. Cut on the pencil lines to make 11 flaps that you can lift. **Do not cut through the back of the flapbook.** After cutting, lift the top flap to reveal the paper underneath. Under the flap write, *There were 10 generations from Adam to Noah (Genesis 5)*. Fold back the flap labeled *1st* and write, *Adam – had 33 sons and 23 daughters. Lived to be 930.* Fold back the flap labeled *2nd* and write, *Seth – son of Adam, studied astronomy. Lived to be 912.* Fold back the flap labeled *3rd* and write, *Enos – son of Seth. Lived to be 905.* Fold back the flap labeled *4th* and write, *Cainan – son of Enos. Lived to be 910.* Save the flapbook for Day 3.

Key Idea: God had to punish Adam and Eve, but along with the penalty came a promise.

Storytime  T

Choose one of the following read aloud options:

★ *Dinosaurs of Eden* p. 12-23

★ Read aloud the next portion of the biography that you selected.

After reading, give each person a white piece of paper or a markerboard and a marker. Set a timer for 3-5 minutes and instruct each person to do a quick outline sketch about the story. Ideas for sketches include settings, characters, actions, important objects, or symbols. When the timer rings, briefly share the sketches.

Key Idea: Use sketching to share the story.

Bible Quiet Time   I

Reading: Choose one option below.

★ *The Illustrated Family Bible* p. 26-29

★ Your own Bible: Genesis chapters 3-4

Scripture Focus: Highlight Genesis 4:6-7.

Prayer Focus: Pray a prayer of confession to admit or acknowledge your sins to God. Begin by reading the highlighted verses out loud as a prayer. End by praying, *I confess to you Lord that I sometimes feel angry too. Forgive me for my anger and help me to do what is right.*

Scripture Memory: Recite Philippians 2:1.
Music: *Philippians 2* CD: Track 1 (verse 1)

Key Idea: The serpent tempted Eve to sin and disobey God's command. She ate from the tree of knowledge, and Adam sinned too.

Independent History Study   I

Open your *Student Notebook* to "Prophecies About Christ". Under "Prophecy" write, *Genesis 3:15*. Read the Scripture from the Bible to discover the prophecy. Under "Fulfillment" write, *1 John 3:8*. Read the fulfillment Scripture. Under "Description", write a few phrases to describe the prophecy about Jesus.

Key Idea: The Son of God would come to crush the serpent's head by destroying the devil's work.

Learning the Basics
Focus: Language Arts, Math, Geography, Bible, and Science

Geography [T]

Read aloud to the students the following pages:

 A Child's Geography Vol. II p. 7-11

Discuss with the students "Field Notes" p. 12.

<u>Key Idea:</u> The stories in the Bible are connected to the earth's geography. The Garden of Eden may have been located in Turkey.

Language Arts [S]

Help students complete one lesson from the following reading program:

 Drawn into the Heart of Reading
— make-up 9/5
Work with the students to complete **one** of the writing options listed below:

 Writing & Rhetoric Book 1: Fable
p. 1 – bottom of p. 4 (Note: Read the text aloud while the students follow along. Save "Talk About It" for Day 3.)

 Your own writing program

<u>Key Idea:</u> Practice language arts skills.

Poetry [I]

Open *Paint Like a Poet* to Lesson 1. Read aloud the poem *"A Late Walk"* by Robert Frost.

Today, you will be painting a yellow backdrop. You will need painting paper, a palette, water, a large flat paintbrush, and yellow paint.

After gathering your supplies, turn to the "Step-by-Step Watercolor Tutorial" for Lesson 1 in *Paint Like a Poet*. Follow steps 1-3 to complete "Part One: Yellow Backdrop". Then, let your background dry. You will complete "Part Two" of the tutorial on Day 3.

<u>Key Idea:</u> Use painting to illustrate poetry.

Math Exploration [S]

Choose **one** of the math options listed below.

 Singapore Primary Mathematics 4A/4B or 5A/5B (see Appendix for schedules), or *Math with Confidence,* or *Apologia Math*

 Your own math program

<u>Key Idea:</u> Use a step-by-step math program.

Science Exploration [I]

 Read *Land Animals of the Sixth Day* p. 1-4. Orally retell or narrate to an adult the portion of text that you read today. Use the *Narration Tips* in the Appendix for help as needed.

Note: Before narrating, please let your parents know that for the upcoming experiment on Day 4, you will need one package of M&M's or Skittles and 21 sheets of colored paper (7 sheets each of 3 different colors, matching 3 of the candy colors). Normally, we do not include experiments that require any supplies that you may not have on hand, however we did include this one from the *Land Animals* book p. 12-14.

<u>Key Idea:</u> On the sixth day, the Bible tells us that God created wild animals, livestock, and creatures that move along the ground.

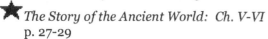

Reading about History

Read about history in the following resource:

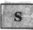 *The Story of the Ancient World: Ch. V-VI* p. 27-29

You will be adding to your timeline in your *Student Notebook* today. In Unit 1 – Box 1, draw and color the earth. Label it, *Creation (4004 B.C.)*. In Box 2, draw and color an ark. Label it, *The Great Flood (2300 B.C.)*. Note: If you are not of the young earth philosophy, you may wish to omit the dates.

Key Idea: The world was filled with sin.

History Project

Get the flapbook that you saved from Day 2. Fold back the flap labeled *5th* and write, *Mahalaleel – son of Cainan. Lived to be 892.* Fold back the flap labeled *6th* and write, *Jared – son of Mahalaleel. Lived to be 962.* Fold back the flap labeled *7th* and write, *Enoch – son of Jared, was a prophet. Taken to heaven without dying when 365.* Fold back the flap labeled *8th* and write, *Methuselah – son of Enoch. Name means, "When he dies, judgment." Died the same year as the Flood. Oldest man – lived to be 969.* Fold back the flap labeled *9th* and write, *Lamech – son of Methuselah. Lived to be 777.* Fold back the flap labeled *10th* and write, *Noah – son of Lamech. Lived through the Flood and to see the birth of Terah (father of Abram) 10 generations later. Lived to be 950.* Glue the back of your flapbook in your *Student Notebook* in Unit 1 – Box 6.

Key Idea: After 10 generations a flood came.

Storytime

Choose one of the following read aloud options:

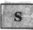 *Dinosaurs of Eden* p. 24-35

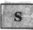 Read aloud the next portion of the biography that you selected.

After the reading, students will give a summary oral narration. The oral narration must be no longer than 5 sentences and should summarize the reading. As students narrate, have them hold up one finger for each sentence shared. Remind students that the focus should be on the big ideas, rather than on the details.

Key Idea: Summarize the story by narrating.

Bible Quiet Time

Reading: Choose one option below.

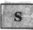 *The Illustrated Family Bible* p. 30-31

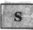 Your own Bible: Genesis chapter 6-7

Scripture Focus: Highlight Genesis 6:9.

Prayer Focus: Pray a prayer of thanksgiving to express gratitude for God's divine goodness. Begin by reading the highlighted verse out loud as a prayer. End by praying, *Thank you Lord for saving Noah and his family so that I can be here today. I am grateful for your word, for Noah's example of living a life in obedience to you, and for...*

Scripture Memory: Recite Philippians 2:1.
Music: *Philippians 2* CD: Track 1 (verse 1)

Key Idea: Noah lived a life pleasing to God.

Independent History Study

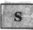 Listen to *What in the World?* Disc 1, Track 3: "Early Man". Then, open your *Student Notebook* to Unit 1. In Box 5, copy in cursive Genesis 6:5 and 6:8.

Key Idea: Adam lived to see 8 generations of his descendents. Noah was 10 generations from Adam.

Learning the Basics

Focus: Language Arts, Math, Geography, Bible, and Science

Bible Study

Read aloud and discuss with the students the following pages:

 The Radical Book for Kids p. 5-9

Key Idea: The Bible contains many different kinds of books. It includes books of poetry, history, law, wisdom, prophecy, Gospel, letters. and more. Each book is written in a certain style. To understand the Bible, it helps to know what kind of book you are reading. Each book has a purpose for your life.

Language Arts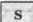

Have students complete one studied dictation exercise (see Appendix for directions and passages).

Work with the students to complete **one** of the writing options listed below:

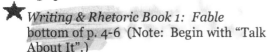*Writing & Rhetoric Book 1: Fable* bottom of p. 4-6 (Note: Begin with "Talk About It".)

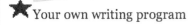Your own writing program

Key Idea: Practice language arts skills.

Poetry

Open *Paint Like a Poet* to Lesson 1. Read aloud the poem *"A Late Walk"* by Robert Frost.

Get the yellow backdrop that you painted on Day 2. Today, you will be adding a tree with a falling leaf. You will need a palette, water, a small flat paintbrush, a toothpick, and brown paint.

After gathering your supplies, turn to the "Step-by-Step Watercolor Tutorial" for Lesson 1 in *Paint Like a Poet*. Follow steps 4-6 to complete "Part Two: Tree with Falling Leaf". When your painting is dry, glue your poetry copywork from Day 1 to your painting. Store your completed artwork in the place you have chosen for it.

Key Idea: Explore poetry moods with painting.

Math Exploration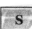

Choose **one** of the math options listed below.

Singapore Primary Mathematics 4A/4B or *5A/5B* (see Appendix for schedules), or *Math with Confidence,* or *Apologia Math*

Your own math program

Key Idea: Use a step-by-step math program.

Science Exploration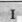

Read *Land Animals of the Sixth Day* p. 5 – middle of p. 8. Write the answer to each numbered question on lined paper. You do not need to copy the question. Use the listed page number as a reference.
1. What was the result of Adam and Eve's sin? (p. 5)
2. If animals weren't designed to eat other animals, then why do they have sharp teeth? (p. 6)
3. Write the words *zoologist* and *habituation* and give their definitions. (p. 6-7)
4. What is the difference between habituating an animal and taming it? (p. 7)
5. What picture does Isaiah 11:6-9 give you of the way that God originally created the animals? (p. 5)

Key Idea: Death and decay entered the world along with the first sin, and this changed God's beautiful creation in sad ways. The animals are affected by death and decay too.

Reading about History | I

Read about history in the following resource:

★ *The Story of the Ancient World:*
  Ch. VII-VIII p. 30 – top of p. 33

You will be writing a narration about *Chapter VII: The Deluge,* which is part of today's history reading.

To prepare for writing your narration, think about the questions below. If you do not know the answers, find them on p. 30 or 31 of *The Story of the Ancient World.* Ask yourself, *Who entered the ark? How was the door to the ark shut? From where did the floodwaters come? How long did the downpour last? What happened to the living creatures on earth? How high did the floodwaters rise? What did the waters carry along with them? How long did the ark float? Why did Noah send out a raven? What happened when Noah sent out the dove? Why was Noah filled with joy when he saw the olive twig? When did Noah come out of the ark?*

After you have thought about the answers to the questions, turn to Unit 1 in your *Student Notebook.* In Box 4, write a 5-8 sentence narration that begins with, *Noah entered the ark...* When you have finished writing, read your sentences out loud to catch any mistakes.

Check for the following things: *Did you include **who** the reading was mainly about? Did you include **what** important thing(s) happened? Did you include **how** it ended? If not, add those things.* Use the *Written Narration Skills* in the Appendix for editing.

Key Idea: Noah was 601 when he came out of the ark. By saving Noah, God kept His promise that He would one day send a Savior.

Storytime | T

Choose one of the following read aloud options:

★ *Dinosaurs of Eden* p. 36-49

★ Read aloud the next portion of the biography that you selected.

After the reading, have each person get a Bible and open it anywhere in Proverbs. Explain, *We will have 5 minutes to skim through the verses in Proverbs to find any connections to today's story. When a connection is found, read the verse out loud and quickly share the connection. At the end of 5 minutes, anyone who has not shared yet must read aloud one verse and make the best connection possible.*

Key Idea: Seek God's word for His guidance.

Bible Quiet Time | I

Reading: Choose one option below.

★ *The Illustrated Family Bible* p. 32-33

★ Your own Bible: Genesis chapter 8; 9:1-17

Scripture Focus: Highlight Genesis 8:21.

Prayer Focus: Pray a prayer of supplication to make a humble and earnest request of God. Begin by reading the highlighted verse out loud as a prayer. End by praying, *I ask you to help me Lord not to follow my heart, which is filled with sin. Instead, help me follow you by...*

Scripture Memory: Copy Philippians 2:1 in your Common Place Book (see Introduction).
Music: *Philippians 2* CD: Track 1 (verse 1)

Key Idea: God made a promise to Noah.

Independent History Study | I

★ Listen to *What in the World?* Disc 1, Track 4: "The Flood". Then, turn to *The Story of the Ancient World* p. 257. Read over the time period between the Flood and Noah's death. What things do you notice?

Key Idea: Noah lived at the time of the Tower of Babel, the Pharaohs, and the building of Babylon and Ur.

3-4 Track

Learning the Basics

Focus: Language Arts, Math, Geography, Bible, and Science

Atlas

Geography   T

Read aloud to the students the following pages:

⭐ *A Child's Geography Vol. II* p. 12-16
Discuss with the students "Field Notes" p. 16.

Key Idea: Turkey is connected with the Biblical account of Eden by the names of two of its rivers, the Tigris and the Euphrates. Due to the changes to the earth's surface made by Noah's Flood, we do not know if these rivers are in the same location as those that bordered Eden.

Language Arts   S

Have students complete one dictation exercise.

Guide students to complete one reading lesson.

⭐ *Drawn into the Heart of Reading*

Help students complete **one** English lesson.

⭐ *Building with Diligence:* Lesson 2
⭐ *Following the Plan:* Lesson 2
⭐ Your own grammar program

Key Idea: Practice language arts skills.

Poetry   I

Open *Paint Like a Poet* to Lesson 1. Today, you will be performing a poetry reading of *"A Late Walk"*. Practice reading the poem aloud with expression that matches the mood of the poem. Then, read the poem aloud in front of your chosen audience. At the end of the reading, share the following, *When I read this poem by Robert Frost, it made me think of...* Call on your audience to share what thoughts the poem brought to their minds. Last, say, *Did you know that Robert Frost was often paid to read his poems at prestigious colleges in the United States? He was even asked to read one of his poems at President J.F.K.'s inauguration.*

Key Idea: Share the poetry of Robert Frost.

w IDad

Math Exploration   S

Choose **one** of the math options listed below.

⭐ *Singapore Primary Mathematics 4A/4B* or *5A/5B* (see Appendix for schedules), or *Math with Confidence,* or *Apologia Math*
⭐ Your own math program

Key Idea: Use a step-by-step math program.

Science Exploration   I

⭐ Read *Land Animals of the Sixth Day* p. 8 – middle of p. 11. Now, skip to the "Experiment" on the bottom of p. 12. Normally, we do not include experiments that require any supplies that you may not have on hand, however we did include this experiment from the Apologia book. You will need one package of M&M's or Skittles and 21 sheets of colored paper (7 sheets each of 3 different colors, matching 3 of the candy colors). Use the same binder or sketchbook you have chosen for science notebooking. Make a science experiment section. For your science experiments, you may either use the Science Lab Form provided in the Appendix of our guide, or write your Lab Form on a blank paper as described below.

At the top of a blank page, write: *How does camouflage make a difference in how well animals survive?* Under the question, write: *'Guess'.* Write down your guess. Follow the directions for the experiment in *Land Animals of the Sixth Day* p. 12-14. Next, on the paper write: *'Procedure'.* Draw the table from p. 13 and fill it in. At the bottom of the paper, write: *'Conclusion'.* Explain what you learned from the experiment.

Key Idea: Camouflage affects which animals survive well in an environment, resulting in natural selection.

Unit 2 - Day 1

Reading about History | I |

Read about history in the following resource:

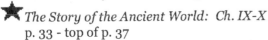 *The Story of the Ancient World:* Ch. IX-X p. 33 - top of p. 37

After the Flood, many people remained in one place and began building a tower to reach the skies. Where could you look to research more about the **Tower of Babel**? Read Genesis 11:1-9 for the most accurate resource on the Tower of Babel. You may also wish to check another resource like www.wikipedia.org.

Answer one or more of the following questions from your research: *Where was the tower built? What was used to build the tower? Why was the tower built? In Genesis 10:8-10, who does it say built the Babylonian empire? What does Nimrod have to do with the tower of Babel? Why did God confuse the people's language? Is the tower still standing today?*

<u>Key Idea</u>: God confused the people's language.

History Project | S |

In this unit you will be making a cylinder seal similar to the ones used by kings in ancient Mesopotamia to "sign" their names. Today you will make the air-dry clay needed to make the cylinder. In a bowl, mix ¼ cup salt with 3/8 cup warm water. Add 1 cup flour to the mixture and stir to combine. With your hands, knead the clay for 5 minutes. Place the clay in an airtight container with a lid for Day 2.

<u>Key Idea</u>: A cylinder seal of King Urukh's has been unearthed. Urukh means "the god Ham".

Storytime | T |

Choose one of the following read aloud options:

 Dinosaurs of Eden p. 50-64

★ Read at least one biography for the next 12 days of plans.

After the reading, students will give a detailed oral narration. Select one paragraph from the story to read out loud to the students. This will be the starting point for the narration. Set a timer for 3-5 minutes. When the timer rings the narration is over, even if it isn't complete. A detailed, descriptive narration is the goal. See *Narration Tips* in the Appendix as needed.

<u>Key Idea</u>: Use oral narration to retell the story.

Bible Quiet Time | I |

Bible Reading: Choose one option below.

★ *The Illustrated Family Bible* p. 34-35 Discuss sidebar "Chapter 9, Verse 29" on p. 34.

★ Your own Bible: Genesis 10:8-12; 11:1-9

Scripture Focus: Highlight Genesis 11:8-9.

Prayer Focus: Pray a prayer of adoration to worship and honor God. Begin by reading the highlighted verses out loud as a prayer. End by praying, *As God, you are worthy of our obedience. I will honor you by...*

Scripture Memory: Recite Philippians 2:2.
Music: *Philippians 2* CD: Track 1 (verses 1-2)

<u>Key Idea</u>: The people disobeyed God at Babel.

Independent History Study | I |

★ Listen to *What in the World?* Disc 1, Track 5: "Descendants of Noah". Then, open your *Student Notebook* to Unit 2. In Box 6, copy in cursive Genesis 11:8-9.

<u>Key Idea</u>: Noah's son Ham had a son named Cush. Cush had a son named Nimrod (which means "rebel"). Nimrod most likely began building the city at Babel in rebellion to God's command to spread out and fill the earth. It is likely that pagan religions also started with Nimrod.

Learning the Basics
Focus: Language Arts, Math, Geography, Bible, and Science

Bible Study   T

Read aloud and discuss with the students the following pages:

 ⭐ *The Radical Book for Kids* p. 10-11 and p. 12-15

<u>Key Idea</u>: The many names of God used in Scripture reveal what He is like. There are straightforward names, compound names, and descriptive names. These names help us learn about God. The gospel is an announcement of what Jesus has done for us through His life, death, and resurrection.

Language Arts   S

Have students complete one studied dictation exercise (see Appendix for directions and passages).

Help students complete one lesson from the following reading program:

⭐ *Drawn into the Heart of Reading*

Work with the students to complete **one** of the English options listed below:

⭐ *Building with Diligence:* Lesson 3

⭐ *Following the Plan:* Lesson 3

⭐ Your own grammar program

<u>Key Idea</u>: Practice language arts skills.

Poetry   I

Open *Paint Like a Poet* to Lesson 2. Read aloud the poem *"The Pasture"*. On a 3 x 5 index card, neatly copy in black ink or in pencil the following highlighted lines from the poem:

I'm going out to clean the pasture spring;
I'll only stop to rake the leaves away
(And wait to watch the water clear, I may):
I sha'n't be gone long. – You come too.
                                   -Robert Frost

Check your work to make sure it is correctly copied. Then, cut around your copywork. You may choose to outline the edge of the cut-out with a dark green marker. Save it for Day 3.

<u>Key Idea</u>: Read and appreciate a variety of classic poetry.

Math Exploration   S

Choose **one** of the math options listed below.

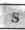 ⭐ *Singapore Primary Mathematics 4A/4B* or *5A/5B* (see Appendix for schedules), or *Math with Confidence*, or *Apologia Math*

⭐ Your own math program

<u>Key Idea</u>: Use a step-by-step math program.

Science Exploration   I

⭐ Read *Land Animals of the Sixth Day* p. 15 – middle of p. 19. Today you will begin a book of animal tracks. You will add to this book throughout the reading of *Land Animals of the Sixth Day*. To make a cover for your book, fold a piece of colored paper in half. Use colored pencils, crayons, or gel or glitter pens to write a title on your book cover. Next, cut a square piece of white paper to glue beneath the title. Before gluing the white paper on the cover, copy Genesis 1:26 on it in cursive. Then, fold 10 sheets of white paper in half and place them inside your cover to make a book. Staple the side of the book to hold it together. On the first page inside the book, draw and label the dog's track as shown in the picture on p. 29. Note: You may choose to use a hardbound blank book with a "Tracks" section for your entries instead.

<u>Key Idea</u>: Mammals are animals that have hair. They are warm-blooded, have vertebrae, and must breathe oxygen from the air. Mammals must sweat to cool off. They also nurse their young.

Learning through History
Focus: The First Cities After the Flood

Reading about History | I

Read about history in the following resource:

⭐ *The Story of the Ancient World: Ch. XI-XII* p. 37 - middle of p. 41

You will be choosing a portion from today's reading that you found memorable or worthy of being reread to copy. Open your *Student Notebook* to Unit 2. In Box 4, carefully copy in cursive the portion from today's reading that you selected. Then, compare your written work to the original. Last, draw a small colorful picture in Box 4 to illustrate your sentences.

Key Idea: After God confused the languages at Babel, the remnant from Babel moved to other cities established by Nimrod.

Storytime | T

Choose one of the following read aloud options:

⭐ *The Golden Bull: Ch. 1-3* p. 1-13

⭐ Read aloud the next portion of the biography that you selected.

After reading, give each person 2 slips of paper. Each person must think of 2 questions to ask about the book and write one question on each slip of paper. Next, fold up the slips of paper and place them in a container. Each person must select at least one question from the container to answer.

Key Idea: Use questioning to share the story.

History Project | S

Take out the air-dry clay that you saved from Day 1. Place a piece of waxed paper on your work surface. Roll part of your clay into a two-inch long cylinder that is less than one inch thick. Cut a small piece of white paper to fit around your cylinder. Decide what picture or symbols you would like on your cylinder to signify your name. Use a dark marker to carefully draw these on your paper. Then, turn the paper over, so your drawing is backward. Wrap it around your cylinder to use as a guide. Use a pencil or the sharp end of a paperclip to carve a deep, wide outline of your design into the clay cylinder. Leave the cylinder out to dry.

Key Idea: Clay tablets that have been unearthed that give a glimpse of Sumerian life.

Bible Quiet Time | I

Reading: Choose the option below.

⭐ Your own Bible: Job chapter 1; 2:1-10; 42

Scripture Focus: Highlight Job 42:2.

Prayer Focus: Pray a prayer of confession to admit or acknowledge your sins to God. Begin by reading the highlighted verse out loud as a prayer. End by praying, *Lord, I confess that I need to trust you more like Job did, even when bad things happen. I'm sorry for…*

Scripture Memory: Recite Philippians 2:2.
Music: *Philippians 2* CD: Track 1 (verses 1-2)

Key Idea: Satan tested Job's faith in God.

Independent History Study | I

⭐ Listen to *What in the World?* Disc 1, Track 6: "Sources and Evidences". Open your *Student Notebook* to "Prophecies About Christ". Under "Prophecy" write, *Job 19:25-27*. Read the Scripture from your Bible to discover the prophecy. Under "Fulfillment" write, *Galatians 4:4-5*. Read the fulfillment Scripture. Under "Description", write a few phrases to describe the prophecy about Jesus.

Key Idea: Job prophecied that he would one day see the promised Redeemer who would come to earth.

Learning the Basics
Focus: Language Arts, Math, Geography, Bible, and Science

Geography [T]

Go to the website link listed under "Bringing It Home" on p. 6 of *A Child's Geography Vol. II*. At the link, select "History & Geography". Then, under "Knowledge Quest" select "ACG2-Extra Activities". Print a copy of the labeled map of **Turkey** on p. 43 and the blank map of **Turkey** on p. 44 for each student. Then, assign students the following page:

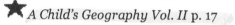 *A Child's Geography Vol. II* p. 17

Note: Do only the "Map Notes" section.

Key Idea: Practice finding and recording the locations of various places on a map of Turkey.

Language Arts [S]

Help students complete one lesson from the following reading program:

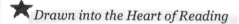 *Drawn into the Heart of Reading*

Work with the students to complete **one** of the writing options listed below:

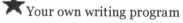 *Writing & Rhetoric Book 1: Fable* p. 8-10 (Note: Omit p. 7. Give students as much help as needed to be successful with the writing assignment.)

★ Your own writing program

Key Idea: Practice language arts skills.

Poetry [I]

Open *Paint Like a Poet* to Lesson 2. Read aloud the poem *"The Pasture"* by Robert Frost.

Today, you will be painting a pasture spring. You will need painting paper, a palette, water, a large flat paintbrush, a small flat paintbrush, a paper towel, and light blue and dark green paint.

After gathering your supplies, turn to the "Step-by-Step Watercolor Tutorial" for Lesson 2 in *Paint Like a Poet*. Follow steps 1-3 to complete "Part One: Pasture Spring". Then, let your background dry. You will complete "Part Two" of the tutorial on Day 3.

Key Idea: Use painting to illustrate poetry.

Math Exploration [S]

Choose **one** of the math options listed below.

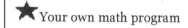 *Singapore Primary Mathematics 4A/4B* or *5A/5B* (see Appendix for schedules), or *Math with Confidence*, or *Apologia Math*

★ Your own math program

Key Idea: Use a step-by-step math program.

Science Exploration [I]

★ Read *Land Animals of the Sixth Day* p. 19 – middle of p. 23. Orally retell or narrate to an adult the portion of text that you read today. Use the *Narration Tips* in the Appendix for help as needed.

Key Idea: Within the order Carnivora there is a group called Caniforms. Some examples of caniforms include dogs, bears, raccoons, and otters. The Canidae family falls under the group Caniform and includes true dogs such as the wolf, the pug, the red fox, the jackal, and the coyote. While dogs can change over time through breeding or natural selection, the kind of creature will remain the same. The Bible says animals reproduce after their own kind.

Learning through History
Focus: The First Cities After the Flood

Reading about History [I]

Read about history in the following resource:

★ *The Story of the Ancient World:* Ch. XIII - XIV p. 41 – middle of p. 44

You will be adding to your timeline in your *Student Notebook* today. In Unit 2 – Box 1, draw and color the Tower of Babel. Label it, *Tower of Babel (2242 B.C.).* In Box 2, draw and color the sun. Label it, *Cushite Shepherd Kings in Egypt (War 2084 B.C.).* In Box 3, draw and color a moon. Label it, *Abram born in Ur (1996 B.C.).*

Key Idea: The city of Ur was known for its moon worship. Abram was born in Ur.

Storytime [T]

Choose one of the following read aloud options:

★ *The Golden Bull:* Ch. 4-6 p. 14-27

★ Read aloud the next portion of the biography that you selected.

After the reading, students will give a summary oral narration. The oral narration must be no longer than 5 sentences and should summarize the reading. As students narrate, have them hold up one finger for each sentence shared. Remind students that the focus should be on the big ideas, rather than on the details.

Key Idea: Summarize the story by narrating.

History Project [S]

Place a piece of waxed paper on your work surface. Use part of your remaining air-dry clay to form a flat clay tablet. Get a pointed pencil or the sharp end of a paperclip to use for etching. Then, etch the cunieform characters shown on p. 41 of *The Story of the Ancient World* into the top half of your clay tablet. Get the cylinder seal that you made on Day 2. Roll your seal across the bottom half of the tablet to "sign" your name. Leave the clay tablet out to air-dry. Using a toothpick, clean any bits of clay out of the grooves in your cylinder seal.

Key Idea: In the Bible Ur is referred to as "Ur of the Chaldeans". Since "Khal'di" was the name for the moon god, the people who worshipped the moon god at Ur came to be known as "Khaldians" or "Chaldeans".

Bible Quiet Time [I]

Reading: Choose one option below.

★ *The Illustrated Family Bible* p. 38-39

★ Your own Bible: Genesis chapter 12

Scripture Focus: Highlight Genesis 12:1-3.

Prayer Focus: Pray a prayer of thanksgiving to express gratitude for God's divine goodness. Begin by reading the highlighted verses out loud as a prayer. End by praying, *Thank you for the blessing of the promised Savior who eventually came from Abram. Thank you...*

Scripture Memory: Recite Philippians 2:2.
Music: *Philippians 2* CD: Track 1 (verses 1-2)

Key Idea: God called Abram to leave Ur.

Independent History Study [I]

★ Listen to *What in the World?* Disc 1, Track 7: "Oldest Cities". Open your *Student Notebook* to "Prophecies About Christ". Under "Prophecy" write, *Genesis 12:3.* Read the Scripture from your Bible to discover the prophecy. Under "Fulfillment" write, *Acts 3:25.* Read the fulfillment Scripture. Under "Description", write a few phrases to describe the prophecy about Jesus.

Key Idea: God promised that through Abram's offspring all people on earth would be blessed. The promised Savior would one day be born from Abram's family tree.

Learning the Basics
Focus: Language Arts, Math, Geography, Bible, and Science

Unit 2 - Day 3

Bible Study   [T]

Read aloud and discuss with the students the following pages:

 The Radical Book for Kids p. 16-18

Key Idea: Christians are to grow in their trust and obedience of Jesus more and more. This growth takes a lifetime! God gives Christians the Holy Spirit to help them grow more like Him. Spiritual disciplines are practices and habits such as reading the Word and praying that help Christians grow in the pursuit of Godliness.

Language Arts   [S]

Have students complete one studied dictation exercise (see Appendix for directions and passages).

Work with the students to complete **one** of the writing options listed below:

 Writing & Rhetoric Book 1: Fable p.11 (Note: If you have one student, your student should read his/her fable aloud to you. Then, help your student edit and correct the fable.)

 Your own writing program

Key Idea: Practice language arts skills.

Poetry   [I]

Open *Paint Like a Poet* to Lesson 2. Read aloud the poem *"The Pasture"* by Robert Frost.

Get the background of the pasture spring that you painted on Day 2. Today, you will be adding twigs in the water. You will need a palette, water, a small flat paintbrush, a toothpick, and brown and black paint.

After gathering your supplies, turn to the "Step-by-Step Watercolor Tutorial" for Lesson 2 in *Paint Like a Poet*. Follow steps 4-6 to complete "Part Two: Twigs in the Water". When your painting is dry, glue your poetry copywork from Day 1 to your painting. Store your completed artwork in the place you have chosen for it.

Key Idea: Explore poetry moods with painting.

Math Exploration   [S]

Choose **one** of the math options listed below.

 Singapore Primary Mathematics 4A/4B or 5A/5B (see Appendix for schedules), or *Math with Confidence,* or *Apologia Math*

 Your own math program

Key Idea: Use a step-by-step math program.

Science Exploration   [I]

Read *Land Animals of the Sixth Day* p. 23-28. Write the answer to each numbered question on lined paper. You do not need to copy the question. Use the listed page to help you answer each question.
1. What are some of the rules of the pack? (p. 23)
2. How does a dog show it's feeling aggressive? (p. 24)
3. Write the words *digitigrade* and *olfactory* and give their definitions. (p. 24-25)
4. Use a globe or a world map to find the locations of the animals in the "Map It" section of p. 29.
5. What picture does John 10:11-12 give you of the wolf?

Key Idea: The alpha male and alpha female are the dominant pair in a pack. This pair has puppies, which are cared for by the pack. A "pecking order" is established among the rest of the pack. The pack hunts.

Unit 2 - Day 4

Reading about History [I]

Read about history in the following resource:

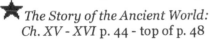 *The Story of the Ancient World:*
Ch. XV - XVI p. 44 - top of p. 48

You will be writing a narration about *Chapter XV: The First War,* which is part of today's history reading.

To prepare for writing your narration, think about the questions below. If you do not know the answers, find them on p. 44-46 of *The Story of the Ancient World.* Ask yourself, *What name was given to Nimrod and his family? How were the Cushites forced to scatter? Why was it rebellion for the Cushites to wander? What did the Cushites establish everywhere that they settled? Whom did they worship? Where was the first war fought on earth? Find Elam and Sumer on the map on p 46. Who ruled in Sumer after the war? Who was King of Elam at the time?*

After you have thought about the answers to the questions, turn to Unit 2 in your *Student Notebook.* In Box 5, write a 5-8 sentence narration that begins with, *The Cushites were descendents of...* When you have finished writing, read your sentences out loud to catch any mistakes.

Check for the following things: *Did you include **who** the reading was mainly about? Did you include **what** important thing(s) happened? Did you include **how** it ended? If not, add those things.* Use the *Written Narration Skills* in the Appendix for editing.

<u>Key Idea</u>: The Cushites brought their false religion to Sumer, Egypt, and the Holy Land.

Storytime [T]

Choose one of the following read aloud options:

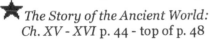 *The Golden Bull: Ch. 7-8 p. 28-40*

★ Read aloud the next part of the biography.

After the reading, have each person get a Bible and open it anywhere in Proverbs. Explain, *We will have 5 minutes to skim through the verses in Proverbs to find any connections to today's story. When a connection is found, read the verse out loud and quickly share the connection. At the end of 5 minutes, anyone who has not shared yet must read aloud one verse and make the best connection possible.*

<u>Key Idea</u>: Seek God's word for His guidance.

Bible Quiet Time [I]

Reading: Choose one option below.

★ *The Illustrated Family Bible* p. 40-41

★ Your own Bible: Genesis 13; 14:11-24; 15

Scripture Focus: Highlight Genesis 15:6.

Prayer Focus: Pray a prayer of supplication to make a humble and earnest request of God. Begin by reading the highlighted verse out loud as a prayer. End by praying, *Help me believe in you more and more like Abram. Guide me to...*

Scripture Memory: Copy Philippians 2:2 in your Common Place Book (see Introduction).
Music: *Philippians 2* CD: Track 1 (verses 1-2)

<u>Key Idea</u>: God called Abram to go to Canaan.

Independent History Study [I]

Open your *Student Notebook* to Unit 2. Write the following generations in the listed box numbers:
7) Noah – lived to be 950. 8) Shem - lived to be 600. Box 9) Arphaxad - lived to be 438. 10) Salah - lived to be 433. 11) Eber - lived to be 464. 12) Peleg - lived to be 239. 13) Reu - lived to be 239. 14) Serug - lived to be 230. 15) Nahor - lived to be 148. 16) Terah - lived to be 205. 17) Abram - lived to be 175.

<u>Key Idea</u>: There were 10 generations from Adam to the Flood and 10 more from Noah to Abram.

Learning the Basics

Focus: Language Arts, Math, Geography, Bible, and Science

Geography 〖T〗

Go to the website link listed on p. 6 of *A Child's Geography Vol. II*. At the link, select "History & Geography". Then, under "Knowledge Quest" select ACG2-Extra Activities". Print the "Travel Log Template" of your choice from p. 39-42. Also, at the link, for older students, print and assign the "Chapter One Review" on p. 67. Assign all students the following page:

★ *A Child's Geography Vol. II* p. 17
Note: Do only the "Travel Notes" section. If desired, play "Music" from the links on p. 18. The "Art" section of p. 18 is an optional extra.

<u>Key Idea</u>: Share three sights from Turkey.

Language Arts 〖S〗

Have students complete one dictation exercise.

Guide students to complete one reading lesson.

★ *Drawn into the Heart of Reading*

Help students complete **one** English lesson.

★ *Building with Diligence:* Lesson 4

★ *Following the Plan:* Lesson 4

★ Your own grammar program

<u>Key Idea</u>: Practice language arts skills.

Poetry 〖I〗

Open *Paint Like a Poet* to Lesson 2. Today, you will be performing a poetry reading of *"The Pasture"*. Practice reading the poem aloud with expression that matches the mood of the poem. Then, read the poem aloud in front of your chosen audience.

At the end of the reading, share the following, *When I read this poem by Robert Frost, it made me think of...* Call on your audience to share what thoughts the poem brought to their minds.

Last, say, *Did you know that Robert Frost often opened his poetry readings by reading "The Pasture"? The poem gave the feeling that he was inviting his listeners to come with him into the world of his poems.*

<u>Key Idea</u>: Share the poetry of Robert Frost.

Math Exploration 〖S〗

Choose **one** of the math options listed below.

★ *Singapore Primary Mathematics 4A/4B* or *5A/5B* (see Appendix for schedules), or *Math with Confidence,* or *Apologia Math*

★ Your own math program

<u>Key Idea</u>: Use a step-by-step math program.

Science Exploration 〖I〗

Turn to the science experiment section in your science binder or sketchbook. For your science experiments, you may either use the Science Lab Form provided in the Appendix of our guide, or write your Lab Form on a blank paper as described below.

At the top of a blank page, write: *How does humans' sense of sight affect their sense of smell?* Under the question, write: *'Guess'*. Write down your guess. Follow the directions for the experiment in *Land Animals of the Sixth Day* p. 30. You may wish to use orange juice or apple juice instead of lemon gelatin for the experiment. Simply add red food coloring to only one glass of juice, leaving the other to remain its regular color. Next, on the paper write: *'Procedure'*. Draw the table from p. 30 and fill it in. If you used juice, write "Yellow Juice" and "Red Juice" as your headings instead. At the bottom of the paper, write: *'Conclusion'*. Explain what you learned from the experiment.

<u>Key Idea</u>: Dogs have a sensitive sense of smell. Often, the humans' sense of smell is affected by their sight.

Learning through History
Focus: God's Covenant with Abraham, Isaac, and Jacob

Reading about History   I

Read about history in the following resource:

★ *The Story of the Ancient World:*
Ch. XVII- XVIII p. 48 - middle of p. 51

God made a covenant with Abraham, Isaac, and Jacob. Where could you look to research more about **Biblical covenants**? Use a Bible, a reference book, or an online resource like www.wikipedia.org to look up *covenants*.

Answer one or more of the following questions from your research: *What is a covenant? Who were some of the people in the Old Testament with whom God made a covenant? What were some of the terms of the covenants? What does Hebrews 9:15 say about a new covenant? How did Christ's death and resurrection begin a new covenant?*

Key Idea: God made a covenent with Abram.

History Project   S

In this unit you will make an optical illusion of stars in a striped background. Cut a piece of white paper to be 6" x 8". Line up a ruler vertically along the short edge of the paper. To make a vertical column, use your pencil to trace along the side of the ruler from the top to the bottom of the paper. Move the ruler and line it up with the new vertical line you drew. Trace the side of the ruler to make a new vertical column. Then, continue this pattern tracing columns across the paper. Save the paper for Day 2.

Key Idea: God promised Abraham that his descendents would be like the stars in the sky.

Storytime   T

Choose one of the following read aloud options:

★ *The Golden Bull:* Ch. 9-10 p. 41-55

★ Read at least one biography for the next 8 days of plans.

After the reading, students will give a detailed oral narration. Select one paragraph from the story to read out loud to the students. This will be the starting point for the narration. Set a timer for 3-5 minutes. When the timer rings the narration is over, even if it isn't complete. A detailed, descriptive narration is the goal. See *Narration Tips* in the Appendix as needed.

Key Idea: Use oral narration to retell the story.

Bible Quiet Time   I

Bible Reading: Choose one option below.

★ *The Illustrated Family Bible* p. 42-45
Optional Extension: p. 36

★ Your own Bible: Genesis 17:15-22; 18; 19:12-29

Scripture Focus: Highlight Genesis 17:1.

Prayer Focus: Pray a prayer of adoration to worship and honor God. Begin by reading the highlighted verse out loud as a prayer. End by praying, *I worship you Lord as the almighty God. You are worthy of praise because...*

Scripture Memory: Recite Philippians 2:3.
Music: *Philippians 2* CD: Track 1 (verses 1-3)

Key Idea: God always keeps His promises.

Independent History Study   I

Open your *Student Notebook* to "Prophecies About Christ". Under "Prophecy" write, *Genesis 17:7.* Read the Scripture from your Bible to discover the prophecy. Under "Fulfillment" write, *Matthew 1:1.* Read the fulfillment Scripture. Under "Description", write a few phrases to describe the prophecy about Jesus.

Key Idea: God promised Abraham that the Savior would be born of his seed and be his descendent.

Bible Study `T`

Read aloud and discuss with the students the following pages:

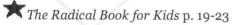 *The Radical Book for Kids* p. 19-23

Key Idea: In the early church, men like Polycarp, Athanasius, and Augustine gave their life for Christ. Polycarp studied under the apostle John and was martyred for his faith. Athanasius was exiled many times in his fight against Aranianism. Augustine heard the gospel from Ambrose and and was forever changed. He wrote over one hundred books.

Language Arts `S`

Have students complete one studied dictation exercise (see Appendix for directions and passages).

Help students complete one lesson from the following reading program:

 Drawn into the Heart of Reading

Work with the students to complete **one** of the English options listed below:

⭐ *Building with Diligence:* Lesson 5

⭐ *Following the Plan:* Lesson 5 (Half)

⭐ Your own grammar program

Key Idea: Practice language arts skills.

Poetry `I`

Open *Paint Like a Poet* to Lesson 3. Read aloud the poem *"A Peck of Gold"*. On a 3 x 5 index card, neatly copy in black ink or in pencil the following highlighted lines from the poem:

All the dust the wind blew high
Appeared like gold in the sunset sky,
But I was one of the children told
Some of the dust was really gold.
                    -Robert Frost

Check your work to make sure it is correctly copied. Then, cut around your copywork. You may choose to outline the edge of the cut-out with a tan or brown marker. Save it for Day 3.

Key Idea: Read and appreciate a variety of classic poetry.

Math Exploration `S`

Choose **one** of the math options listed below.

⭐ *Singapore Primary Mathematics 4A/4B* or *5A/5B* (see Appendix for schedules), or *Math with Confidence*, or *Apologia Math*

⭐ Your own math program

Key Idea: Use a step-by-step math program.

Science Exploration `I`

⭐ Read *Land Animals of the Sixth Day* p. 31 – top of p. 36. Get your book about animal tracks that you began last unit. At the top of the next page in your book, copy in cursive 1 Samuel 17:37. Beneath the verse, draw and label the black bear, brown bear, and polar bear tracks as shown in the "Track It" drawings on p. 49.

Key Idea: Bears are in the family Ursidae and are considered caniforms. Bears can stand on two legs and are plantigrades, meaning they don't walk on their toes. They are mostly vegetarians, even though their teeth place them in the order Carnivora. Polar bears, however, mainly eat meat. Bears are dormant during the winter but can awaken easily from their winter rest. It's important for people not to feed bears, or the bears become habituated. It's also important to know what to do if you are ever faced with a bear.

Reading about History | I

Read about history in the following resource:

 The Story of the Ancient World:
Ch. XIX- XX p. 51-54

You will be choosing a portion from today's reading that you found memorable or worthy of being reread to copy. Open your *Student Notebook* to Unit 3. In Box 4, carefully copy in cursive the portion from today's reading that you selected. Then, compare your written work to the original. Last, draw a small colorful picture in Box 4 to illustrate your sentences.

Key Idea: Isaac was born to Abraham and Sarah when Abraham was 100 years old! Sarah wanted Hagar and Ishmael sent away. God told Abraham to listen to Sarah, as Isaac was God's chosen heir. God promised that Ishmael would also become a great nation.

History Project | S

Get a clean sheet of white paper, and cut it to be 6" x 8". Draw 4 different-sized star shapes on the paper. Then, cut out the 4 stars. Get the striped paper that you saved from Day 1. Lay the stars on your striped paper so that the stars are not touching one another. Use your pencil to carefully trace around each star shape. Save your paper for Day 3.

Key Idea: Abraham trusted God would provide an heir for him. He knew God would keep His promise, even though God was asking him to sacrifice Isaac. Abraham did not withhold anything from God. As a result of his faith, God richly blessed Abraham with descendents as numerous as the stars.

Storytime | T

Choose one of the following read aloud options:

 The Golden Bull: Ch. 11-12 p. 56-67

Read aloud the next portion of the biography that you selected.

After reading, work with the students to plan a 3 minute skit with simple props to act out part of today's reading. Set a timer for 3 minutes to quickly prepare for the skit. Make sure that you participate in the skit along with the students. When the timer rings, set it again for 3 minutes and perform the skit. You do not need an audience, as the goal is the retelling.

Key Idea: Use a skit to retell part of the story.

Bible Quiet Time | I

Reading: Choose one option below.

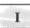 *The Illustrated Family Bible* p. 46-47

Your own Bible: Genesis 21:1-20; 22:1-19

Scripture Focus: Highlight Genesis 22:12.

Prayer Focus: Pray a prayer of confession to admit or acknowledge your sins to God. Begin by reading the highlighted verse out loud as a prayer. End by praying, *I confess to you Lord that sometimes I withhold things from you. Help me to remember that everything I have belongs to you.*

Scripture Memory: Recite Philippians 2:3.
Music: *Philippians 2* CD: Track 1 (verses 1-3)

Key Idea: God tested Abraham through Isaac.

Independent History Study | I

Open your *Student Notebook* to "Prophecies About Christ". Under "Prophecy" write, *Genesis 22:17-18*. Read the Scripture to discover the prophecy. Under "Fulfillment" write, *Galatians 3:16*. Read the fulfillment Scripture. Under "Description", write a few phrases to describe the prophecy about Jesus.

Key Idea: God repeated His promise to Abraham that all nations on earth would be blessed through him.

Learning the Basics

Focus: Language Arts, Math, Geography, Bible, and Science

Geography | T |

Read aloud to the students the following pages:

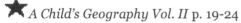 *A Child's Geography Vol. II* p. 19-24

Discuss with the students "Field Notes" p. 24.

<u>Key Idea</u>: Mount Ararat is the highest mountain in Turkey. It is mentioned in the Bible as the landing place of Noah's Ark after the Flood. In Turkey, you can also visit the very salty Lake Van and the village of Haran. Haran is mentioned in the Bible as the place where God called Abraham to the Promised Land and where Jacob worked for Laban.

Language Arts | S |

Help students complete one lesson from the following reading program:

 Drawn into the Heart of Reading

Work with the students to complete **one** of the writing options listed below:

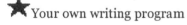 *Writing & Rhetoric Book 1: Fable* p. 12-14 (Note: Read the text aloud while the students follow along. You will read the fable on Day 3.)

★ Your own writing program

<u>Key Idea</u>: Practice language arts skills.

Poetry | I |

Open *Paint Like a Poet* to Lesson 3. Read aloud the poem *"A Peck of Gold"* by Robert Frost.

Today, you will be painting a sky backdrop. You will need painting paper, a palette, water, a large flat paintbrush, and light blue, rose, and yellow paint.

After gathering your supplies, turn to the "Step-by-Step Watercolor Tutorial" for Lesson 3 in *Paint Like a Poet*. Follow steps 1-3 to complete "Part One: Sky Backdrop". Then, let your background dry. You will complete "Part Two" of the tutorial on Day 3.

<u>Key Idea</u>: Use painting to illustrate poetry.

Math Exploration | S |

Choose **one** of the math options listed below.

★ *Singapore Primary Mathematics 4A/4B or 5A/5B* (see Appendix for schedules), or *Math with Confidence,* or *Apologia Math*

★ Your own math program

<u>Key Idea</u>: Use a step-by-step math program.

Science Exploration | I |

★ Read *Land Animals of the Sixth Day* p. 36 – middle of p. 41. Orally retell or narrate to an adult the portion of text that you read today. Use the *Narration Tips* in the Appendix for help as needed. Then, use a globe or a world map to find the locations of polar bears, brown bears, American black bears, pandas, and sun bears listed in the "Map It" section of p. 50.

<u>Key Idea</u>: A brown bear has a large hump above its shoulders. Brown bears are very aggressive bears and are dangerous to people. Black bears are the most common bears in North America. They are often smaller than brown bears. Polar bears are actually black skinned and are very large carnivores. Sun bears are omnivores and are nocturnal, sleeping during the day. Pandas prefer to eat bamboo and are quite docile. They are an endangered species.

Learning through History
Focus: God's Covenant with Abraham, Isaac, and Jacob

Unit 3 - Day 3

Reading about History | I |

Read about history in the following resource:

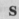 *The Story of the Ancient World: Ch. XXI- XXII* p. 55 - middle of p. 58

You will be adding to your timeline in your *Student Notebook* today. In Unit 3 – Box 1, draw and color a fire. Label it, *Destruction of Sodom and Gomorrah (1897 B.C.)*. In Box 2, draw and color the number 100. Label it, *Birth of Isaac (1896 B.C.)*. In Box 3, draw and color a hand grabbing the heel of a foot. Label it, *Birth of Jacob and Esau (1836 B.C.)*.

Key Idea: Eliezer prayed for God to bless his mission for Abraham by showing him a suitable wife for Isaac. God brought Rebekah.

Storytime | T |

Choose one of the following read aloud options:

★ *The Golden Bull: Ch. 13-14* p. 68-81

★ Read aloud the next portion of the biography that you selected.

After the reading, students will give a summary oral narration. The oral narration must be no longer than 5 sentences and should summarize the reading. As students narrate, have them hold up one finger for each sentence shared. Remind students that the focus should be on the big ideas, rather than on the details.

Key Idea: Summarize the story by narrating.

History Project | S |

Get your striped paper that you saved from Day 2. Choose **one** colored marker to use for creating your illusion. Use your marker to color the first column, however any part of a star that is inside the first column should be left white. The second column will be left white, however any part of a star that is inside the second column should be colored. The third column will be colored, with any star parts within the column staying white. Continue across the paper one column at a time, alternating colored columns with white columns and white star parts with colored star parts. Glue your illusion in your *Student Notebook* in Unit 3 – Box 7.

Key Idea: God told Isaac that He would make Isaac's descendents as numerous as the stars.

Bible Quiet Time | I |

Reading: Choose one option below.

★ *The Illustrated Family Bible* p. 48-49

★ Your own Bible: Genesis 24:1-27; 25:19-34

Scripture Focus: Highlight Genesis 24:1.

Prayer Focus: Pray a prayer of thanksgiving to express gratitude for God's divine goodness. Begin by reading the highlighted verse out loud as a prayer. End by praying, *Thank you for the many blessings you have given me, such as...*

Scripture Memory: Recite Philippians 2:3.
Music: *Philippians 2* CD: Track 1 (verses 1-3)

Key Idea: God told Rebekah and Isaac that their older son would serve their younger son.

Independent History Study | I |

Open your *Student Notebook* to "Prophecies About Christ". Under "Prophecy" write, *Genesis 26:2-4*. Read the Scripture from your Bible to discover the prophecy. Under "Fulfillment" write, *Matthew 1:1-2*. Read the fulfillment Scripture. Under "Description", write a few phrases to describe the prophecy about Jesus. Open your *Student Notebook* to Unit 3. In Box 6, copy in cursive Genesis 25:23.

Key Idea: God passed the covenant from Abraham to Isaac that the Savior would be born of Isaac's seed.

Bible Study T

Read aloud and discuss with the students the following pages:

 The Radical Book for Kids p. 24-28

Key Idea: Often we get angry because we **either** want something someone else has **or** we have lost something we desired to keep. If you feel angry, pray and ask God for help to stay calm. Wait to talk until you are calm. Then, seek to show love instead of anger. If you lose your temper, repent to God and man. After genuinely asking for forgiveness, search your heart for the source of the anger.

Language Arts S

Have students complete one studied dictation exercise (see Appendix for directions and passages).

Work with the students to complete **one** of the writing options listed below:

 Writing & Rhetoric Book 1: Fable p. 15-18 (Note: Read the text aloud while the students follow along. Then, discuss.)

 Your own writing program

Key Idea: Practice language arts skills.

Poetry I

Open *Paint Like a Poet* to Lesson 3. Read aloud the poem *"A Peck of Gold"* by Robert Frost.

Get the sky backdrop that you painted on Day 2. Today, you will be adding dusty clouds. You will need a palette, water, a large flat paintbrush, and light blue, rose, and yellow paint.

After gathering your supplies, turn to the "Step-by-Step Watercolor Tutorial" for Lesson 3 in *Paint Like a Poet*. Follow steps 4-6 to complete "Part Two: Dusty Clouds". When your painting is dry, glue your poetry copywork from Day 1 to your painting. Store your completed artwork in the place you have chosen for it.

Key Idea: Explore poetry moods with painting.

Math Exploration S

Choose **one** of the math options listed below.

 Singapore Primary Mathematics 4A/4B or *5A/5B* (see Appendix for schedules), or *Math with Confidence*, or *Apologia Math*

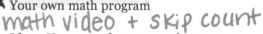 Your own math program   *math video + skip count songs*

Key Idea: Use a step-by-step math program.

Science Exploration I

Read *Land Animals of the Sixth Day* p. 41 – middle of p. 46. Write the answer to each numbered question on lined paper. You do not need to copy the question. Use the listed page(s) to help you.

1. What are some of the characteristics of mustelids? (p. 42-43)
2. Write the words *romp* and *holt* and give their definitions. (p. 43)
3. Describe what you learned about skunks. (p. 45-46)
4. Use a globe or a world map to find the locations of river otters, sea otters, skunks, and raccoons listed in the "Map It" section of p. 50.
5. On a clean page in your book of animal tracks, draw and label raccoon tracks as shown on p. 49.

Key Idea: The members of the Mustelidae family, also called the weasel family, are often known for their soft fur and their odor. In spite of their odor, skunks are now categorized in their own family, Mephitidae.

Learning through History
Focus: God's Covenant with Abraham, Isaac, and Jacob

Unit 3 - Day 4

Reading about History I

Read about history in the following resource:

★ *The Story of the Ancient World:* Ch. XXIII p. 58 - top of p. 60

You will be writing a narration about *Chapter XXIII: The Brothers' Rivalry*, which is part of today's history reading.

To prepare for writing your narration, think about the questions below. If you do not know the answers, find them on p. 58-60 of *The Story of the Ancient World*. Ask yourself, *What was the blessing that Isaac would give his heir? When did the Lord share that the blessing would be Jacob's? Why did Isaac intend to give the blessing to Esau? What did Rebekah do about this? When Esau found out that Jacob had received the blessing of the covenant, what was his reaction? How did Rebekah keep Jacob safe? Why did Esau marry a daughter of Ishmael's?*

After you have thought about the answers to the questions, turn to Unit 3 in your *Student Notebook*. In Box 5, write a 5-8 sentence narration that begins with, *As the time came for Isaac to give the blessing of the covenant...* When you have finished writing, read your sentences out loud to catch any mistakes.

Check for the following things: *Did you include **who** the reading was mainly about? Did you include **what** important thing(s) happened? Did you include **how** it ended? If not, add those things.* Use the *Written Narration Skills* in the Appendix for editing.

Key Idea: Isaac did not intend to give the blessing of the covenant to Jacob. Yet, Jacob received the blessing as God had foretold.

Storytime T

Choose one of the following read aloud options:

★ *The Golden Bull:* Ch. 15-16 p. 82-94

★ Read aloud the next part of the biography.

After the reading, have each person get a Bible and open it anywhere in Proverbs. Explain, *We will have 5 minutes to skim through the verses in Proverbs to find any connections to today's story. When a connection is found, read the verse out loud and quickly share the connection. At the end of 5 minutes, anyone who has not shared yet must read aloud one verse and make the best connection possible.*

Key Idea: Seek God's word for His guidance.

Bible Quiet Time I

Reading: Choose one option below.

★ *The Illustrated Family Bible* p. 50-51

★ Your own Bible: Genesis 27:1-46

Scripture Focus: Highlight Genesis 26:34.

Prayer Focus: Pray a prayer of supplication to make a humble and earnest request of God. Begin by reading the highlighted verse out loud as a prayer. End by praying, *I see the trouble that Esau got into for marrying pagan women. Please help me marry a person who loves you and is pleasing to you.*

Scripture Memory: Copy Philippians 2:3 in your Common Place Book (see Introduction).
Music: *Philippians 2* CD: Track 1 (verses 1-3)

Key Idea: Esau's life was not pleasing to God.

Independent History Study I

Open your *Student Notebook* to Unit 3. In Box 8, copy in cursive Genesis 26:4-5.

Key Idea: God passed the covenant that He had made with Abraham onto His chosen heir, Isaac. God was keeping His promise to Abraham, and passing it onto Isaac. Eventually, God made the same covenant with Jacob.

Learning the Basics
Focus: Language Arts, Math, Geography, Bible, and Science

Geography | T |

Read aloud to the students the following pages:

 A Child's Geography Vol. II p. 25-29

Discuss with the students "Field Notes" p. 29.

<u>Key Idea</u>: Tarsus is a busy city in Turkey. In Bible times, Tarsus was a bustling sea port on the Mediterranean Sea. Today, it is located inland. Tarsus was the birthplace of Apostle Paul. In the region of Cappadocia, New Testament Christians lived in underground cities built within basalt rock Fairy Chimneys.

Language Arts | S |

Have students complete one dictation exercise.

Guide students to complete one reading lesson.

⭐ *Drawn into the Heart of Reading*

Help students complete **one** English lesson.

⭐ *Building with Diligence:* Lesson 6

⭐ *Following the Plan:* Lesson 5 (Last half)

⭐ Your own grammar program

<u>Key Idea</u>: Practice language arts skills.

Poetry | I |

Open *Paint Like a Poet* to Lesson 3. Today, you will be performing a poetry reading of *"A Peck of Gold"*. Practice reading the poem aloud with expression that matches the mood of the poem. Then, read the poem aloud in front of your chosen audience.

At the end of the reading, share the following, *When I read this poem by Robert Frost, it made me think of...* Call on your audience to share what thoughts the poem brought to their minds. Last, say, *Did you know that Robert Frost was born in San Francisco, California, home of the Golden Gate Bridge? What insight does that give you about his poem "A Peck of Gold"?*

<u>Key Idea</u>: Share the poetry of Robert Frost.

Math Exploration | S |

Choose **one** of the math options listed below.

⭐ *Singapore Primary Mathematics 4A/4B* or *5A/5B* (see Appendix for schedules), or *Math with Confidence,* or *Apologia Math*

⭐ Your own math program

<u>Key Idea</u>: Use a step-by-step math program.

Science Exploration | I |

⭐ Read *Land Animals of the Sixth Day* p. 46 – top of p. 49. Now, skip to the "Experiment" on p. 50. Turn to the science experiment section in your science binder or sketchbook. At the top of a blank page, write: *How does a polar bear's black skin help keep it warm?* Under the question, write: *'Guess'.* Write down your guess. Follow the directions for the experiment in *Land Animals of the Sixth Day* on p. 50. If you do not have white and dark trash bags or two thermometers, then do the alternate experiment below.

Get two similar-sized ice cubes and two plastic bags. Place one ice cube in each bag. Close the bags. Place the bags on an aluminum cookie sheet or in an aluminum cake pan. Place a black square of paper or fabric over one bag, and a white square of paper or fabric over the other bag. Make sure the squares are the same size. Set the cookie sheet or cake pan of ice cubes outside in full sun. Wait 10-20 minutes and check the ice cubes. Which color absorbed more light, causing more melting? Next, on the paper write: *'Procedure'.* Draw a picture of the experiment. At the bottom, write: *'Conclusion'.* Explain what you learned.

<u>Key Idea</u>: When exposed to the sun, dark colors generally absorb more light. The polar bear's dark skin absorbs light well, which helps it to stay warm.

Learning through History
Focus: Egypt at the Time of Joseph

Reading about History $\boxed{\text{I}}$

Read about history in the following resource:

⭐ *The Story of the Ancient World:*
Ch. XXIV-XXV p. 60 - middle of p. 64

When God made a covenant with Abraham, He promised Abraham (and later Isaac and Jacob) the land described in Genesis 15:18-20. Where could you look to research more about the **Promised Land** or the **Land of Canaan**? Use a Bible, an online resource like www.wikipedia.org, or a reference book.

Answer one or more of the following questions from your research: *Between which two rivers was the Promised Land located? Point to this area on a globe or a map. What were some of the names of the groups of people living in the Promised Land at the time of Abraham? Why was the Promised Land also called the Land of Canaan? Who was Canaan?*

Key Idea: Jacob went to Haran to find a wife. He later returned to the Promised Land.

History Project $\boxed{\text{S}}$

In this unit you will make a shepherd's headband and head covering. Measure and cut two pieces of string (or yarn) that are each 1 yard long. Lay the pieces of string on top of one another, and then knot the strings together about 7 inches from one end. Cut a straw into 10-12 one inch pieces. Choose a large light-weight towel, scarf, or tablecloth to fold into a triangular shape for a head covering.

Key Idea: Jacob was a shepherd for Laban.

Storytime $\boxed{\text{T}}$

Choose one of the following read aloud options:

⭐ *The Golden Bull:* Ch. 17-18 p. 95-107

⭐ Read at least one biography for the next 4 days of plans.

After the reading, students will give a detailed oral narration. Select one paragraph from the story to read out loud to the students. This will be the starting point for the narration. Set a timer for 3-5 minutes. When the timer rings the narration is over, even if it isn't complete. A detailed, descriptive narration is the goal. See *Narration Tips* in the Appendix as needed.

Key Idea: Use oral narration to retell the story.

Bible Quiet Time $\boxed{\text{I}}$

Bible Reading: Choose one option below.

⭐ *The Illustrated Family Bible* p. 52-55

⭐ Your own Bible: Genesis 28:10-22; 29:14-30

Scripture Focus: Highlight Genesis 28:15.

Prayer Focus: Pray a prayer of adoration to worship and honor God. Begin by reading the highlighted verse out loud as a prayer. End by praying, *I praise you Lord for always being with me and watching over me wherever I go.*

Scripture Memory: Recite Philippians 2:4.
Music: *Philippians 2* CD: Track 1 (verses 1-4)

Key Idea: God spoke to Jacob in a dream.

Independent History Study $\boxed{\text{I}}$

Open your *Student Notebook* to "Prophecies About Christ". Under "Prophecy" write, *Genesis 28:13-14.* Read the Scripture to discover the prophecy. Under "Fulfillment" write, *Luke 1:31-33.* Read the fulfillment Scripture. Under "Description", write a few phrases to describe the prophecy about Jesus.

Key Idea: The Savior would be born of the seed of Jacob, and all people would be blessed through Him.

Learning the Basics
Focus: Language Arts, Math, Geography, Bible, and Science

Bible Study [T]

Read aloud and discuss with the students the following pages:

⭐ *The Radical Book for Kids* p. 29-31

Key Idea: The first five books of the Bible contain God's laws. These laws were given to the people of Israel. The laws were summed up by Jesus in Mark 12:29-31. We are to love God with all our heart, soul, and mind. We are also to love our neighbor as ourself. These books of the Bible are called the Pentateuch or the Books of the Law.

Language Arts [S]

Have students complete one studied dictation exercise (see Appendix for directions and passages).

Help students complete one lesson from the following reading program:

⭐ *Drawn into the Heart of Reading*

Work with the students to complete **one** of the English options listed below:

⭐ *Building with Diligence:* Lesson 7

⭐ *Following the Plan:* Lesson 6

⭐ Your own grammar program

Key Idea: Practice language arts skills.

Poetry [I]

Open *Paint Like a Poet* to Lesson 4. Read aloud the poem *"A Passing Glimpse"*. On a 3 x 5 index card, neatly copy in black ink or in pencil the following highlighted lines from the poem:

I often see flowers from a passing car
That are gone before I can tell what they are.
I want to get out of the train and go back
To see what they were beside the track.
                                    -Robert Frost

Check your work to make sure it is correctly copied. Then, cut around your copywork. You may choose to outline the edge of the cut-out with a yellow marker. Save it for Day 3.

Key Idea: Read and appreciate a variety of classic poetry.

Math Exploration [S]

Choose **one** of the math options listed below.

⭐ *Singapore Primary Mathematics 4A/4B* or *5A/5B* (see Appendix for schedules), or *Math with Confidence*, or *Apologia Math*

⭐ Your own math program

Key Idea: Use a step-by-step math program.

Science Exploration [I]

⭐ Read *Land Animals of the Sixth Day* p. 51 – top of p. 57. Get your book about animal tracks that you began in Unit 2. At the top of the next page in your book of tracks, copy Proverbs 28:1 in cursive. Beneath the verse, draw and label an American wildcat's tracks as shown in the "Track It" drawing on p. 68. Then, use a globe or a world map to find the locations of the animals listed in the first column of the "Map It" section on p. 68.

Key Idea: Cats belong to the family Felidae. They purr, often have retractable claws, and have very flexible skeletons. Their eyes are acutely sensitive to light, helping them to see well even at night. Their whiskers act as sensors, sensing slight movements in the air. Wild cats like lions, cougars, and tigers are camouflaged by their fur coats. Big cats are not afraid of people. They are dangerous predators.

Reading about History | I

Read about history in the following resource:

★ *The Story of the Ancient World:*
Ch. XXVI-XXVII p. 64 - middle of p. 67

You will be choosing a portion from today's reading that you found memorable or worthy of being reread to copy. Open your *Student Notebook* to Unit 4. In Box 4, carefully copy in cursive the portion from today's reading that you selected. Then, compare your written work to the original. Last, draw a small colorful picture in Box 4 to illustrate your sentences.

Key Idea: In revenging their sister Dinah, Simeon and Levi lost their right to inherit the blessing of the covenant from Jacob. Jacob favored his son Joseph and hoped to bless him.

Storytime | T

Choose one of the following read aloud options:

★ *The Golden Bull: Ch. 19-20 p. 108-120*

★ Read aloud the next portion of the biography that you selected.

After reading, give students a few minutes to prepare a short advertisement speech for the book. During the speech, students should hold up the book and say the book title and the name of the author. The wording of the advertisement should provide a peek into the book without giving away the ending. The goal should be for listeners to feel like they've "Got to Have This Book"!

Key Idea: Use an ad speech to share the story.

History Project | S

Get out the string, pieces of straw, and the head covering. Wrap the ends of the two pieces of string with tape to make threading easier. Thread one end of string through a piece of straw. Then, entering from the opposite end, thread the other string through the same piece of straw. Pull the ends of both strings to move the straw close to the knotted end. It should form a loop. Repeat the steps with a new piece of straw. After all the pieces of straw have been looped, tie a knot at the end to hold the straws in place. Remove the tape and knot each of the 4 ends of string. Fold your cloth head covering into a triangular shape. Lay the covering on top of your head, holding the two points next to your ears (with one point in back). Tie the headband around your head covering to keep it in place. Save it to wear on Day 3.

Key Idea: Jacob's sons were shepherds.

Bible Quiet Time | I

Reading: Choose one option below.

★ *The Illustrated Family Bible* p. 56-57

★ Your own Bible: Genesis chapters 32-33

Scripture Focus: Highlight Genesis 32:11.

Prayer Focus: Pray a prayer of confession to admit or acknowledge your sins to God. Begin by reading the highlighted verse out loud as a prayer. End by praying, *I confess to you Lord that I sometimes feel afraid too. Help me not to be afraid of...*

Scripture Memory: Recite Philippians 2:4.
Music: *Philippians 2* CD: Track 1 (verses 1-4)

Key Idea: God changed Jacob's name to Israel on his return to the Holy Land. Jacob (or Israel) settled in Shechem with his family.

Independent History Study | I

Open your *Student Notebook* to Unit 4. Look at the map and trace with your finger Abraham's journeys, Eliezer's journey for Isaac, and Jacob's flight to Haran. In Box 6, copy Genesis 32:9-10.

Key Idea: God took care of Jacob and was with him, just as He had promised. Esau forgave Jacob.

Learning the Basics
Focus: Language Arts, Math, Geography, Bible, and Science

Geography [T]

Have students get both the blank map and the labeled map of **Turkey** that they began in Unit 3.

Then, assign students the following page:

★ *A Child's Geography Vol. II* p. 31

Geo 25-24

Note: Do only the "Map Notes" section.

<u>Key Idea</u>: Practice finding and recording the locations of various places on a map of Turkey.

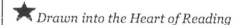

Language Arts [S]

Help students complete one lesson from the following reading program:

★ *Drawn into the Heart of Reading*

Work with the students to complete **one** of the writing options listed below:

★ *Writing & Rhetoric Book 1: Fable* p. 20-21 (Note: Omit p. 19. Guide students through the lesson, so they are successful writing a summary.)

★ Your own writing program

<u>Key Idea</u>: Practice language arts skills.

Poetry [I]

Open *Paint Like a Poet* to Lesson 4. Read aloud the poem *"A Passing Glimpse"* by Robert Frost.

Today, you will be painting a field backdrop. You will need painting paper, a palette, water, a large flat paintbrush, a small flat paintbrush, a paper towel, and blue, brown, yellow, and green paint.

After gathering your supplies, turn to the "Step-by-Step Watercolor Tutorial" for Lesson 4 in *Paint Like a Poet*. Follow steps 1-2 to complete "Part One: Field Backdrop". Then, let your background dry. You will complete "Part Two" of the tutorial on Day 3.

<u>Key Idea</u>: Use painting to illustrate poetry.

Math Exploration [S]

Choose **one** of the math options listed below.

★ *Singapore Primary Mathematics 4A/4B* or *5A/5B* (see Appendix for schedules), or *Math with Confidence*, or *Apologia Math*

★ Your own math program

<u>Key Idea</u>: Use a step-by-step math program.

Science Exploration [I]

★ Read *Land Animals of the Sixth Day* p. 57 – middle of p. 62. Orally retell or narrate to an adult the portion of text that you read today. Use the *Narration Tips* in the Appendix for help as needed. Choose either the "Try This" on p. 58 or on p. 60 to do.

<u>Key Idea</u>: Tigers prefer to live in the jungle where their coats help them blend in with their surroundings. They stalk large prey and can swim and jump. Many tigers live in India. Wild cats live all over the world. The North American cats include the bobcat, cougar, and Canada lynx. Hyenas are in the feliform family called Hyaenidae and are not true cats.

Learning through History
Focus: Egypt at the Time of Joseph

Reading about History [I]

Read about history in the following resource:

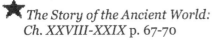 *The Story of the Ancient World: Ch. XXVIII-XXIX* p. 67-70

You will be adding to your timeline in your *Student Notebook* today. In Unit 4 – Box 1, draw and color a pyramid. Label it, *Amosis drives Cushites out of Egypt (1824 B.C.).* In Box 2, draw and color a ladder going into the clouds. Label it, *Jacob's Ladder (1759 B.C.).* In Box 3, draw and color a pair of handcuffs. Label it, *Joseph sold into slavery.*

Key Idea: The first king of Egypt was a son of Ham named Mizraim (or Menes). Mizraim diverted the Nile River and built the city of Memphis.

History Project [S]

Have a parent help you plan a simple "Hebrew" meal for today. This usually included white cheese (but yellow cheese can be used intead), a choice of fruit (such as grapes, figs, dates or raisins), a choice of vegetable (beans, peas, onions, lettuce, or cucumbers), bread (dipped in vinegar or spread with honey or jam), choice of drink (water, milk, or grape juice), and may include yogurt, almonds or porridge. Spread a blanket on the floor as your table. Wash your hands with water before eating. Then, say a blessing. Arrange the food on platters or plates in the center of the blanket. Eat your meal squatting around the platters. Use your fingers to put food from the platters into your own bowl. Make sure to wear your shepherd's headdress.

Key Idea: The Shepherd Kings were Cushites.

Storytime [T]

Choose one of the following read aloud options:

 The Golden Bull: Ch. 21-22 p. 121-138

Read aloud the next portion of the biography that you selected.

After the reading, students will give a summary oral narration. The oral narration must be no longer than 5 sentences and should summarize the reading. As students narrate, have them hold up one finger for each sentence shared. Remind students that the focus should be on the big ideas, rather than on the details.

Key Idea: Summarize the story by narrating.

Bible Quiet Time [I]

Reading: Choose one option below.

⭐ *The Illustrated Family Bible* p. 58-59

⭐ Your own Bible: Genesis chapter 37

Scripture Focus: Highlight Genesis 37:9-11.

Prayer Focus: Pray a prayer of thanksgiving to express gratitude for God's divine goodness. Begin by reading the highlighted verses out loud as a prayer. End by praying, *I am so grateful Lord that you have a plan for my life. Help me to keep in mind that nothing surprises you. Guide me to....*

Scripture Memory: Recite Philippians 2:4.
Music: *Philippians 2* CD: Track 1 (verses 1-4)

Key Idea: Joseph's brothers sold him to Ishmaelite traders who were going to Egypt.

Independent History Study [I]

⭐ Listen to *What in the World?* Disc 2, Track 1: "Historical Chronology".

Key Idea: The Cushites brought their pagan worship to Egypt. They worshipped Am'on-Ra, or the sun god Ham. They also worshipped the moon, the stars, and their ancestors such as Nimrod.

Learning the Basics
Focus: Language Arts, Math, Geography, Bible, and Science

Bible Study $\boxed{T}$

Read aloud and discuss with the students the following pages:

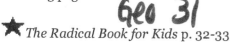
Geo 31

★ *The Radical Book for Kids* p. 32-33

<u>Key Idea</u>: Remember the following steps for cleaning your room: 1) Make your bed. 2) Make sure everything has a place and is put in its place. 3) Leave nothing on the floor that does not belong there. 4) Leave nothing in your room that belongs in different room. 5) Place clothes in the hamper, or hang them in the closet, or fold them and put them in your dresser drawer, or set them out for the next day. 6) Empty the trash.

Language Arts $\boxed{S}$

Have students complete one studied dictation exercise (see Appendix for directions and passages).

Work with the students to complete **one** of the writing options listed below:

 Writing & Rhetoric Book 1: Fable p. 22-23

 Your own writing program

<u>Key Idea</u>: Practice language arts skills.

Poetry $\boxed{I}$

Open *Paint Like a Poet* to Lesson 4. Read aloud the poem *"A Passing Glimpse"* by Robert Frost.

Get the field backdrop that you painted on Day 2. Today, you will be adding grass and flowers. You will need a palette, water, a small round paintbrush, toothpicks, and brown, green, dark green, and purple paint.

After gathering your supplies, turn to the "Step-by-Step Watercolor Tutorial" for Lesson 4 in *Paint Like a Poet*. Follow steps 3-5 to complete "Part Two: Grass and Flowers". When your painting is dry, glue your poetry copywork from Day 1 to your painting. Store your completed artwork in the place you have chosen for it.

<u>Key Idea</u>: Explore poetry moods with painting.

Math Exploration $\boxed{S}$

Choose **one** of the math options listed below.

 Singapore Primary Mathematics 4A/4B or 5A/5B (see Appendix for schedules), or *Math with Confidence,* or *Apologia Math*

 Your own math program

<u>Key Idea</u>: Use a step-by-step math program.

Science Exploration $\boxed{I}$

★ Read *Land Animals of the Sixth Day* p. 62 – middle of p. 67. Write the answer to each numbered question on lined paper. You do not need to copy the question. Use the listed page(s) to help you.
1. What is the difference between *mutation* and *natural selection*? (p. 62)
2. Describe one of the following: aardwolf, Asian cat, mongoose, or meerkat. (p. 64-66)
3. Write the words *diurnal* and *nocturnal* and give their definitions. (p. 66)
4. Use a globe or a world map to find the locations of the animals in the second column of the "Map It" section of p. 68.
5. In Psalm 104:20-21, how does God provide for animals?

<u>Key Idea</u>: Along with sin, mutations, diseases, and deformities came into the world. These affect animals.

Reading about History [I]

Read about history in the following resource:

★ *The Story of the Ancient World:*
Ch. XXX-XXXI p. 71-73

You will be writing a narration about *Chapter XXX: The Theban Revolt,* which is part of today's history reading.

To prepare for writing your narration, think about the questions below. If you do not know the answers, find them on p. 71-72 of *The Story of the Ancient World.* Ask yourself, *Where did the Shepherd Kings build their capital city? Even though the Shepherd Kings had conquered all of Egypt, how was their treatment of Lower Egypt diffeeent from their treatment of Upper Egypt? Where was the capital city in Upper Egypt? Why did the Theban prince Rasekenen take up arms and fight the Shepherd Kings? What was the outcome of this battle? Whem Amosis became the leader in Egypt, what did he do? How did the assault against the city of Avaris end? Who built Jerusalem?*

After you have thought about the answers to the questions, turn to Unit 4 in your *Student Notebook.* In Box 5, write a 5-8 sentence narration that begins with, *After the Shepherd Kings conquered Egypt...* When you have finished writing, read your sentences out loud to catch any mistakes.

Check for the following things: *Did you include **who** the reading was mainly about? Did you include **what** important thing(s) happened? Did you include **how** it ended? If not, add those things.* Use the *Written Narration Skills* in the Appendix for editing.

Key Idea: The Shepherd Kings conquered Egypt, until Amosis was victorious over them.

Storytime [T]

Choose one of the following read aloud options:

★ *The Golden Bull:* Ch. 23-25 p. 139-154

★ Read aloud the next portion of the biography that you selected.

After the reading, have each person get a Bible and open it anywhere in Proverbs. Explain, *We will have 5 minutes to skim through the verses in Proverbs to find any connections to today's story. When a connection is found, read the verse out loud and quickly share the connection. At the end of 5 minutes, anyone who has not shared yet must read aloud one verse and make the best connection possible.*

Key Idea: Seek God's word for His guidance.

Bible Quiet Time [I]

Reading: Choose the option below.

★ Your own Bible: Genesis chapter 39

Scripture Focus: Highlight Genesis 39:3-4.

Prayer Focus: Pray a prayer of supplication to make a humble and earnest request of God. Begin by reading the highlighted verse out loud as a prayer. End by praying, *Be with me Lord, just as you were with Joseph. Help me to find favor in your eyes and to have success in...*

Scripture Memory: Copy Philippians 2:4 in your Common Place Book.
Music: *Philippians 2* CD: Track 1 (verses 1-4)

Key Idea: Even though Joseph was a slave and was in prison in Egypt, God was with Joseph.

Independent History Study [I]

★ Listen to *What in the World?* Disc 2, Track 2: "Problems with the Chronology".

Key Idea: There are problems in determining the order and length of each Pharaoh's reign in Egypt.

Learning the Basics

Focus: Language Arts, Math, Geography, Bible, and Science

Geography 〔 T 〕

Go to the website link listed on p. 6 of *A Child's Geography Vol. II*. At the link, select "History & Geography". Then, under "Knowledge Quest" select ACG2-Extra Activities". Print the "Travel Log Template" of your choice from p. 39-42. Also at the link, for older students, print and assign the "Chapter Two Review" on p. 68. Assign all students the following page:

★ *A Child's Geography Vol. II* p. 31
Note: Do only the "Travel Notes" section. If desired, peruse the "Books" and read the "Poetry" on p. 30 as an optional extra.

<u>Key Idea</u>: Share three sights from Turkey.

Language Arts 〔 S 〕

Have students complete one dictation exercise.

Guide students to complete one reading lesson.

★ *Drawn into the Heart of Reading*

Help students complete **one** English lesson.

★ *Building with Diligence:* Lesson 8

★ *Following the Plan:* Lesson 7

★ Your own grammar program

<u>Key Idea</u>: Practice language arts skills.

Poetry 〔 I 〕

Open *Paint Like a Poet* to Lesson 4. Today, you will be performing a poetry reading of "*A Passing Glimpse*". Practice reading the poem aloud with expression that matches the mood of the poem. Then, read the poem aloud in front of your chosen audience. At the end of the reading, share the following, *When I read this poem by Robert Frost, it made me think of...* Call on your audience to share what thoughts the poem brought to their minds. Last, say, *Did you know that when Robert Frost was born in 1874, trains were used for travel? The automobile was unheard of, and Henry Ford didn't mass-produce it until 1914. So, the "passing car" Frost is referring to in today's poem was a train car.*

<u>Key Idea</u>: Share the poetry of Robert Frost.

Math Exploration 〔 S 〕

Choose **one** of the math options listed below.

 ★ *Singapore Primary Mathematics 4A/4B* or *5A/5B* (see Appendix for schedules), or *Math with Confidence,* or *Apologia Math*

★ Your own math program

<u>Key Idea</u>: Use a step-by-step math program.

Science Exploration 〔 I 〕

Turn to the science experiment section in your science binder or sketchbook. At the top of a blank page, write: *How do cougars and deer affect one another?* Under the question, write: *'Guess'*. Write down your guess.

Follow the directions for the experiment in *Land Animals of the Sixth Day* p. 69-70. You may choose to use index cards instead of cardboard for the experiment. You may also choose to print pictures of the cougar from www.wikipedia.org. If so, type "cougar" in the search. Click on the picture of the cougar to enlarge it. Print it 6 times. You may either choose to repeat the steps to print the "deer", or choose to write "deer" on 20 small papers instead.

Next, on the paper write: *'Procedure'*. Draw the table from p. 70 and fill it in. At the bottom of the paper, write: *'Conclusion'*. Explain what you learned from the experiment.

<u>Key Idea</u>: The relationship between predator and prey keeps the cougar and deer population balanced.

Learning through History
Focus: The Pharaohs of Ancient Egypt

Unit 5 - Day 1

Reading about History | I |

Read about history in the following resource:

★ *The Story of the Ancient World: Ch. XXXII-XXXIII p. 74 – middle of p. 77*

Pharaoh allowed Joseph's father, Jacob, and his brothers with their families to settle in Goshen. Where could you look to research more about the **Land of Goshen**? Read the Bible passage Genesis 46:31-34 and Genesis 47:6, 11 for the most accurate resource on the Land of Goshen. You may also wish to check another resource such as www.wikipedia.org.

Answer one or more of the following questions from your research: *Where was the Land of Goshen located? What river watered the land in Goshen? Near which ancient city was Goshen located? What do you remember about the Shepherd Kings (Cushites)? Why were shepherds detestable to the Egyptians? How long did the Israelites live in Goshen?*

Key Idea: God gave Pharaoh two dreams.

History Project | S |

In this unit you will make Egyptian Palace Bread. You will need 5 slices of white bread. Wheat bread will work as a substitute, however it will result in a denser Egyptian bread. Neatly cut off the crusts of the bread slices. Pour one cup of honey into a large lidded container. Dip both sides of each bread slice in honey until covered. Place the lid on the container. Soak the bread in honey to use on Day 2.

Key Idea: During the famine, Joseph's brothers came to see him at Pharaoh's palace in order to buy food. They did not recognize him.

Storytime | T |

Choose one of the following read aloud options:

★ *The Golden Bull: Ch. 26-27 p. 155-167*

★ Read at least one adventure for the next 16 days of plans (see Appendix for suggestions).

After the reading, students will give a detailed oral narration. Select one paragraph from the story to read out loud to the students. This will be the starting point for the narration. Set a timer for 3-5 minutes. When the timer rings the narration is over, even if it isn't complete. A detailed, descriptive narration is the goal. See *Narration Tips* in the Appendix as needed.

Key Idea: Use oral narration to retell the story.

Bible Quiet Time | I |

Bible Reading: Choose one option below.

★ *The Illustrated Family Bible* p. 60-61

★ Your own Bible: Genesis chapters 40-41

Scripture Focus: Highlight Genesis 41:16.

Prayer Focus: Pray a prayer of adoration to worship and honor God. Begin by reading the highlighted verse out loud as a prayer. End by praying, *I give you adoration for being able to do all things. Nothing is too hard for you. I praise you for helping me with...*

Scripture Memory: Recite Philippians 2:5.
Music: *Philippians 2* CD: Track 2 (verse 5)

Key Idea: God revealed the meaning of dreams to Joseph. The dreams were prophecies of what was to come.

Independent History Study | I |

Open your *Student Notebook* to Unit 5. In Box 6, copy in cursive Genesis 41:25, 32.

Key Idea: God revealed His plans to Pharaoh in two different dreams. God used Joseph to interpret the dreams for Pharaoh. There would be seven years of abundance followed by seven years of famine.

Learning the Basics

Focus: Language Arts, Math, Geography, Bible, and Science

Bible Study   [T]

Read aloud and discuss with the students the following pages:

 The Radical Book for Kids p. 34-37

Key Idea: How do we know the Bible is true? God has preserved thousands of Old and New Testament manuscripts for thousands of years. These manuscripts precisely match one another. In this way, we can know exactly what God's Word says. God has protected His Word as He promised.

Language Arts   [S]

Have students complete the first studied dictation exercise (see Appendix).

Help students complete one lesson from the following reading program:

 Drawn into the Heart of Reading

Work with the students to complete **one** of the English options listed below:

★ *Building with Diligence:* Lesson 9

★ *Following the Plan:* Lesson 8

★ Your own grammar program

Key Idea: Practice language arts skills.

Poetry   [I]

Open *Paint Like a Poet* to Lesson 5. Read aloud the poem *"One Step Backward Taken"*. On a 3 x 5 index card, neatly copy in black ink or in pencil the following highlighted lines from the poem:

Not only sands and gravels
Were once more on their travels,
But gulping muddy gallons
Great boulders off their balance
Bumped heads together dully
And started down the gully.
                    -Robert Frost

Check your work to make sure it is correctly copied. Then, cut around your copywork. You may choose to outline the edge of the cut-out with a dark brown marker. Save it for Day 3.

Key Idea: Read and appreciate classic poetry.

Math Exploration   [S]

Choose **one** of the math options listed below.

★ *Singapore Primary Mathematics 4A/4B* or *5A/5B* (see Appendix for schedules), or *Math with Confidence*, or *Apologia Math*

★ Your own math program

Key Idea: Use a step-by-step math program.

Science Exploration   [I]

★ Read *Land Animals of the Sixth Day* p. 71 – middle of p. 76. Follow the directions for "Try This" on p. 73. To do "Try This", print a world map at one of the following links:

www.printableworldmap.net

http://en.wikipedia.org/wiki/File:Winkel-tripel-projection.jpg

Today you will add to your science notebook. At the top of an unlined paper, copy Psalm 95:3-5 in cursive. Beneath the verse, glue the continents you cut out from the map to make one piece of land.

Key Idea: At one time the continents may have been one big piece of land, and they may have broken apart during or after the Flood. The Ice Age may have created land bridges, which would explain how animals and people came to be spread out on other continents.

Reading about History | I |

Read about history in the following resource:

 The Story of the Ancient World:
Ch. XXXIV-XXXV p. 77 – middle of p. 80

You will be choosing a portion from today's reading that you found memorable or worthy of being reread to copy. Open your *Student Notebook* to Unit 5. In Box 4, carefully copy in cursive the portion from today's reading that you selected. Then, compare your written work to the original. Last, draw a small colorful picture in Box 4 to illustrate your sentences.

Key Idea: Joseph's brothers came to Egypt in search of food. Joseph tested his brothers to see if they had changed. When Judah offered himself in place of Benjamin, Joseph knew they were different and that they were sorry.

History Project | S |

Today you will finish making Egyptian Palace Bread. Ask an adult for help in preheating the oven to 250 degrees. Then, lightly grease a small deep baking dish. Using a spatula, pile the honey-soaked slices of bread neatly one on top of another in the baking dish. Ask an adult to help you place the baking dish in the oven. Bake the bread for 45 minutes. After 45 minutes, have an adult remove the bread from the oven and let it cool slightly before placing it in the refrigerator to chill for at least 15 minutes. Serve the bread by cutting it into very small slices and topping it with whipped cream, sweetened heavy cream, or ice cream.

Key Idea: Joseph was second only to Pharaoh.

Storytime | T |

Choose one of the following read aloud options:

 The Golden Bull: Ch. 28-30 p. 168-184

★ Read aloud the next portion of the adventure that you selected.

After reading, give each person a white piece of paper or a markerboard and a marker. Set a timer for 3-5 minutes and instruct each person to do a quick outline sketch about the story. Ideas for sketches include settings, characters, actions, important objects, or symbols. When the timer rings, briefly share the sketches.

Key Idea: Use sketching to share the story.

Bible Quiet Time | I |

Reading: Choose one option below.

★ *The Illustrated Family Bible* p. 62-63

★ Your own Bible: Genesis chapters 42-43

Scripture Focus: Highlight Genesis 45:5.

Prayer Focus: Pray a prayer of confession to admit or acknowledge your sins to God. Begin by reading the highlighted verse out loud as a prayer. End by praying, *I confess that sometimes I get distressed or angry when bad things happen. Please forgive me for my distress about _____ and help me place my trust in you.*

Scripture Memory: Recite Philippians 2:5.
Music: *Philippians 2* CD: Track 2 (verse 5)

Key Idea: Joseph trusted God with his life.

Independent History Study | I |

Open your *Student Notebook* to "Prophecies About Christ". Under "Prophecy" write, *Genesis 49:8-10.* Read the Scripture to discover the prophecy. Under "Fulfillment" write, *Matthew 1:1-3.* Read the fulfillment Scripture. Under "Description", write a few phrases to describe the prophecy about Jesus.

Key Idea: The ruling sceptor will not depart from Judah, because Christ will be born of the tribe of Judah.

Learning the Basics

Focus: Language Arts, Math, Geography, Bible, and Science

Geography [T]

Read aloud to the students the following pages:

 A Child's Geography Vol. II p. 32 – first two paragraphs on p. 35

Discuss with the students "Field Notes" p. 35.

<u>Key Idea</u>: The once-busy city of Ephesus in Turkey is now a ghost town. Many tourists come to visit the site of this ancient city yearly. The ruins at Ephesus include a three-story library, an amphitheater, and one marble column from the Temple at Artemis built for the false goddess Diana.

Language Arts [S]

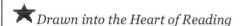

Help students complete one lesson from the following reading program:

⭐ *Drawn into the Heart of Reading*

Work with the students to complete **one** of the writing options listed below:

⭐ *Writing & Rhetoric Book 1: Fable* p. 24-27 (Note: Read aloud the text while the students follow along. Then, discuss.)

⭐ Your own writing program

<u>Key Idea</u>: Practice language arts skills.

Poetry [I]

Open *Paint Like a Poet* to Lesson 5. Read aloud the poem *"One Step Backward Taken"* by Robert Frost.

Today, you will be painting a rocky backdrop. You will need painting paper, a palette, water, a large flat paintbrush, a pencil, and tan or peach paint.

After gathering your supplies, turn to the "Step-by-Step Watercolor Tutorial" for Lesson 5 in *Paint Like a Poet*. Follow steps 1-3 to complete "Part One: Rocky Backdrop". Then, let your background dry. You will complete "Part Two" of the tutorial on Day 3.

<u>Key Idea</u>: Use painting to illustrate poetry.

Math Exploration [S]

Choose **one** of the math options listed below.

 ⭐ *Singapore Primary Mathematics 4A/4B* or *5A/5B* (see Appendix for schedules), or *Math with Confidence,* or *Apologia Math*

⭐ Your own math program

<u>Key Idea</u>: Use a step-by-step math program.

Science Exploration [I]

⭐ Read *Land Animals of the Sixth Day* from the middle of p. 76-80. Orally retell or narrate to an adult the portion of text that you read today. Use the *Narration Tips* in the Appendix for help as needed.

<u>Key Idea</u>: Most marsupials have a special pouch in which their babies develop. Kangaroos, wallabies, wombats, koalas, and possums are all marsupials. Wallabies are small kangaroos. There are many different species of wallabies. Koalas are marsupials that are able to eat the usually poisonous eucalyptus leaves. The koalas have a special chemical that allows them to eat the leaves without being poisoned.

Reading about History   [I]

Read about history in the following resource:

⭐ *The Story of the Ancient World:*
   Ch. XXXVI p. 80 – top of p. 82

You will be adding to your timeline in your *Student Notebook* today. In Unit 5 – Box 1, draw and color a dream cloud with 7 fat sheaves of grain and 7 thin ones. Label it, *Joseph interprets Pharaoh's dreams (1715 B.C.).* In Box 2, draw and color an Egyptian ship. Label it, *Hatshepsut, His Majesty Herself.* In Box 3, draw and color a pyramid. Label it, *Thutmosis the Conqueror.*

<u>Key Idea</u>: Hatshepsut was a female Pharaoh.

Storytime   [T]

Choose one of the following read aloud options:

⭐ *The Golden Bull:* *Ch. 31-33* p. 185-200

⭐ Read aloud the next portion of the adventure that you selected.

After the reading, students will give a summary oral narration. The oral narration must be no longer than 5 sentences and should summarize the reading. As students narrate, have them hold up one finger for each sentence shared. Remind students that the focus should be on the big ideas, rather than on the details.

<u>Key Idea</u>: Summarize the story by narrating.

History Project   [S]

Use an index card or a recipe card to copy the recipe for Egyptian Palace Bread listed below.
Ingredients:
5 slices of white bread
1 cup of honey
Whipped cream, sweetened cream, or ice cream

Directions:
Neatly cut off the crusts of the slices of bread. Pour the honey into a large bowl. Soak the bread in the honey for at least 30 minutes. Preheat the oven to 250 degrees. Grease a baking dish. Use a spatula to pile the slices of bread one on top of the other. Bake the bread at 250 degrees for 45 minutes. Cool the bread in the refrigerator for 15 minutes. Cut the bread into small slices and serve with your choice of cream.

<u>Key Idea</u>: Egyptians enjoyed various breads.

Bible Quiet Time   [I]

Reading: Choose one option below.

⭐ *The Illustrated Family Bible* p. 64

⭐ Your own Bible: Genesis chapter 44-45: 46:1-6

Scripture Focus: Highlight Genesis 46:3-4.

Prayer Focus: Pray a prayer of thanksgiving to express gratitude for God's divine goodness. Begin by reading the highlighted verses out loud as a prayer. End by praying, *I am so grateful that I am never truly alone, because you are always with me. Thank you for...*

Scripture Memory: Recite Philippians 2:5.
Music: *Philippians 2* CD: Track 2 (verse 5)

<u>Key Idea</u>: God spoke to Jacob and told him to go to Egypt. Jacob obeyed and settled there.

Independent History Study   [I]

Open your *Student Notebook* to Unit 5. Begin writing the names of Jacob's children in order next to their mother by using the listed numbers: 1) Reuben 2) Simeon 3) Levi 4) Judah 5) Dan 6) Naphtali

<u>Key Idea</u>: It is difficult to know which Pharaoh was ruling when the Israelites moved to Goshen in Egypt.

Learning the Basics
Focus: Language Arts, Math, Geography, Bible, and Science

Bible Study   [T]

Read aloud and discuss with the students the following pages:

 The Radical Book for Kids p. 38-41

<u>Key Idea</u>: God designed us in His image. Yet, with sin in the world, we need rescuing from our sin. The Bible is filled with stories of rescue. God rescued Israel from Goliath and fought for David. He sent Jonah to rescue the Ninevites, and then rescued Jonah when Jonah ran. He sent Jesus to rescue us from sin, Satan, and death. The Bible is filled with people who made good decisions and bad decisions, but God Himself is the hero of the story.

Language Arts   [S]

Have students complete one studied dictation exercise (see Appendix for directions and passages).

Work with the students to complete **one** of the writing options listed below:

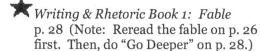 *Writing & Rhetoric Book 1: Fable* p. 28 (Note: Reread the fable on p. 26 first. Then, do "Go Deeper" on p. 28.)

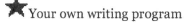 Your own writing program

<u>Key Idea</u>: Practice language arts skills.

Poetry   [I]

Open *Paint Like a Poet* to Lesson 5. Read aloud the poem *"One Step Backward Taken"* by Robert Frost.

Get the rocky backdrop that you painted on Day 2. Today, you will be adding details and shadows. You will need a palette, water, a small round paintbrush, a toothpick, a pencil, and brown, tan or peach, grey, and white paint.

After gathering your supplies, turn to the "Step-by-Step Watercolor Tutorial" for Lesson 5 in *Paint Like a Poet*. Follow steps 4-6 to complete "Part Two: Details and Shadows". When your painting is dry, glue your poetry copywork from Day 1 to your painting. Store your completed artwork in the place you have chosen for it.

<u>Key Idea</u>: Explore poetry moods with painting.

Math Exploration   [S]

Choose **one** of the math options listed below.

 Singapore Primary Mathematics 4A/4B or 5A/5B (see Appendix for schedules), or *Math with Confidence,* or *Apologia Math*

 Your own math program

<u>Key Idea</u>: Use a step-by-step math program.

Science Exploration   [I]

 Read *Land Animals of the Sixth Day* p. 81-86. Write the answer to each numbered question on lined paper. You do not need to copy the question. Use the listed page to help you answer each question.
1. Describe one of the following: Marsupial mole, Tasmanian devil, or Tasmanian tiger. (p. 81-82)
2. Write the words *prehensile* and *omnivore* and give their definitions. (p. 83)
3. What does a Virginia opossum do to defend itself when it cannot escape? (p. 85)
4. Use a globe or a world map to find the locations of the animals in the "Map It" section of p. 86.
5. On a clean page in your book of animal tracks, draw and label opossum tracks as shown on p. 87.

<u>Key Idea</u>: Marsupial moles spend their lives digging. Tasmanian devils are marsupials that are mostly scavengers. The Virginia opossum plays dead when it is unable to escape.

Learning through History
Focus: The Pharaohs of Ancient Egypt

Reading about History [I]

Read about history in the following resource:

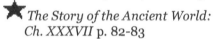 *The Story of the Ancient World:*
Ch. XXXVII p. 82-83

You will be writing a narration about *Chapter XXXVII: Thutmosis the Conqueror,* which is part of today's history reading.

To prepare for writing your narration, think about the questions below. If you do not know the answers, find them on p. 82 or 83 of *The Story of the Ancient World.* Ask yourself, *Why was Thutmosis one of Egypt's greatest Pharaohs? What did Thutmosis do in the first year of his reign? How did Pharaoh Thutmosis attack the Canaanites in Megiddo? When Pharaoh was victorious, what did he bring back to Egypt? Describe the pattern that Pharaoh set after this. What did Thutmosis establish at Karnak? Where were the Israelites during Thutmosis' campaigns?*

After you have thought about the answers to the questions, turn to Unit 5 in your *Student Notebook.* In Box 5, write a 5-8 sentence narration that begins with, *In the first year of Thutmosis' reign...* When you have finished writing, read your sentences out loud to catch any mistakes.

Check for the following things: *Did you include **who** the reading was mainly about? Did you include **what** important thing(s) happened? Did you include **how** it ended? If not, add those things.* Use the *Written Narration Skills* in the Appendix for editing.

<u>Key Idea</u>: As Pharaoh, Thutmosis conquered many lands and expanded Egypt's rule. He also made sure that conquered cities continued paying tribute to Egypt.

Storytime [T]

Choose one of the following read aloud options:

 Boy of the Pyramids: Ch. 1 p. 5-14

Read aloud the next portion of the adventure that you selected.

After the reading, have each person get a Bible and open it anywhere in Proverbs. Explain, *We will have 5 minutes to skim through the verses in Proverbs to find any connections to today's story. When a connection is found, read the verse out loud and quickly share the connection. At the end of 5 minutes, anyone who has not shared yet must read aloud one verse and make the best connection possible.*

<u>Key Idea</u>: Seek God's word for His guidance.

Bible Quiet Time [I]

Reading: Choose one option below.

Illustrated Family Bible Stories p. 66

Your own Bible: Exodus chapter 1

Scripture Focus: Highlight Exodus 1:12.

Prayer Focus: Pray a prayer of supplication to make a humble and earnest request of God. Begin by reading the highlighted verse out loud as a prayer. End by praying, *I ask you to be with Christians everywhere who are oppressed. Help me be strong for you by...*

Scripture Memory: Copy Philippians 2:5 in your Common Place Book.
Music: *Philippians 2* CD: Track 2 (verse 5)

<u>Key Idea</u>: The Hebrew people were oppressed.

Independent History Study [I]

Open your *Student Notebook* to Unit 5. Finish writing the names of Jacob's children in order next to their mother by using the listed numbers: 7) Gad 8) Asher 9) Issachar 10) Zebulun 11) Dinah 12) Joseph (His sons become two half-tribes: Manassah and Ephraim) 13) Benjamin

<u>Key Idea</u>: As time passed, a new pharaoh rose up in Egypt who did not remember Joseph.

Learning the Basics
Focus: Language Arts, Math, Geography, Bible, and Science

Geography [T]

Read aloud to the students the following pages:

★ *A Child's Geography Vol. II* – Read the last two paragraphs on p. 35 – p. 41. Discuss with the students "Field Notes" p. 41.

Key Idea: Oil wrestling, camel wrestling, and Children's Day are events that are important in Turkey. The Hagia Sophia, or the Church of the Holy Wisdom, can be seen in Istanbul. It was originally a Christian church and later a mosque for Muslims. Now, it is a museum. Many of the people in Turkey are Muslims, following the religion of Islam.

Language Arts [S]

Have students complete one dictation exercise.

Guide students to complete one reading lesson.

★ *Drawn into the Heart of Reading*

Help students complete **one** English lesson.

★ *Building with Diligence:* Lesson 10

★ *Following the Plan:* Lesson 9

★ Your own grammar program

Key Idea: Practice language arts skills.

Poetry [I]

Open *Paint Like a Poet* to Lesson 5. Today, you will be performing a poetry reading of *"One Step Backward Taken"*. Practice reading the poem aloud with expression that matches the mood of the poem. Then, read the poem aloud in front of your chosen audience. At the end of the reading, share the following, *When I read this poem by Robert Frost, it made me think of...* Call on your audience to share what thoughts the poem brought to their minds. Last, say, *Did you know that Robert Frost's father was originally from the South? But then, he moved to New Hampshire and later to California during the Civil War. Robert Frost was named after the famous southern general Robert E. Lee.*

Key Idea: Share the poetry of Robert Frost.

Math Exploration [S]

Choose **one** of the math options listed below.

★ *Singapore Primary Mathematics 4A/4B* or *5A/5B* (see Appendix for schedules), or *Math with Confidence*, or *Apologia Math*

★ Your own math program

Key Idea: Use a step-by-step math program.

Science Exploration [I]

Turn to the science experiment section in your science binder or sketchbook. At the top of a blank page, write: *What are some differences you notice among animal tracks that help to identify one animal track from another?* Under the question, write: *'Guess'.* Write down your guess. Follow the directions for the project in *Land Animals of the Sixth Day* p. 87-88. If you do not have the supplies for the project on p. 87-88, then do the alternate activity below instead.

Make air dry clay for carving animal tracks. To make the clay, stir together 1 cup flour and ½ cup salt. Add ½ cup hot water and stir. Knead the dough for 5 minutes. Then, wrap foil around a cake pan lid or a cookie sheet and roll the clay out onto the foil. Using the illustrations from your tracking book as a guide, carve the imprint of various tracks into the clay with a toothpick, spoon, and butter knife. Allow the tracks to dry. Next, on the paper write: *'Procedure'.* Draw a picture of the activity. At the bottom of the paper, write: *'Conclusion'.* Explain what you learned. When the tracks are dry, check to see if another family member can identify them using your tracking book for help.

Key Idea: Each animal track has its own shape, size, and pattern that helps to differentiate it from others.

Learning through History
Focus: God's Judgment Upon Egypt

Unit 6 - Day 1

Reading about History   I

Read about history in the following resource:

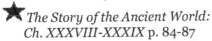 *The Story of the Ancient World:*
Ch. XXXVIII-XXXIX p. 84-87

The discovery of the undisturbed tomb of Pharaoh **Tutankhamun**, later labeled "**KV62**", gave archaeologists a spectacular glimpse of life in ancient Egypt. Use an encyclopedia, reference book, or online resource like www.wikipedia.org to research it.

Answer one or more of the following questions from your research: *When was "King Tut" or Tutankhamen's tomb discovered? Where was it located? Who discovered it? What did the archaeologists find as they entered the tomb? Why hadn't Tutankhamen's tomb been found earlier? Where are the items from the tomb today? Why did Tutankhamen or "King Tut" become so famous?*

Key Idea: Tutankhamen was originally named Tutankhaten in honor of Aten. His name was changed to reflect worship of Amon instead.

History Project   S

In this unit you will be making a column like those found in Egypt at the Temple of Karnak. See the picture on p. 86 of *A Story of the Ancient World.* To make your column, roll an 8½" x 11" white sheet of paper into a hollow cylinder about 2" wide. Tape the cylinder inside so that it doesn't unroll. Add glitter to white paint thinned with water to paint the outside of the column. Let it dry until Day 2.

Key Idea: The columns of the Temple of Amon-Ra at Karnak are still standing today.

Storytime   T

Choose one of the following read aloud options:

⭐ *Boy of the Pyramids:* Ch. 2 p. 15-28

⭐ Read at least one adventure for the next 12 days of plans.

After the reading, students will give a detailed oral narration. Select one paragraph from the story to read out loud to the students. This will be the starting point for the narration. Set a timer for 3-5 minutes. When the timer rings the narration is over, even if it isn't complete. A detailed, descriptive narration is the goal. See *Narration Tips* in the Appendix as needed.

Key Idea: Use oral narration to retell the story.

Bible Quiet Time   I

Bible Reading: Choose one option below.

⭐ *The Illustrated Family Bible* p. 67-69

⭐ Your own Bible: Exodus chapters 2-3

Scripture Focus: Highlight Exodus 3:5-7.

Prayer Focus: Pray a prayer of adoration to worship and honor God. Begin by reading the highlighted verses out loud as a prayer. End by praying, *I worship you for your holiness, Lord, and bow down before your presence like Moses. You alone are...*

Scripture Memory: Recite Philippians 2:6.
Music: *Philippians 2* CD: Track 2 (vs. 5-6)

Key Idea: God used an Egyptian princess to save Moses. Later, God spoke to Moses.

Independent History Study   I

⭐ Listen to *What in the World?* Disc 2, Half of Track 3: "Egyptian History". Pause after 8 minutes or so. Then, open your *Student Notebook* to Unit 6. In Box 6, copy in cursive Exodus 1:8-9 and 11.

Key Idea: Tutankhamen, son of Akhenaten, became Pharaoh as a young boy and died as a young man.

Learning the Basics
Focus: Language Arts, Math, Geography, Bible, and Science

Bible Study $\boxed{T}$

Read aloud and discuss with the students the following pages:

 The Radical Book for Kids p. 42-43

<u>Key Idea</u>: God sent the shepherd boy David to defeat the giant Goliath. David used a sling to fight Goliath. Follow the included directions to make a simple sling.

Language Arts $\boxed{S}$

Have students complete one studied dictation exercise (see Appendix for directions and passages).

Help students complete one lesson from the following reading program:

 Drawn into the Heart of Reading

Work with the students to complete **one** of the English options listed below:

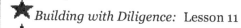 *Building with Diligence:* Lesson 11

 Following the Plan: Lesson 10 (Half)

★ Your own grammar program

<u>Key Idea</u>: Practice language arts skills.

Poetry $\boxed{I}$

Open *Paint Like a Poet* to Lesson 6. Read aloud the poem *"Fireflies in the Garden"*. On a 3 x 5 index card, neatly copy in black ink or in pencil the following highlighted lines from the poem:

Here come real stars to fill the upper skies,
And here on earth come emulating flies,
That though they never equal stars in size,
(And they were never really stars at heart)
Achieve at times a very star-like start.
Only, of course, they can't sustain the part.
                                        -Robert Frost

Check your work to make sure it is correctly copied. Then, cut around your copywork. You may choose to outline the edge of the cut-out with a black marker. Save it for Day 3.

<u>Key Idea</u>: Read and appreciate classic poetry.

Math Exploration $\boxed{S}$

Choose **one** of the math options listed below.

 Singapore Primary Mathematics 4A/4B or 5A/5B (see Appendix for schedules), or *Math with Confidence,* or *Apologia Math*

 Your own math program

<u>Key Idea</u>: Use a step-by-step math program.

Science Exploration $\boxed{I}$

★ Read *Land Animals of the Sixth Day* p. 89 – middle of p. 95. Today you will add to your science notebook. At the top of an unlined paper, copy 1 Corinthians 15:39 in cursive. Beneath the verse, draw the chart shown at the top of p. 95 in *Land Animals of the Sixth Day*. You will refer to this chart as you're reading the pages for this unit's science lesson.

<u>Key Idea</u>: Primates are mammals with forward-facing eyes, which gives them good depth perception for jumping. They usually have opposable thumbs and often have opposable toes. These help primates grasp tree limbs. Many primates are omnivores. Primates have fairly large brains and form groups called troops. Troops have an alpha male and an alpha female. Man is different from the primates, because we were created in God's image.

Reading about History | I |

Read about history in the following resource:

 ★ *The Story of the Ancient World:* Ch. XL-XLI p. 88 – top of p. 93

You will be choosing a portion from today's reading that you found memorable or worthy of being reread to copy. Open your *Student Notebook* to Unit 6. In Box 4, carefully copy in cursive the portion from today's reading that you selected. Then, compare your written work to the original. Last, draw a small colorful picture in Box 4 to illustrate your sentences.

<u>Key Idea</u>: Moses was the great-grandson of Levi, son of Jacob (or Israel). Moses had two older siblings, Miriam and Aaron.

Storytime | T |

Choose one of the following read aloud options:

★ *Boy of the Pyramids:* Ch. 3 p. 29-36

★ Read aloud the next portion of the adventure that you selected.

After reading, give each person 2 slips of paper. Each person must think of 2 questions to ask about the book and write one question on each slip of paper. Next, fold up the slips of paper and place them in a container. Each person must select at least one question from the container to answer.

<u>Key Idea</u>: Use questioning to share the story.

History Project | S |

Take out the temple column that you saved from Day 1. The lotus flower was a sacred Egyptian flower. Look at the flower painted on the wall in the picture on p. 76 of *The Story of the Ancient World*. Cut only the top edges of your temple column to resemble the petals of a lotus flower. Then, roll the edges of the flower around your pencil to get them to bend out. Next, outline the edges of the flower petals in gold. Under the flower petals, use a blue marker to draw several thin blue lines in a circle around the outside of your column. Save your column for Day 3.

<u>Key Idea</u>: God used Moses' upbringing in an Egyptian palace and his time of living in the desert to prepare him for God's calling.

Bible Quiet Time | I |

Reading: Choose one option below.

★ *The Illustrated Family Bible* p. 70-71

★ Your own Bible: Exodus chapters 4-5

Scripture Focus: Highlight Exodus 4:13.

Prayer Focus: Pray a prayer of confession to admit or acknowledge your sins to God. Begin by reading the highlighted verse out loud as a prayer. End by praying, *I confess Lord that sometimes I want someone else to do what you ask, instead of me. Help me to obey...*

Scripture Memory: Recite Philippians 2:6.
Music: *Philippians 2* CD: Track 2 (vs. 5-6)

<u>Key Idea</u>: God used Moses to save his people.

Independent History Study | I |

★ Listen to *What in the World?* Disc 2, Last Half of Track 3: "Egyptian History". Open your *Student Notebook* to "Prophecies About Christ". Under "Prophecy" write, *Exodus 3:13-15*. Read the Scripture from your Bible to discover the prophecy. Under "Fulfillment" write, *John 13:19*. Read the fulfillment Scripture. Under "Description", write a few phrases to describe the prophecy about Jesus.

<u>Key Idea</u>: God told Moses "I AM WHO I AM", meaning Jehovah or the one who will deliver His people.

Learning the Basics
Focus: Language Arts, Math, Geography, Bible, and Science

Geography [T]

Have students get both the blank map and the labeled map of **Turkey** that they began in Unit 3.

Then, assign students the following page:

 A Child's Geography Vol. II p. 42

Note: Do only the "Map Notes" section.

Key Idea: Practice finding and recording the locations of various places on a map of Turkey.

Language Arts [S]

Help students complete one lesson from the following reading program:

 Drawn into the Heart of Reading

Work with the students to complete **one** of the writing options listed below:

 Writing & Rhetoric Book 1: Fable p. 30-32 (Note: Omit p. 29. Guide students through the lesson, so they are successful writing an amplification.)

Your own writing program

Key Idea: Practice language arts skills.

Poetry [I]

Open *Paint Like a Poet* to Lesson 6. Read aloud the poem *"Fireflies in the Garden"* by Robert Frost.

Today, you will be painting a night sky backdrop. You will need painting paper, a palette, water, a large flat paintbrush, masking tape, a paper towel, and dark blue and purple paint.

After gathering your supplies, turn to the "Step-by-Step Watercolor Tutorial" for Lesson 6 in *Paint Like a Poet*. Follow steps 1-3 to complete "Part One: Night Sky Backdrop". Then, let your background dry. You will complete "Part Two" of the tutorial on Day 3.

Key Idea: Use painting to illustrate poetry.

Math Exploration [S]

Choose **one** of the math options listed below.

 Singapore Primary Mathematics 4A/4B or 5A/5B (see Appendix for schedules), or *Math with Confidence,* or *Apologia Math*

 Your own math program

Key Idea: Use a step-by-step math program.

Science Exploration [I]

Read *Land Animals of the Sixth Day* middle of p. 95 – bottom of p. 100. Orally retell or narrate to an adult the portion of text that you read today. Use the *Narration Tips* in the Appendix for help as needed.

Key Idea: Lemurs, bushbabies, lorises, and aye-ayes are in the suborder Strepsirrhini. These are primates with wet noses that are nocturnal and often eat insects and plants. The suborder Haplorrhini includes dry-nosed primates such as mandrills, tamarins, and tarsiers.

Learning through History
Focus: God's Judgment Upon Egypt

Unit 6 - Day 3

Reading about History | I

Read about history in the following resource:

⭐ *The Story of the Ancient World:*
Ch. XLII-XLIII p. 93 – middle of p. 97

You will be adding to your timeline in your *Student Notebook* today. In Unit 6 – Box 1, draw and color a sun disc. Label it, *Akhenaten – Pharaoh of one god*. In Box 2, draw and color a crook and flail. Label it, *Tutankhamun (1616 B.C.)*. In Box 3, draw and color a burning bush. Label it, *Moses – 10 Plagues (1491 B.C.)*.

Key Idea: God hardened Pharaoh's heart, so all of Egypt would see through God's miraculous signs that there is only one true God.

Storytime | T

Choose one of the following read aloud options:

⭐ *Boy of the Pyramids:* Ch. 4 p. 37-54

⭐ Read aloud the next portion of the adventure that you selected.

After the reading, students will give a summary oral narration. The oral narration must be no longer than 5 sentences and should summarize the reading. As students narrate, have them hold up one finger for each sentence shared. Remind students that the focus should be on the big ideas, rather than on the details.

Key Idea: Summarize the story by narrating.

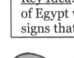

History Project | S

Take out the temple column that you saved from Day 2. Today, you will draw small symbols to stand for the 10 plagues. For the first plague, draw a red river. For the second plague, draw a green frog. For the third plague, draw a swarm of gnats and lice. For the fourth plague, draw flies. For the fifth plague, draw a crossed out cow or bull. For the sixth plague, draw boils or sores on beasts or man. For the seventh plague, draw hail. For the eighth plague, draw locusts or grasshoppers. For the ninth plague, draw darkness. For the tenth plague, draw a gravestone for the firstborn son.

Key Idea: Through 9 plagues, Pharaoh refused to obey God. After the 10th plague, Pharaoh sent a message to Moses in the middle of the night telling the Israelites to leave Egypt. The angel of death had passed over the Israelites.

Bible Quiet Time | I

Reading: Choose one option below.

⭐ *The Illustrated Family Bible* p. 72-75

⭐ Your own Bible: Exodus chapter 7:14-22; 8:1-7, 16-24; chapters 9-11

Scripture Focus: Highlight Exodus 12:26-27.

Prayer Focus: Pray a prayer of thanksgiving to express gratitude for God's divine goodness. Begin by reading the highlighted verses out loud as a prayer. End by praying, *I worship you for sparing the Israelites. Thank you for sparing me through Christ.*

Scripture Memory: Recite Philippians 2:6.
Music: *Philippians 2* CD: Track 2 (vs. 5-6)

Key Idea: God sent 10 plagues upon Egypt.

Independent History Study | I

Open your *Student Notebook* to Unit 6 and copy the plague on the numbered line and next to it the Egyptian god who was judged. 1) water turned to blood – Nile River worshipped as god of life 2) frogs – frogs worshipped as goddess of the land 3) gnats & lice – gnats, symbol of god of the earth 4) flies - scarab beetle, god of insects 5) disease on livestock – bull and cow worshipped as sacred

Key Idea: God used the ten plagues as a judgment against Egypt's false gods. There is only one true God.

Learning the Basics
Focus: Language Arts, Math, Geography, Bible, and Science

Bible Study | T |

Read aloud and discuss with the students the following pages:

 The Radical Book for Kids p. 44-46

<u>Key Idea</u>: J.C. Ryle was an English pastor, church leader, and author. His book *Thoughts for Young Men* is over 100 years old, yet it is still read today. The book includes advice for young people who want to follow Jesus. Ryle advises young people to have a clear view of sin, to get to know Jesus personally, to remember your soul will spend eternity somewhere, to look for ways to serve God now, and to make the Bible your guide.

Language Arts | S |

Have students complete one studied dictation exercise (see Appendix for directions and passages).

Work with the students to complete **one** of the writing options listed below:

 Writing & Rhetoric Book 1: Fable p. 33-34 (Note: Guide students through the lesson, so they are successful writing a summary.)

 Your own writing program

<u>Key Idea</u>: Practice language arts skills.

Poetry | I |

Open *Paint Like a Poet* to Lesson 6. Read aloud the poem *"Fireflies in the Garden"* by Robert Frost.

Get the night sky backdrop that you painted on Day 2. Today, you will be adding fireflies and a tree. You will need a palette, water, a small flat paintbrush, a toothpick, and yellow and black paint.

After gathering your supplies, turn to the "Step-by-Step Watercolor Tutorial" for Lesson 6 in *Paint Like a Poet*. Follow steps 4-6 to complete "Part Two: Fireflies and Tree". When your painting is dry, glue your poetry copywork from Day 1 to your painting. Store your completed artwork in the place you have chosen for it.

<u>Key Idea</u>: Explore poetry moods with painting.

Math Exploration | S |

Choose **one** of the math options listed below.

 Singapore Primary Mathematics 4A/4B or 5A/5B (see Appendix for schedules), or *Math with Confidence*, or *Apologia Math*

 Your own math program

<u>Key Idea</u>: Use a step-by-step math program.

Science Exploration | I |

 Read *Land Animals of the Sixth Day* from the bottom of p. 100 – top of p. 105. Write the answer to each numbered question on lined paper. You do not need to copy the question. Refer to the listed pages.
1. What are some of the differences between monkeys and apes? (p. 101)
2. On your notebooking page from Day 1, add two boxes below Catarrhini labeled *Old World Monkeys* and *Apes*. Under *Old World Monkeys,* add two more boxes labeled *Colobinae* and *Cercopithecinae*. Under *Apes,* add two boxes labeled *Great Apes* and *Lesser Apes*. (p. 101, 103)
3. Write the words *proboscis* and *brachiation* and give their definitions. (p. 101 and p. 104)
4. Use a globe or a world map to find the locations of the animals in the "Map It" section of p. 109.
5. After reading Genesis 1:26-27, how can we be sure that we are not descended from apes?

<u>Key Idea</u>: Monkeys and apes are both primates, yet they are different from one another.

Reading about History | I

Read about history in the following resource:

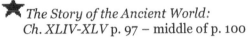 *The Story of the Ancient World:*
Ch. XLIV-XLV p. 97 – middle of p. 100

You will be writing a narration about *Chapter XLV: The Unexpected Battle,* which is part of today's history reading.

To prepare for writing your narration, think about the questions below. If you do not know the answers, find them on p. 99-100 of *The Story of the Ancient World.* Ask yourself, *Who were the Amalekites? What news about the Israelites spread everywhere? Why did the Amalekites choose to make war against the Israelites? How did the Amalekites attack them? Why did the Israelites panic? What did Moses encourage them to do? While Joshua and the Israelites fought the Amalekites, what did Moses do? Why did Moses have Aaron and Hur support his arms? How did this victory bless the Israelites?*

After you have thought about the answers to the questions, turn to Unit 6 in your *Student Notebook.* In Box 5, write a 5-8 sentence narration that begins with, *In the second month after the Israelites escaped from Egypt...* When you have finished writing, read your sentences out loud to catch any mistakes.

Check for the following things: *Did you include **who** the reading was mainly about? Did you include **what** important thing(s) happened? Did you include **how** it ended? If not, add those things.* Use the *Written Narration Skills* in the Appendix for editing.

Key Idea: The Amelekites, who descended from Ham, were wandering Cushite nomads who attacked the Israelites. God helped Israel.

Storytime | T

Choose one of the following read aloud options:

 Boy of the Pyramids: Ch. 5 p. 55-70

★ Read aloud the next part of the adventure.

After the reading, have each person get a Bible and open it anywhere in Proverbs. Explain, *We will have 5 minutes to skim through the verses in Proverbs to find any connections to today's story. When a connection is found, read the verse out loud and quickly share the connection. At the end of 5 minutes, anyone who has not shared yet must read aloud one verse and make the best connection possible.*

Key Idea: Seek God's word for His guidance.

Bible Quiet Time | I

Reading: Choose one option below.

★ *The Illustrated Family Bible* p. 76-79

★ Your own Bible: Exodus 12:31-42; 14; 15:22-27

Scripture Focus: Highlight Exodus 13:21.

Prayer Focus: Pray a prayer of supplication to make a humble and earnest request of God. Begin by reading the highlighted verse out loud as a prayer. End by praying, *I pray for you to lead me like you did the Israelites. Show me what you want me to do and where to go.*

Scripture Memory: Copy Philippians 2:6 in your Common Place Book.
Music: *Philippians 2* CD: Track 2 (vs. 5-6)

Key Idea: God led the Israelites in the desert.

Independent History Study | I

Open your *Student Notebook* to Unit 6. Copy the plague on the numbered line and next to it the Egyptian god who was judged. 6) boils – god of wisdom and medicine 7) hail – sky goddess 8) locusts – false gods who protect crops 9) darkness – sun god Amon 10) death of first born – Pharaoh, embodiment of Amon

Key Idea: After God's judgment against Egypt, it never again returned to its former glory.

Learning the Basics
Focus: Language Arts, Math, Geography, Bible, and Science

Geography   T

Go to the website link listed on p. 6 of *A Child's Geography Vol. II.* At the link, select "History & Geography". Then, under "Knowledge Quest" select ACG2-Extra Activities". Print the "Travel Log Template" of your choice from p. 39-42. Also at the link, for older students, print and assign the "Chapter Three Review" on p. 69. Assign all students the page below.

★ *A Child's Geography Vol. II* p. 42

Note: Do the "Travel Notes" section on p. 42.

<u>Key Idea:</u> Share three sights from Turkey.

Language Arts   S

Have students complete one dictation exercise.

Guide students to complete one reading lesson.

★ *Drawn into the Heart of Reading*

Help students complete **one** English lesson.

★ *Building with Diligence:* Lesson 12

★ *Following the Plan:* Lesson 10 (Last half)

★ Your own grammar program

<u>Key Idea:</u> Practice language arts skills.

Poetry   I

Open *Paint Like a Poet* to Lesson 6. Today, you will be performing a poetry reading of *"Fireflies in the Garden"*. Practice reading the poem aloud with expression that matches the mood of the poem. Then, read the poem aloud in front of your chosen audience. At the end of the reading, share the following, *When I read this poem by Robert Frost, it made me think of...* Call on your audience to share what thoughts the poem brought to their minds. Last, say, *Did you know that when Robert Frost was eleven years old his father died of tuberculosis? His father had requested to be buried in New England. So in 1885, Robert's family returned to the New England area. Lacking money to return to the West, they lived with his grandfather in Massachusetts. Much of Robert's poetry would be written about life in the New England states.*

<u>Key Idea:</u> Share the poetry of Robert Frost.

Math Exploration   S

Choose **one** of the math options listed below.

★ *Singapore Primary Mathematics 4A/4B* or *5A/5B* (see Appendix for schedules), or *Math with Confidence,* or *Apologia Math*

★ Your own math program

<u>Key Idea:</u> Use a step-by-step math program.

Science Exploration   I

★ Read *Land Animals of the Sixth Day* p. 105 – middle of p. 109. Now, skip to the "Experiment" on p. 110. Turn to the science experiment section in your science binder or sketchbook. At the top of a blank page, write: *Why is depth perception a needed skill for both humans and primates?* Under the question, write: *'Guess'*. Write down your guess.

Follow the directions for the experiment in *Land Animals of the Sixth Day* p. 110. Next, on the paper write: *'Procedure'*. Draw a chart similar to the one shown on p. 110 and fill it in with your own objects and distances. At the bottom of the paper, write: *'Conclusion'*. Explain what you learned from the experiment.

<u>Key Idea:</u> Depth perception helps you guess how near or far away things are. Judging distances is an important skill for primates to have as they leap from one branch to the next!

Learning through History
Focus: God's Chosen People Rebel

Reading about History [I]

Read about history in the following resource:

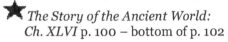 *The Story of the Ancient World:*
  Ch. XLVI p. 100 – bottom of p. 102

As priest, Aaron was to wear an ephod. Where could you look to research more about the **ephod** and **breastplate**? Read Exodus 28 as the most accurate resource on God's instructions for the design of these garments.

Answer one or more of the following questions from your research: *What is an ephod? What was fastened on the shoulder pieces of the ephod? Why were onyx stones fastened on the shoulder pieces of the ephod? Describe the breastplate. What were the Urim and the Thummim? Why did Aaron have bells on the hem of his gown? From which tribe were the priests?*

<u>Key Idea:</u> In Moses' absence, Aaron failed.

History Project [S]

In this unit you will be making a breastplate like the High Priest Aaron wore. Open your *Student Notebook* to Unit 7 to see the gemstones that you will be making for the breastplate. Mix together 4 Tbsp. white glue, 8 Tbsp. cornstarch, 2 Tbsp. water, and 2 Tbsp. toothpaste to make air dry clay. Roll the clay into 12 "gemstones" that are the same size as those in the *Student Notebook* and are flat on the back. Allow the gemstones to dry over-night. Also, make 12 smaller "rocks" for Unit 8.

<u>Key Idea:</u> God gave the Israelites very specific instructions. The people needed to obey.

Storytime [T]

Choose one of the following read aloud options:

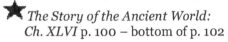 *Boy of the Pyramids:* Ch. 6 p. 71-82

★ Read at least one adventure for the next 8 days of plans.

After the reading, students will give a detailed oral narration. Select one paragraph from the story to read out loud to the students. This will be the starting point for the narration. Set a timer for 3-5 minutes. When the timer rings the narration is over, even if it isn't complete. A detailed, descriptive narration is the goal. See *Narration Tips* in the Appendix as needed.

<u>Key Idea:</u> Use oral narration to retell the story.

Bible Quiet Time [I]

Bible Reading: Choose one option below.

★ *The Illustrated Family Bible* p. 80-83
  Optional extension: p. 65

★ Your own Bible: Exodus 20:1-21; 32

Scripture Focus: Highlight Exodus 20:1-3.

Prayer Focus: Pray a prayer of adoration to worship and honor God. Begin by reading the highlighted verses out loud as a prayer. End by praying, *I praise you as the one true God who has always been and always will be.*

Scripture Memory: Recite Philippians 2:7.
Music: *Philippians 2* CD: Track 2 (vs. 5-7)

<u>Key Idea:</u> The people returned to idol worship.

Independent History Study [I]

Open your *Student Notebook* to "Prophecies About Christ". Under "Prophecy" write, *Hosea 11:1.* Read the Scripture from your Bible to discover the prophecy. Under "Fulfillment" write, *Matthew 2:13-15.* Read the fulfillment Scripture. Under "Description", write a few phrases to describe the prophecy about Jesus.

<u>Key Idea:</u> Hosea prophecied that out of Egypt God would call His Son. God did this with the nation of Israel and did it again with His only Son, Jesus, when He called Him back from Egypt upon Herod's death.

Learning the Basics

Focus: Language Arts, Math, Geography, Bible, and Science

Bible Study [T]

Read aloud and discuss with the students the following pages:

 The Radical Book for Kids p. 47-50

Key Idea: Many phrases we use in everyday conversation come from the Bible. Often, people don't even realize they are quoting Scripture when they use certain everyday phrases. On the other hand, some everyday phrases attributed to the Bible aren't actually in God's Word. You have to read and study Scripture to know what is really in God's Word.

Language Arts [S]

Have students complete one studied dictation exercise (see Appendix for directions and passages).

Help students complete one lesson from the following reading program:

 Drawn into the Heart of Reading

Work with the students to complete **one** of the English options listed below:

 Building with Diligence: Lesson 13

 Following the Plan: Lesson 11 (Half)

Your own grammar program

Key Idea: Practice language arts skills.

Poetry [I]

Open *Paint Like a Poet* to Lesson 7. Read aloud the poem *"Gathering Leaves"*. On a 3 x 5 index card, neatly copy in black ink or in pencil the following highlighted lines from the poem:

Spades take up leaves
No better than spoons,
And bags full of leaves
Are light as balloons.

                    -Robert Frost

Check your work to make sure it is correctly copied. Then, cut around your copywork. You may choose to outline the edge of the cut-out with an orange marker. Save it for Day 3.

Key Idea: Read and appreciate a variety of classic poetry.

Math Exploration [S]

Choose **one** of the math options listed below.

 Singapore Primary Mathematics 4A/4B or *5A/5B* (see Appendix for schedules), or *Math with Confidence,* or *Apologia Math*

 Your own math program

Key Idea: Use a step-by-step math program.

Science Exploration [I]

Read *Land Animals of the Sixth Day* p. 111 – bottom of p. 115.

Get your book about animal tracks that you began last unit. At the top of the next page in your book, copy in cursive Psalm 8:6-7. Beneath the verse, draw and label the beaver tracks, rabbit tracks, and armadillo tracks as shown in the "Track It" drawings on p. 129.

Key Idea: Rodents thrive everywhere in the world. They are usually small, have short limbs, and are plantigrades. Many rodents have long tails. Rodents also have special teeth for gnawing and often eat plants. The three main groups of rodents are squirrel-like rodents, mouse-like rodents, and cavy-like rodents.

Reading about History [I]

Read about history in the following resource:

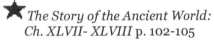 *The Story of the Ancient World:*
Ch. XLVII- XLVIII p. 102-105

You will be choosing a portion from today's reading that you found memorable or worthy of being reread to copy. Open your *Student Notebook* to Unit 7. In Box 3, carefully copy in cursive the portion from today's reading that you selected. Then, compare your written work to the original. Last, draw a small colorful picture in Box 3 to illustrate your sentences.

Key Idea: As Moses pleaded with the Lord, God forgave the Israelites for their idol worship. However, their sin was not without consequences. As the Israelites began work on the tabernacle, according to God's specific plans, they learned to follow God's laws.

History Project [S]

Get the 12 large stones that you made on Day 1. Read the Biblical description of the 12 stones used on the breastplate in Exodus 28:16-21. You will paint your stones so that they resemble the 12 gemstones pictured in your *Student Notebook* in Unit 7. Wait to write the Hebrew names of the tribes on the stones until Day 3. When you you have finished painting, lay the gemstones flat to dry until Day 3. Do not paint the 12 smaller stones, but instead save them for Unit 8.

Key Idea: The Israelites needed to learn to fear the Lord because He is just and holy. To be His chosen people, they needed to understand that He is different from pagan idols and gods.

Storytime [T]

Choose one of the following read aloud options:

 Boy of the Pyramids: Ch. 7 p. 83-94

Read aloud the next portion of the adventure that you selected.

After reading, work with the students to plan a 3 minute skit with simple props to act out part of today's reading. Set a timer for 3 minutes to quickly prepare for the skit. Make sure that you participate in the skit along with the students. When the timer rings, set it again for 3 minutes and perform the skit. You do not need an audience, as the goal is the retelling.

Key Idea: Use a skit to retell part of the story.

Bible Quiet Time [I]

Reading: Choose one option below.

The Illustrated Family Bible p. 86-87

Your own Bible: Numbers chapters 11-12

Scripture Focus: Highlight Numbers 11:1.

Prayer Focus: Pray a prayer of confession to admit or acknowledge your sins to God. Begin by reading the highlighted verse out loud as a prayer. End by praying, *I confess to you Lord that sometimes I complain about things too. Forgive me for my complaining about... Help me take my problems to you instead.*

Scripture Memory: Recite Philippians 2:7.
Music: *Philippians 2* CD: Track 2 (vs. 5-7)

Key Idea: The Israelites complained often.

Independent History Study [I]

Open your *Student Notebook* to "Prophecies About Christ". Under "Prophecy" write, *Deuteronomy 18:18-19.* Read the Scripture to discover the prophecy. Under "Fulfillment" write, *John 6:14.* Read the fulfillment Scripture. Under "Description", write a few phrases to describe the prophecy about Jesus.

Key Idea: Moses prophecied that the Savior would be a Prophet, like him, who would speak God's words.

Learning the Basics
Focus: Language Arts, Math, Geography, Bible, and Science

Geography [T]

Have Turkish tea with the students following the directions in the "Food" section of p. 43. Any type of tea may be used.

While having your tea, read aloud the prayer with the students on the following page:

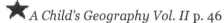 *A Child's Geography Vol. II* p. 46

As an optional extra, choose to make Turkish Delight or Noah's Pudding as directed on p. 44-45.

<u>Key Idea</u>: It's important to pray for those in other countries who need to know the Lord.

Language Arts [S]

Help students complete one lesson from the following reading program:

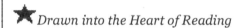 *Drawn into the Heart of Reading*

Work with the students to complete **one** of the writing options listed below:

★ *Writing & Rhetoric Book 1: Fable* p. 35-39 (Note: Read the text aloud while the students follow along. Then, discuss.)

★ Your own writing program

<u>Key Idea</u>: Practice language arts skills.

Poetry [I]

Open *Paint Like a Poet* to Lesson 7. Read aloud the poem *"Gathering Leaves"* by Robert Frost.

Today, you will be painting a yellow backdrop. You will need painting paper, a palette, water, a large flat paintbrush, and yellow paint.

After gathering your supplies, turn to the "Step-by-Step Watercolor Tutorial" for Lesson 7 in *Paint Like a Poet*. Follow steps 1-3 to complete "Part One: Yellow Backdrop". Then, let your background dry. You will complete "Part Two" of the tutorial on Day 3.

<u>Key Idea</u>: Use painting to illustrate poetry.

Math Exploration [S]

Choose **one** of the math options listed below.

★ *Singapore Primary Mathematics 4A/4B or 5A/5B* (see Appendix for schedules), or *Math with Confidence,* or *Apologia Math*

★ Your own math program

<u>Key Idea</u>: Use a step-by-step math program.

Science Exploration [I]

★ Read *Land Animals of the Sixth Day* bottom of p. 115 – top of p. 120. Orally retell or narrate to an adult the portion of text that you read today. Use the *Narration Tips* in the Appendix for help as needed. Then, use a globe or a world map to find the locations of the animals in the first column of the "Map It" section of p. 129.

<u>Key Idea</u>: Beavers are rodents that build dams. These dams create a wetland habitat for many species that are endangered. Their dams also purify the water downstream. Hedgehogs, shrews, and moles are examples of animals that are in the order Insectivora. These animals eat insects and don't fit well in any other order.

Reading about History — I

Read about history in the following resource:

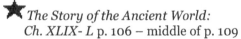 *The Story of the Ancient World:*
Ch. XLIX- L p. 106 – middle of p. 109

You will be adding to your timeline in your *Student Notebook* today. In Unit 7 – Box 1, draw and color two stone tablets. Label it, *Ten Commandments (1491 B.C.).* In Box 2, draw and color purple grapes on a vine. Label it, *12 Spies enter Canaan – 40 years of wandering (1490 B.C.).*

Key Idea: At God's command, Moses sent 12 spies (one from each tribe) to spy out the land of Canaan. Although the land was beautiful and fertile, 10 of the spies doubted whether they could take the land. They were doubting God.

History Project — S

Choose an 8" x 12" red, blue, or purple piece of construction paper to be your breastplate. Then, cut an 8" x 6" piece of yellow paper and glue it in the middle of your breastplate. Following the gemstone picture in your *Student Notebook* as a guide, use a black permanent marker to write the matching Hebrew name for the tribe on the corresonding colored gemstone. Then, glue the stones on the yellow part of the breastplate, according to the order shown in your *Student Notebook*.

Key Idea: Only two spies believed God would help them take Canaan. The two spies were Joshua, of the tribe of Ephraim, and Caleb, of the tribe of Judah. Ephraim was Joseph's son, and Judah's line would one day include Jesus.

Storytime — T

Choose one of the following read aloud options:

 Boy of the Pyramids: Ch. 8 p. 95-112

⭐ Read aloud the next portion of the adventure that you selected.

After the reading, students will give a summary oral narration. The oral narration must be no longer than 5 sentences and should summarize the reading. As students narrate, have them hold up one finger for each sentence shared. Remind students that the focus should be on the big ideas, rather than on the details.

Key Idea: Summarize the story by narrating.

Bible Quiet Time — I

Reading: Choose one option below.

⭐ *The Illustrated Family Bible* p. 88-89

⭐ Your own Bible: Numbers 13:1-2, 26-33; 14

Scripture Focus: Highlight Numbers 13:27.

Prayer Focus: Pray a prayer of thanksgiving to express gratitude for God's divine goodness. Begin by reading the highlighted verse out loud as a prayer. End by praying, *Thank you for allowing me grow up in a free country that is flowing with milk and honey too, due to its abundant blessings of...*

Scripture Memory: Recite Philippians 2:7.
Music: *Philippians 2* CD: Track 2 (vs. 5-7)

Key Idea: The Promised Land was all that God promised it would be.

Independent History Study — I

⭐ Listen to *What in the World?* Disc 2, Track 4: "Abraham Through Moses". Then, open your *Student Notebook* to Unit 7. In Box 5, copy in cursive Numbers 14:11.

Key Idea: The people doubted the Lord's help in taking the Promised Land, even after all of His miracles.

Learning the Basics
Focus: Language Arts, Math, Geography, Bible, and Science

Bible Study   [T]

Read aloud and discuss with the students the following pages:

 The Radical Book for Kids p. 51-55

Key Idea: In 1452, the invention of the printing press led Gutenberg to print Bibles and make them available to the common man. Today, the Bible is available in 2500 different languages. When you read God's Word, it is important to have a good translation or version of the Bible. Next, it is important to have a plan and a time and place to read the Bible. As you read, ask God for help to understand His Word. Take your time as you read and try to learn more about God. Then, think about what you read.

Language Arts   [S]

Have students complete one studied dictation exercise (see Appendix for directions and passages).

Work with the students to complete **one** of the writing options listed below:

 Writing & Rhetoric Book 1: Fable p. 41-43 (Note: Omit p. 40. Guide students through the lesson, so they are successful writing a summary.)

 Your own writing program

Key Idea: Practice language arts skills.

Poetry   [I]

Open *Paint Like a Poet* to Lesson 7. Read aloud the poem *"Gathering Leaves"* by Robert Frost.

Get the yellow backdrop that you painted on Day 2. Today, you will be adding an autumn tree. You will need a palette, water, a dropper, a small flat paintbrush, paper towels (or a sponge), and brown, orange, and yellow paint.

After gathering your supplies, turn to the "Step-by-Step Watercolor Tutorial" for Lesson 7 in *Paint Like a Poet*. Follow steps 4-6 to complete "Part Two: Autumn Tree". When your painting is dry, glue your poetry copywork from Day 1 to your painting. Store your completed artwork in the place you have chosen for it.

Key Idea: Explore poetry moods with painting.

Math Exploration   [S]

Choose **one** of the math options listed below.

 Singapore Primary Mathematics 4A/4B or 5A/5B (see Appendix for schedules), or *Math with Confidence*, or *Apologia Math*

 Your own math program

Key Idea: Use a step-by-step math program.

Science Exploration   [I]

Read *Land Animals of the Sixth Day* middle of p. 120 – top of p. 126. Write the answer to each numbered question on lined paper. You do not need to copy the question. Use the listed pages for help.
1. What are some differences between rabbits and hares? (p. 121)
2. Write the words *patagium* and *viviparous* and give their definitions. (p. 122-123)
3. Which two egg-laying animals were difficult for scientists to classify as mammals? (p. 123-124)
4. Use a globe or a world map to find the locations of the animals listed in the second column of the "Map It" section of p. 129.
5. What does Job 12:7-10 teach us about our Maker?

Key Idea: Each mammal has its own God-given characteristics that help identify it from other mammals.

Reading about History | I

Read about history in the following resource:

The Story of the Ancient World:
   Ch. LI-LII p. 109 – top of p. 113

You will be writing a narration about *Chapter LI: The Bronze Serpent,* which is part of today's history reading.

To prepare for writing your narration, think about the questions below. If you do not know the answers, find them on p. 109-111 of *The Story of the Ancient World.* Ask yourself, *When the Israelites complained in the desert, what came among them? What did God tell Moses to make in response? How were the people to be healed? What lesson did the bronze serpent represent later? How did treating the bronze serpent as a relic become a problem for the Israelite nation later? Where do we see the emblem of the serpent wrapped around a pole today? When the Amorites would not allow the Israelites to pass through their country, what happened? Whom did the Israelites fight next? What was the result of the battle with Og?*

After you have thought about the answers to the questions, turn to Unit 7 in your *Student Notebook.* In Box 4, write a 5-8 sentence narration that begins with, *As the Israelites were wandering in the desert...* When you have finished writing, read your sentences out loud to catch any mistakes. Check for the following things: *Did you include **who** the reading was mainly about? Did you include **what** important thing(s) happened? Did you include **how** it ended? If not, add those things.* Then, edit with the *Narration Skills.*

<u>Key Idea:</u> The Israelites wandered 40 years.

Storytime | T

Choose one of the following read aloud options:

Boy of the Pyramids: Ch. 9 p. 113-122

Read aloud the next part of the adventure.

After the reading, have each person get a Bible and open it anywhere in Proverbs. Explain, *We will have 5 minutes to skim through the verses in Proverbs to find any connections to today's story. When a connection is found, read the verse out loud and quickly share the connection. At the end of 5 minutes, anyone who has not shared yet must read aloud one verse and make the best connection possible.*

<u>Key Idea:</u> Seek God's word for His guidance.

Bible Quiet Time | I

Reading: Choose one option below.

The Illustrated Family Bible p. 90-91
   Optional extension: p. 85

Your own Bible: Numbers 22; 23:1-12

Scripture Focus: Highlight Numbers 22:20.

Prayer Focus: Pray a prayer of supplication to make a humble and earnest request of God. Begin by reading the highlighted verse out loud as a prayer. End by praying, *Help me to do what you tell me to do no matter how great or small. Help me heed your word, the Bible.*

Scripture Memory: Copy Philippians 2:7 in your Common Place Book.
Music: *Philippians 2* CD: Track 2 (vs. 5-7)

<u>Key Idea:</u> Balaam blessed the Israelites.

Independent History Study | I

Open your *Student Notebook* to "Prophecies About Christ". Under "Prophecy" write, *Numbers 21:8-9.* Read the Scripture to discover the prophecy. Under "Fulfillment" write, *John 3:14-15.* Read the fulfillment Scripture. Under "Description", write a few phrases to describe the prophecy about Jesus.

<u>Key Idea:</u> Like the bronze serpent in the desert, the Son of Man would be lifted up on the cross to save us.

Learning the Basics
Focus: Language Arts, Math, Geography, Bible, and Science

Geography   [T]

Read aloud to the students the following pages:

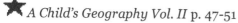 *A Child's Geography Vol. II* p. 47-51

Discuss with the students "Field Notes" p. 52.

Key Idea: Jews, Christians, and Muslims claim Israel as the holy land. The twelve tribes of Israel (Jacob) settled in this land thousands of years before Christ's birth. However, after the Romans destroyed Jerusalem in 70 A.D., the Jewish people were scattered. In 1948, Israel became a country once more. Many Jews from all over the world chose to return home.

Language Arts   [S]

Have students complete one dictation exercise.

Guide students to complete one reading lesson.

 Drawn into the Heart of Reading

Help students complete **one** English lesson.

★ *Building with Diligence:* Lesson 14 (Half)

★ *Following the Plan:* Lesson 11 (Last half)

★ Your own grammar program

Key Idea: Practice language arts skills.

Poetry   [I]

Open *Paint Like a Poet* to Lesson 7. Today, you will be performing a poetry reading of "Gathering Leaves". Practice reading the poem aloud with expression that matches the mood of the poem. Then, read the poem aloud in front of your chosen audience.

At the end of the reading, share the following, *When I read this poem by Robert Frost, it made me think of...* Call on your audience to share what thoughts the poem brought to their minds. Last, say, *Did you know that Robert Frost's grandfather owned a mill, and Robert worked as a bobbin boy in the mill? He didn't like the job or how strict his grandfather was. So, he was relieved when his mother got a job teaching in Salem, and they moved.*

Key Idea: Share the poetry of Robert Frost.

Math Exploration   [S]

Choose **one** of the math options listed below.

★ *Singapore Primary Mathematics 4A/4B* or *5A/5B* (see Appendix for schedules), or *Math with Confidence*, or *Apologia Math*

★ Your own math program

Key Idea: Use a step-by-step math program.

Science Exploration   [I]

★ Read *Land Animals of the Sixth Day* p. 126-128. At the top of a blank page, write: *What special adaptations did God give the anteater to help it get the food it needs?* Under the question, write: *'Guess'.* Write down your guess. **Activity 1:** Follow the directions for "Try This" on p. 127 in *Land Animals of the Sixth Day.* Anteaters flick their tongues about 150 times a minute. Why does the anteater need to have such a fast tongue? **Activity 2:** Measure the length of your tongue by laying a piece of string or yarn on your tongue and marking the string at the tip your tongue. Then, measure the yarn to the mark. An anteater's tongue is 2 feet long. Cut a piece of string or yarn that is 2' long. Why does an anteater need such a long tongue? **Activity 3:** Place raisins or chocolate chips on a plate to be ants. Use your tongue to try to lick up the ants. You may not use your lips. Then, use your 2' string or yarn as the anteater's tongue. coat part of it with honey. Use it to pick up the ants. Why does the anteater need a sticky tongue? Next, on the paper write: *'Procedure'.* Draw all three activities. Write: *'Conclusion'.* Explain what you learned. **Note:** The owl pellet experiment on p. 130 is optional. Choose whether to complete it on your own.

Key Idea: God gave anteaters long, sticky tongues that can be flicked quickly to catch and eat insects.

Learning through History
Focus: God's Chosen People Enter Canaan

Reading about History `I`

Read about history in the following resource:

★ *The Story of the Ancient World:*
Ch. LIII-LIV p. 113 - top of p. 117

A horn called a **shofar** is mentioned quite a few times in the Bible. Use a Bible, a reference book, or an online resource like www.wikipedia.org to look up *shofar*.

Answer one or more of the following questions from your research: *What is a shofar? When was a shofar used? Give some examples from the Bible of times when shofars are mentioned. How was a shofar made? What kind of sound did a shofar make? How was it blown? Are shofars still used today? Explain.*

Key Idea: At God's command, the shofars were blown at the fall of Jericho. Shofars were often used in religious festivals and also during battle to show that the battle belonged to God.

History Project `S`

Fold a blue piece of paper in half like a hamburger bun. Open the paper and cut on the fold-line to make two pieces. Hold one blue paper the long way and cut 1" strips halfway through the paper. Repeat this with the second sheet. Next, roll each strip around your pencil to curl it. Then, glue the two pieces of blue paper onto a piece of brown paper to show the waters of the Jordan River rolling back, leaving a strip of brown down the middle as a path for the Israelites to cross. (Save for Day 2)

Key Idea: God parted the waters of the Jordan River, just as He'd parted the Red Sea.

Storytime `T`

Choose one of the following read aloud options:

★ Your own Bible: Ruth chapter 1

★ Read at least one adventure for the next 4 days of plans.

After the reading, students will give a detailed oral narration. Select one paragraph from the story to read out loud to the students. This will be the starting point for the narration. Set a timer for 3-5 minutes. When the timer rings the narration is over, even if it isn't complete. A detailed, descriptive narration is the goal. See *Narration Tips* in the Appendix as needed.

Key Idea: Use oral narration to retell the story.

Bible Quiet Time `I`

Bible Reading: Choose one option below.

★ *The Illustrated Family Bible* p. 92-95

★ Your own Bible: Joshua chapters 1-3

Scripture Focus: Highlight Joshua 2:11.

Prayer Focus: Pray a prayer of adoration to worship and honor God. Begin by reading the highlighted verse out loud as a prayer. End by praying, *Lord, as the maker of heaven and earth, you deserve adoration. I worship you...*

Scripture Memory: Recite Philippians 2:8.
Music: *Philippians 2* CD: Track 2 (vs. 5-8)

Key Idea: God fulfilled His promise to Abraham, Isaac, and Jacob when He brought their descendents into the land of Canaan.

Independent History Study `I`

Open your *Student Notebook* to "Prophecies About Christ". Under "Prophecy" write, *Psalm 89:3-4.* Read the Scripture to discover the prophecy. Under "Fulfillment" write, *Acts 13:22-23.* Read the fulfillment Scripture. Under "Description", write a few phrases to describe the prophecy about Jesus.

Key Idea: Rahab was the mother of Boaz, great-grandfather of David. Christ would be of the line of David.

Learning the Basics

Focus: Language Arts, Math, Geography, Bible, and Science

Bible Study [T]

Read aloud and discuss with the students the following pages:

 The Radical Book for Kids p. 56-57

<u>Key Idea</u>: The Old Testament is mainly written in Hebrew. Hebrew is read from right to left. The original Hebrew alphabet did not contain any vowels. Those who spoke Hebrew knew which vowels went with each word automatically. Hebrew also does not have any capital letters. All letters are the same size.

Language Arts [S]

Have students complete one studied dictation exercise (see Appendix for directions and passages).

Help students complete one lesson from the following reading program:

 Drawn into the Heart of Reading

Work with the students to complete **one** of the English options listed below:

★ *Building with Diligence:* Lesson 14 (Half)

★ *Following the Plan:* Lesson 12

★ Your own grammar program

<u>Key Idea</u>: Practice language arts skills.

Poetry [I]

Choose one of Robert Frost's poems from Lessons 1-7 in *Paint Like a Poet* to memorize.

You will have 2 weeks (units) to memorize the entire poem. So, you should have half of your chosen poem memorized by Day 4 of this unit.

After you have chosen your poem to memorize, read it three times, adding actions to help you remember the words.

<u>Key Idea</u>: Read and appreciate classic poetry.

Math Exploration [S]

Choose **one** of the math options listed below.

 Singapore Primary Mathematics 4A/4B or 5A/5B (see Appendix for schedules), or *Math with Confidence*, or *Apologia Math*

 Your own math program

<u>Key Idea</u>: Use a step-by-step math program.

Science Exploration [I]

★ Read *Land Animals of the Sixth Day* p. 131 – middle of p. 137. Get your book about animal tracks that you began in Unit 2. At the top of the next page in your book of tracks, copy in cursive Job 39:19-21. Beneath the verse, draw and label horse and donkey tracks as shown in the "Track It" drawings on p. 149.

Then, use a globe or a world map to find the locations of the animals listed in the "Map It" section on p. 149.

<u>Key Idea</u>: Beasts of burden, or livestock, are hoofed creatures that are ungulates. Some examples of ungulates are horses, deer, sheep, cows, goats, camels, elephants, and giraffes. Some ungulates are domesticated, while others are wild.

Learning through History
Focus: God's Chosen People Enter Canaan

Reading about History [I]

Read about history in the following resource:

★ *The Story of the Ancient World:*
   Ch. LV-LVI p. 117 - bottom of p. 120

You will be choosing a portion from today's reading that you found memorable or worthy of being reread to copy. Open your *Student Notebook* to Unit 8. In Box 4, carefully copy in cursive the portion from today's reading that you selected. Then, compare your written work to the original. Last, draw a small colorful picture in Box 4 to illustrate your sentences.

Key Idea: God fought on the side of Israel as long as they obeyed Him. God lengthened a day so Joshua and Israel could overcome 5 Canaanite kings. In doing so, God showed He is greater than the gods the Canaanites worshipped, which were the sun and moon.

History Project [S]

Today, you will make a cut out of the Ark of the Covenant to add to your model of the crossing of the Jordan River that you made on Day 1. On a 4" x 4" square of yellow paper, make a sketch of the Ark of the Covenant. Use the picture of the Ark of the Covenant in Unit 8 of your *Student Notebook* for help in drawing your sketch. When you are finished drawing, cut your sketch of the Ark of the Covenant out of the yellow paper. Save it for Day 3.

Key Idea: When the feet of the priests carrying the Ark of the Covenant touched the water of the Jordan River, it parted to let the entire Israelite nation pass through on dry ground.

Storytime [T]

Choose one of the following read aloud options:

★ Your own Bible: Ruth chapter 2

★ Read aloud a portion of the adventure.

After reading, give students a few minutes to prepare a short advertisement speech for the book. During the speech, students should hold up the book and say the book title and the name of the author. The wording of the advertisement should provide a peek into the book without giving away the ending. The goal should be for listeners to feel like they've "Got to Have This Book"!

Key Idea: Use an ad speech to share the story.

Bible Quiet Time [I]

Reading: Choose one option below.

★ *The Illustrated Family Bible* p. 96-97
   Optional extension: p. 84

★ Your own Bible: Joshua 5:13-15; 6; 12:7-24

Scripture Focus: Highlight Joshua 6:2.

Prayer Focus: Pray a prayer of confession to admit or acknowledge your sins to God. Begin by reading the highlighted verse out loud as a prayer. End by praying, *I confess I need to trust you more for the outcomes of my life. The battles are yours and so is the glory.*

Scripture Memory: Recite Philippians 2:8.
Music: *Philippians 2* CD: Track 2 (vs. 5-8)

Key Idea: Achan did not obey God's command, and he brought trouble upon the Israelites.

Independent History Study [I]

Open your *Student Notebook* to Unit 8. In Box 6, copy in cursive one or more of the following facts about Joshua: 1) Joshua and Caleb were the only two survivors of the Egyptian plagues and exodus to settle in Canaan. 2) Joshua was Moses' personal helper for 40 years. 3) Joshua was one of only two spies who trusted God to help Israel conquer Canaan.

Key Idea: God promised to be with Joshua and never leave him, just like He was with Moses.

Geography　　T

Read aloud to the students the following pages:

 A Child's Geography Vol. II p. 52 (second column) – p. 56

Discuss with the students "Field Notes" p. 56.

Key Idea: Israel's western coastal plain is near the Mediterranean Sea. The sea keeps the climate mild with dry summers and wet winters. The majority of Israel's population lives in this area. The port city of Joppa, or Jaffe today, is no longer a port. Its coast has been "silted up". Haifa is now Israel's major port city.

Language Arts　　S

Help students complete one lesson from the following reading program:

 Drawn into the Heart of Reading

Work with the students to complete **one** of the writing options listed below:

★ *Writing & Rhetoric Book 1: Fable* p. 44 (Note: Reread the fable on p. 36 first. Then, brainstorm ideas with students for today's lesson. Read aloud the example in the Teacher's Guide p. 44 for help.)

★ Your own writing program

Key Idea: Practice language arts skills.

Poetry　　I

Today, you will copy half of the Robert Frost poem from *Paint Like a Poet* that you chose to memorize this week.

At the top of a clean page in your *Common Place Book*, copy the title and the author of the poem. Then, copy half of the poem in cursive, leaving the rest of the page blank.

You will copy the remaining half of the poem during the next unit.

Practice the portion of the poem that you copied today by reading it aloud.

Key Idea: Copy and memorize classic poetry.

Math Exploration　　S

Choose **one** of the math options listed below.

★ *Singapore Primary Mathematics 4A/4B or 5A/5B* (see Appendix for schedules), or *Math with Confidence*, or *Apologia Math*

★ Your own math program

Key Idea: Use a step-by-step math program.

Science Exploration　　I

★ Read *Land Animals of the Sixth Day* middle of p. 137 - 142. Orally retell or narrate to an adult the portion of text that you read today. Use the *Narration Tips* in the Appendix for help as needed.

Key Idea: Mastodons and wooly mammoths have similar skeletons. Both mastodons and mammoths are extinct. Horses, donkeys, rhinos, and tapirs are in the order Perissodactyla. They walk on their toes and have a large middle toe. The horse family is called Equidae. Horses are herbivores, have excellent hearing, and often form herds. They can also sleep standing up! There are many different breeds of horses.

Reading about History   I

Read about history in the following resource:

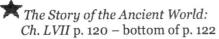 *The Story of the Ancient World:*
Ch. LVII p. 120 – bottom of p. 122

You will be adding to your timeline in your *Student Notebook* today. In Unit 8 – Box 1, draw and color a pile of rocks. Label it, *Fall of Jericho (1451 B.C.).* In Box 2, draw and color an iron chariot. Label it, *Sisera is killed (1285 B.C.).* In Box 3, draw and color a burning torch. Label it, *Gideon called by God (1245 B.C.).*

Key Idea: After the death of Joshua, the Israelites turned their backs on God and began to worship the idols of the people in the land of Canaan.

Storytime   T

Choose one of the following read aloud options:

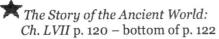 Your own Bible: Ruth chapter 3

⭐ Read aloud the next portion of the adventure that you selected.

After the reading, students will give a summary oral narration. The oral narration must be no longer than 5 sentences and should summarize the reading. As students narrate, have them hold up one finger for each sentence shared. Remind students that the focus should be on the big ideas, rather than on the details.

Key Idea: Summarize the story by narrating.

History Project   S

Get the 12 small unpainted stones that you saved from Unit 7. Scatter the 12 stones in the center of the brown paper path that you made on Day 1. Reread the story of the parting of the Jordan River in Joshua 3:9-17 and 4:1-18. Next, use the cutout of the Ark of the Covenant that you made on Day 2 to act out the story. As you move the Ark of the Covenant to the center of the brown path, pick up the stones one at a time and carry them out of the riverbed. Then, move the Ark of the Covenant out of the water. Last, set up the 12 stones as a memorial to remember how God parted the river before the 12 tribes. Use your model to tell the story to someone else.

Key Idea: How could God's people forget Him after all of His miraculous signs?

Bible Quiet Time   I

Reading: Choose one option below.

⭐ *The Illustrated Family Bible* p. 100-101
Optional extension: p. 98

⭐ Your own Bible: Judges chapter 4

Scripture Focus: Highlight Judges 4:14-15.

Prayer Focus: Pray a prayer of thanksgiving to express gratitude for God's divine goodness. Begin by reading the highlighted verses out loud as a prayer. End by praying, *Thank you for going before me, Lord, and for always having a plan. I'm so glad that...*

Scripture Memory: Recite Philippians 2:8.
Music: *Philippians 2* CD: Track 2 (vs. 5-8)

Key Idea: Each time God's people repented, He sent them a judge to deliver them.

Independent History Study   I

Open your *Student Notebook* to Unit 8. In Box 7, copy in cursive one or more of the following facts about Deborah: 1) Deborah, wife of Lappidoth, was a prophetess and a leader of Israel. 2) She predicted that Sisera would be killed by a woman (Jael). 3) She marched with Barak against Sisera's 900 iron chariots.

Key Idea: God used Deborah to free Israel from the Canaanite king, Jabin, and his general Sisera.

Learning the Basics
Focus: Language Arts, Math, Geography, Bible, and Science

Bible Study [T]

Read aloud and discuss with the students the following pages:

 The Radical Book for Kids p. 58-61

Key Idea: There are 66 books in the Bible. The Old Testament books can be categorized as books of history & law, books of poetry & wisdom, books of major prophets, and books of minor prophets.

Language Arts [S]

Have students complete one studied dictation exercise (see Appendix for directions and passages).

Work with the students to complete **one** of the writing options listed below:

 Writing & Rhetoric Book 1: Fable p. 45-46 (Note: Have students choose only **one** section to memorize, either the beginning, the middle, or the end. You will read aloud the other 2 sections for the recitation.)

 Your own writing program

Key Idea: Practice language arts skills.

Poetry [I]

Practice reading aloud half of the poem that you chose to memorize from *Paint Like a Poet*, using the actions that you added to help you remember the words. Do this 2 times.

Then, recite half of the poem without looking at the words.

You have 2 weeks (units) to memorize the entire poem. So, you should have half of your chosen poem memorized by Day 4 of this unit.

Key Idea: Memorize classic poetry.

Math Exploration [S]

Choose **one** of the math options listed below.

 Singapore Primary Mathematics 4A/4B or *5A/5B* (see Appendix for schedules), or *Math with Confidence,* or *Apologia Math*

⭐ Your own math program

Key Idea: Use a step-by-step math program.

Science Exploration [I]

⭐ Read *Land Animals of the Sixth Day* p. 143-148. Write the answer to each numbered question on lined paper. You do not need to copy the question. Use the listed page to help you answer each question.
1. How are horses measured? (p. 143)
2. Write the words *foal, yearling, filly, colt, mare,* and *stallion* and give their definitions. (p. 143)
3. What is unique about each zebra? (p. 145)
4. How do oxpeckers help rhinos? (p. 146)
5. When the Israelites returned to Jerusalem from captivity in Babylon, what does Ezra 2:66-67 say they had with them?

Key Idea: As evidenced by the Bible, ungulates have been beasts of burden through much of history.

Unit 8 - Day 4

Reading about History $\boxed{I}$

Read about history in the following resource:

 The Story of the Ancient World:
Ch. LVIII-LIX p. 122 – middle of p. 126

You will be writing a narration about *Chapter LIX: Defeat of the Midianites,* which is part of today's history reading.

To prepare for writing your narration, think about the questions below. If you do not know the answers, find them on p. 124-126 of *The Story of the Ancient World.* Ask yourself, *Why did God want Gideon to have only a small army? What did God tell Gideon to do? When the army was still too large, what did God tell Gideon to do next? How many men did Gideon take to meet the Midianites? When God sent Gideon to spy on the enemy, what did Gideon hear? How did Gideon arm his men? When did they attack? What was the result? Why did Gideon refuse to be king? What reward did Gideon accept? How did this reward become an idol? When Gideon died, what did the Israelites do?*

After you have thought about the answers to the questions, turn to Unit 8 in your *Student Notebook.* In Box 5, write a 5-8 sentence narration that begins with, *Even though Gideon had a large army, God...* When you have finished writing, read your sentences out loud to catch any mistakes. Check for the following things: *Did you include **who** the reading was mainly about? Did you include **what** important thing(s) happened? Did you include **how** it ended? If not, add those things.* Use the *Written Narration Skills* in the Appendix to guide in editing the narration.

<u>Key Idea</u>: When the Israelites repented, God sent the judge Gideon to deliver them.

Storytime $\boxed{T}$

Choose one of the following read aloud options:

 Your own Bible: Ruth chapter 4

★ Read aloud a portion of the adventure.

After the reading, have each person get a Bible and open it anywhere in Proverbs. Explain, *We will have 5 minutes to skim through the verses in Proverbs to find any connections to today's story. When a connection is found, read the verse out loud and quickly share the connection. At the end of 5 minutes, anyone who has not shared yet must read aloud one verse and make the best connection possible.*

<u>Key Idea</u>: Seek God's word for His guidance.

Bible Quiet Time $\boxed{I}$

Reading: Choose one option below.

★ *The Illustrated Family Bible* p. 102-103

★ Your own Bible: Judges chapters 6-7

Scripture Focus: Highlight Judges 6:12-14.

Prayer Focus: Pray a prayer of supplication to make a humble and earnest request of God. Begin by reading the highlighted verse out loud as a prayer. End by praying, *I ask you to help me do your will and go where you send me. Help my strength to be in you and not in...*

Scripture Memory: Copy Philippians 2:8 in your Common Place Book.
Music: *Philippians 2* CD: Track 2 (vs. 5-8)

<u>Key Idea</u>: God used Gideon and a small army to defeat the Midianites. The battle was God's.

Independent History Study $\boxed{I}$

Open your *Student Notebook* to Unit 8. In Box 8, copy in cursive one or more of the following facts about Gideon: 1) Gideon was from the tribe of Manasseh, son of Joseph. 2) Gideon's first task from God was to tear down the altar of Baal in Israel. 3) With only 300 men, the Lord used Gideon to beat the Midianites.

<u>Key Idea</u>: Gideon was Israel's fifth judge. God called him to defeat the Midianites with only 300 men.

Geography   T

Go to the website link listed under "Bringing It Home" on p. 6 of *A Child's Geography Vol. II*. At the link, select "History & Geography". Then, under "Knowledge Quest" select ACG2-Extra Activities". Print a copy of the labeled map of **Israel & Jordan** on p. 45 and the blank map of **Israel & Jordan** on p. 46 for each student. Then, assign the following page:

★ *A Child's Geography Vol. II* p. 57
Note: Do only the "Map Notes" section. If desired, play "Music" from the links on p. 58.

Key Idea: Practice finding and recording the locations of various places on a map of Israel.

Poetry   I

Practice reading aloud half of the poem that you chose to memorize from *Paint Like a Poet*, using the actions that you added to help you remember the words. Do this 2 times.

Then, recite half of the poem without looking at the words.

You have 2 weeks (units) to memorize the entire poem. So, you should have half of your chosen poem memorized by today.

Key Idea: Memorize classic poetry.

Language Arts   S

Have students complete one dictation exercise.

Guide students to complete one reading lesson.

★ *Drawn into the Heart of Reading*

Help students complete **one** English lesson.

★ *Building with Diligence:* Lesson 15

★ *Following the Plan:* Lesson 13

★ Your own grammar program

Key Idea: Practice language arts skills.

Math Exploration   S

Choose **one** of the math options listed below.

★ *Singapore Primary Mathematics 4A/4B* or *5A/5B* (see Appendix for schedules), or *Math with Confidence*, or *Apologia Math*

★ Your own math program

Key Idea: Use a step-by-step math program.

Science Exploration   I

Turn to the science experiment section in your science binder or sketchbook. At the top of a blank page, write: *What are some of the different gaits, or ways in which a horse walks?* Under the question, write: 'Guess'. Write down your guess. Look at the four most common gaits shown on p. 142 of *Land Animals of the Sixth Day*. Use four fingers to follow the numbered movements to tap out each gait. Do this by placing both hands in front of you with fingers upraised, as if you are getting ready to play the piano. Next, fold all fingers up toward your palm, except for your two thumbs and two index fingers. Place these 4 fingers like the pictures on p. 142 to tap out each gait in correct sequence. If you have access to the internet, go to the course website listed on p. vii and click on Lesson 8. View the video links of a horse walking, trotting, cantering, and galloping. Next, on the paper write: 'Procedure'. Draw the numbered gaits from p. 142 and label them. At the bottom of the paper, write: 'Conclusion'. Explain what you learned from this activity.

Note: The Review Game on p. 149-150 is optional. Choose whether to complete it on your own.

Key Idea: Horses have four common gaits. They usually walk, trot, canter, or gallop.

Unit 9 - Day 1

Reading about History | I |

Read about history in the following resource:

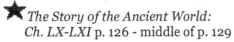 *The Story of the Ancient World: Ch. LX-LXI p. 126 - middle of p. 129*

After the death of Moses and Joshua, Israel was ruled by judges. Where could you look to research more about the **judges of Israel**? Use a Bible, a reference book, or an online resource like www.wikipedia.org to look up *judges of Israel*.

Answer one or more of the following questions from your research: *What is a judge? How did a person become a judge in Israel? Who were some of the judges after the time of Moses and Joshua? Who was Israel's last judge before the Isralites begged for a king? Why did God appoint judges in Israel? How did the Israelites respond to the judges?*

Key Idea: After Gideon's death, his son Abimelech killed all but one of Gideon's descendents in order to be king.

History Project | S |

In this unit you will make a Philistine helmet. Cut two long strips of yellow paper that are each 2" wide. Use clear tape to tape the two strips together to make one long strip of paper. Wrap the long strip around your head to get the correct size for the helmet. Make sure not to make the fit too tight. After sizing, cut off any excess paper from the strip that is not needed. Next, use red, blue, and purple paint to paint designs on one side of the yellow strip. Lay it flat to dry for Day 2.

Key Idea: The Philistines conquered Israel.

Storytime | T |

Choose one of the following read aloud options:

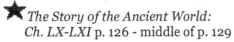 *Jashub's Journal: Shebat* p. 7-16

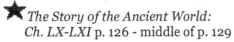 Read at least one historical fiction book for the next 16 days of plans (see Appendix).

After the reading, students will give a detailed oral narration. Select one paragraph from the story to read out loud to the students. This will be the starting point for the narration. Set a timer for 3-5 minutes. When the timer rings the narration is over, even if it isn't complete. A detailed, descriptive narration is the goal. See *Narration Tips* in the Appendix as needed.

Key Idea: Use oral narration to retell the story.

Bible Quiet Time | I |

Bible Reading: Choose the option below.

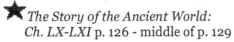 *The Illustrated Family Bible* p. 104-105 Optional extension: p. 99

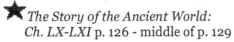 Your own Bible: Judges chapter 11

Scripture Focus: Highlight Judges 11:30-31.

Prayer Focus: Pray a prayer of adoration to worship and honor God. Begin by reading the highlighted verses out loud as a prayer. End by praying, *A vow to the Lord is very special. Help me not to make quick promises, but instead to give you honor with my words by...*

Scripture Memory: Recite Philippians 2:9.
Music: *Philippians 2* CD: Track 2 (vs. 5-9)

Key Idea: Jephthah was a judge and a warrior.

Independent History Study | I |

Open your *Student Notebook* to Unit 9. In Box 5, copy Judges 11:27 in cursive.

Key Idea: The Ammonites and Moabites were descendents of Lot, Abraham's nephew. The Ammonites wrongly accused Israel of stealing their land. Israel's ninth judge, Jephthah, knew God was the real judge.

Learning the Basics

Focus: Language Arts, Math, Geography, Bible, and Science

Bible Study [T]

Read aloud and discuss with the students the following pages:

 The Radical Book for Kids p. 62-64

Key Idea: There are 66 books in the Bible. The New Testament books can be categorized as Gospels, history, Paul's epistles or letters to the churches, Paul's epistles or letters to individuals, general epistles or letters, and apocalyptic writing.

Language Arts [S]

Have students complete one studied dictation exercise (see Appendix for directions and passages).

Help students complete one lesson from the following reading program:

 Drawn into the Heart of Reading

Work with the students to complete **one** of the English options listed below:

★ *Building with Diligence:* Lesson 16

★ *Following the Plan:* Lesson 14

★ Your own grammar program

Key Idea: Practice language arts skills.

Poetry [I]

Continue memorizing the Robert Frost poem that you chose from *Paint Like a Poet* in Unit 8. You should have half of your chosen poem memorized already.

You should memorize the rest of the poem by Day 4 of this unit.

Today, read the entire poem 3 times, adding actions to the last half of the poem to help you memorize the words more easily.

Key Idea: Read and appreciate a variety of classic poetry.

Math Exploration [S]

Choose **one** of the math options listed below.

★ *Singapore Primary Mathematics 4A/4B* or *5A/5B* (see Appendix for schedules), or *Math with Confidence,* or *Apologia Math*

★ Your own math program

Key Idea: Use a step-by-step math program.

Science Exploration [I]

★ Read *Land Animals of the Sixth Day* p. 151 – top of p. 155. Get your book about animal tracks that you began in Unit 2. At the top of the next page in your book of tracks, copy 2 Samuel 22:33-34 in cursive. Beneath the verse, draw and label deer tracks and cattle tracks as shown in the "Track It" drawings on p. 169.

Key Idea: There are over 200 species of even-toed ungulates. Even-toed ungulates do not have a middle toe. Many of these species use a process called rumination for eating. Ruminants chew their cud. Cattle, sheep, bison, deer, antelopes, goats, giraffes, buffalo and llamas are examples of ruminants. In India, Hindus do not eat cattle, even though many people are starving, because they believe cattle are sacred.

Learning through History
Focus: The Israelites Suffer from Idolatry

Reading about History [I]

Read about history in the following resource:

⭐ *The Story of the Ancient World:*
Ch. LXII p. 129 - middle of p. 131

You will be choosing a portion from today's reading that you found memorable or worthy of being reread to copy. Open your *Student Notebook* to Unit 9. In Box 3, carefully copy in cursive the portion from today's reading that you selected. Then, compare your written work to the original. Last, draw a small colorful picture in Box 3 to illustrate your sentences.

Key Idea: In a time of famine, Naomi and her husband left Bethlehem and went to Moab to live. Their two sons married Moabite women. When Naomi's husband and sons died, she went back home. Her daughter-in-law Ruth went with her.

History Project [S]

Today you will continue making your Philistine helmet. You will need two 9" x 12" pieces of construction paper that are the same color. Either blue, red, or purple is best. On the long side of each paper, measure and draw a line running 2" above the bottom edge of the paper. You will not make any cuts in this 2" section of the page. Next, use your scissors to cut fringes from the top of the paper down to meet the line you drew. Make sure to cut the fringes neatly and evenly. These will be your helmet's feathered tufts which will be held in place by your decorative yellow band on Day 3.

Key Idea: The Philistines came from Egypt.

Storytime [T]

Choose one of the following read aloud options:

⭐ *Jashub's Journal: Adar* p. 17-26

⭐ Read aloud the next portion of the historical fiction book that you selected.

After reading, give each person a white piece of paper or a markerboard and a marker. Set a timer for 3-5 minutes and instruct each person to do a quick outline sketch about the story. Ideas for sketches include settings, characters, actions, important objects, or symbols. When the timer rings, briefly share the sketches.

Key Idea: Use sketching to share the story.

Bible Quiet Time [I]

Reading: Choose one option below.

⭐ *The Illustrated Family Bible* p. 112-115

⭐ Your own Bible: Ruth 1; 2:1-12; 3:10-11; 4:13-22

Scripture Focus: Highlight Ruth 3:10-11.

Prayer Focus: Pray a prayer of confession to admit or acknowledge your sins to God. Begin by reading the highlighted verses out loud as a prayer. End by praying, *I confess that it may be hard to wait for you to show me who I should marry one day. Help me to be like Ruth and be patient and of noble character.*

Scripture Memory: Recite Philippians 2:9.
Music: *Philippians 2* CD: Track 2 (vs. 5-9)

Key Idea: Ruth married Boaz, son of Rahab.

Independent History Study [I]

Open your *Student Notebook* to the "Prophecies About Christ". Under "Prophecy" write, *Isaiah 9:6-7*. Read the Scripture to discover the prophecy. Under "Fulfillment" write, *Matthew 1:1-6*. Read the fulfillment Scripture. Under "Description", write a few phrases to describe the prophecy about Jesus.

Key Idea: David was the great-grandson of Boaz. The Savior would one day be born of the line of David.

Learning the Basics
Focus: Language Arts, Math, Geography, Bible, and Science

Geography   [T]

Go to the website link listed on p. 6 of *A Child's Geography Vol. II*. At the link, select "History & Geography". Then, under "Knowledge Quest" select ACG2-Extra Activities". Print the "Travel Log Template" of your choice from p. 39-42. Also at the link, for older students, print and assign the "Chapter Four Review" on p. 70. Assign all students the following page:

 A Child's Geography Vol. II p. 57

Note: Do only the "Travel Notes" section. The "Art" section of p. 58 is an optional extra.

Key Idea: Share three sights from Israel.

Poetry   [I]

Today, you will copy the last half of the Robert Frost poem from *Paint Like a Poet* that you chose to memorize this week.

Beneath the first part of the poem that you copied in the last unit, copy the rest of the poem in cursive in your *Common Place Book*.

Practice the portion of the poem that you copied today by reading it aloud.

Key Idea: Copy and memorize classic poetry.

Language Arts   [S]

Help students complete one lesson from the following reading program:

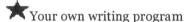 *Drawn into the Heart of Reading*

Work with the students to complete **one** of the writing options listed below:

 Writing & Rhetoric Book 1: Fable
p. 47 – top of p. 51 (Note: Read the text aloud while the students follow along. Then, discuss.)

 Your own writing program

Key Idea: Practice language arts skills.

Math Exploration   [S]

Choose **one** of the math options listed below.

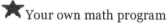 *Singapore Primary Mathematics 4A/4B or 5A/5B (see Appendix for schedules), or Math with Confidence,* or *Apologia Math*

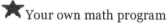 Your own math program

Key Idea: Use a step-by-step math program.

Science Exploration   [I]

 Read *Land Animals of the Sixth Day* p. 155 – middle of p. 158. Orally retell or narrate to an adult the portion of text that you read today. Use the *Narration Tips* in the Appendix for help as needed.

Key Idea: At the time of the Lewis and Clark Expedition, there were too many bison to count in North America. By the 1900's, fewer than 1,000 bison were left! At that time, bison became endangered animals and were protected by laws. Today, bison are not endangered anymore. Caprines are a group in the family Bovidae. Goats, duikers, sheep, and chamois are examples of caprines. They are often raised for their meat and their milk.

Learning through History
Focus: The Israelites Suffer from Idolatry

Unit 9 - Day 3

Reading about History   I

Read about history in the following resource:

⭐ *The Story of the Ancient World:*
Ch. LXIII-LXIV p. 131 - top of p. 136

You will be adding to your timeline in your *Student Notebook* today. In Unit 9 – Box 1, draw and color an arm with muscles. Label it, *Samson is born (1155 B.C.).* In Box 2, draw and color a golden box with carrying poles. Label it, *Ark of Covenant captured by Philistines (1117 B.C.).*

Key Idea: At the time when Samson was judge in Israel, the Philistines were oppressing Israel. Samson loved two different Philistine women who both contributed to his downfall.

Storytime   T

Choose one of the following read aloud options:

⭐ *Jashub's Journal: Abib* p. 27-38

⭐ Read aloud the next portion of the historical fiction book that you selected.

After the reading, students will give a summary oral narration. The oral narration must be no longer than 5 sentences and should summarize the reading. As students narrate, have them hold up one finger for each sentence shared. Remind students that the focus should be on the big ideas, rather than on the details.

Key Idea: Summarize the story by narrating.

History Project   S

Get the long yellow strip of paper you made on Day 1 and the two fringed papers you made on Day 2. Tape the two fringed papers together to make one long strip with the fringes at the top. Next, tape the fringed strip to the unpainted side of your yellow strip with clear tape. Then, join the two ends of the strips together and tape them to form a circular helmet. Roll the tips of the fringes around your pencil to bend them out. Place the helmet on your head. Next, cut one more strip of yellow paper 1" wide and 9" long as a chin strap. Attach the strap to the helmet with clear tape in front of your ears on both sides, so the strap runs under your chin. Your helmet is now complete.

Key Idea: After Samson had been captured by the Philistines, God used Samson once more to push down their temple upon them.

Bible Quiet Time   I

Reading: Choose one option below.

⭐ *The Illustrated Family Bible* p. 106-111

⭐ Your own Bible: Judges 13; 16:4-31

Scripture Focus: Highlight Judges 13:24-25.

Prayer Focus: Pray a prayer of thanksgiving to express gratitude for God's divine goodness. Begin by reading the highlighted verses out loud as a prayer. End by praying, *Thank you for your Spirit that lives within me. Help me listen when...*

Scripture Memory: Recite Philippians 2:9.
Music: *Philippians 2* CD: Track 2 (vs. 5-9)

Key Idea: Samson was a Nazarite, set apart by God for a special purpose. As a symbol of his vow to God, he was not to cut his hair.

Independent History Study   I

Open your *Student Notebook* to Unit 9. Look at the map in Box 6. Find the cities that were ruled by the Philistines at the time of Samson: Gaza, Ashkelon, Ashdod, Ekron, and Gath. Find Dan on the map, which is the tribe from which Samson was born. Note the red box on the globe to see where these cities were.

Key Idea: When Samson was born at the time of Eli as priest, the Philistines had ruled Israel for 40 years.

Learning the Basics

Focus: Language Arts, Math, Geography, Bible, and Science

Bible Study [T]

Read aloud and discuss with the students the following pages:

 The Radical Book for Kids p. 65-71

Key Idea: In Bible times, Jewish men were required to travel to Jerusalem for Passover, Pentecost, and the Feast of Booths. The Day of Atonement was the most holy day of the year. The Feast of Booths was a time for the Israelites to remember the way God cared for them during their forty years in the wilderness. Passover was a time for the Israelites to celebrate God's rescue of His people from Egypt. Pentecost was a time to thank God for a bountiful harvest.

Poetry [I]

Using the actions that you added on Day 1, practice reading aloud the poem from *Paint Like a Poet* that you chose to memorize. Do this 2 times.

Then, recite the poem without looking at the words.

You should have your chosen poem memorized by Day 4 of this unit.

Key Idea: Memorize classic poetry.

Language Arts [S]

Have students complete one studied dictation exercise (see Appendix for directions and passages).

Work with the students to complete **one** of the writing options listed below:

 Writing & Rhetoric Book 1: Fable p. 52-56 (Note: Omit "Writing Time" p. 51. Guide students through the lesson, so they are successful writing an amplification.)

 Your own writing program

Key Idea: Practice language arts skills.

Math Exploration [S]

Choose **one** of the math options listed below.

 Singapore Primary Mathematics 4A/4B or 5A/5B (see Appendix for schedules), or *Math with Confidence*, or *Apologia Math*

 Your own math program

Key Idea: Use a step-by-step math program.

Science Exploration [I]

 Read *Land Animals of the Sixth Day* middle of p. 158-162. Write the answer to each numbered question on lined paper. You do not need to copy the question. Use the listed pages for help.

1. What special adaptations do camels have to help them survive in the desert? (p. 158-159)
2. Write the words *spar* and *musk* and give their definitions. (p. 160)
3. Why is the giraffe's blood pressure complicated to figure out? (p. 161)
4. Use a globe or a world map to find the locations of the animals in the "Map It" section of p. 169.
5. For what purposes did the queen of Sheba use the camels in 2 Chronicles 9:1?

Key Idea: God gave camels special adaptations for life in the desert. He also made the giraffe's heart with special adaptations for regulating its blood pressure within its long neck.

Reading about History | I |

Read about history in the following resource:

The Story of the Ancient World:
Ch. LXV-LXVI p. 136 – top of p. 140

You will be writing a narration about *Chapter LXVI: The Ark Captured,* which is part of today's history reading.

To prepare for writing your narration, think about the questions below. If you do not know the answers, find them on p. 138-140 of *The Story of the Ancient World.* Ask yourself, *At this time, who were the Israelites fighting? Why did Eli's sons bring the Ark of the Covenant into the camp? What was the outcome? When the news of the defeat reached Eli, what happened? Why did the wife of Phinehas name her son Ichabod? Where did the Philistines take the Ark? What happened to the statue of their god, Dagon? Why did the Philistines decide to send the Ark back to the Israelites? How did they send it back? What happened to the men who looked within the Ark? Where did the Ark end up?*

After you have thought about the answers to the questions, turn to Unit 9 in your *Student Notebook.* In Box 4, write a 5-8 sentence narration that begins with, *When the Israelites were fighting the Philistines...* When you have finished writing, read your sentences out loud to catch any mistakes.

Check for the following things: *Did you include **who** the reading was mainly about? Did you include **what** important thing(s) happened? Did you include **how** it ended? If not, add those things.* Use the *Written Narration Skills* in the Appendix for editing.

<u>Key Idea</u>: Eli's sons were killed as prophecied.

Storytime | T |

Choose one of the following read aloud options:

Jashub's Journal: Ziv p. 39-50

Read aloud the next portion of the historical fiction book that you selected.

After the reading, have each person get a Bible and open it anywhere in Proverbs. Explain, *We will have 5 minutes to skim through the verses in Proverbs to find any connections to today's story. When a connection is found, read the verse out loud and quickly share the connection. At the end of 5 minutes, anyone who has not shared yet must read aloud one verse and make the best connection possible.*

<u>Key Idea</u>: Seek God's word for His guidance.

Bible Quiet Time | I |

Reading: Choose one option below.

The Illustrated Family Bible p. 116-119

Your own Bible: 1 Samuel 1; 3:19-21; 4

Scripture Focus: Highlight 1 Samuel 3:10.

Prayer Focus: Pray a prayer of supplication to make a humble and earnest request of God. Begin by reading the highlighted verse out loud as a prayer. End by praying, *Help me listen to your words in the Bible and live to serve you like Samuel by...*

Scripture Memory: Copy Philippians 2:9 in your Common Place Book.
Music: *Philippians 2* CD: Track 2 (vs. 5-9)

<u>Key Idea</u>: Samuel was a judge and a prophet.

Independent History Study | I |

Open your *Student Notebook* to Unit 9. Use the map in Box 6 to find Shiloh. This was the location of the Tabernacle where Samuel served the Lord. Find the names of the twelve tribes of Israel (except Levi).

<u>Key Idea</u>: The Levites were chosen by God to be priests. Eli was the high priest when Samuel was a boy.

Geography [T]

Read aloud to the students the following pages:

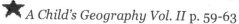 *A Child's Geography Vol. II* p. 59-63

Discuss with the students "Field Notes" p. 64.

Key Idea: Beersheba was once the home of Abraham and his flocks of sheep. Today, it is a bustling city. Bedouin tribes make their home in the Negev Desert. Israeli farmers use the loess soil of the desert to grow tomatoes, grapes, strawberries, and melons. Elat is located on the shores of the Red Sea. This is Israel's southernmost city.

Language Arts [S]

Have students complete one dictation exercise.

Guide students to complete one reading lesson.

★ *Drawn into the Heart of Reading*

Help students complete **one** English lesson.

★ *Building with Diligence:* Lesson 17

★ *Following the Plan:* Lesson 15

★ Your own grammar program

Key Idea: Practice language arts skills.

Poetry [I]

Today, you will be performing a poetry recitation of the Robert Frost poem that you chose to memorize from *Paint Like a Poet.* You will recite your poem to an audience of your choosing, without looking at the words.

Before reciting, practice saying the poem aloud using an expression that matches the mood of the poem. Then, stand and recite the poem aloud in front of your chosen audience.

At the end of the recitation, share the following, *I decided to choose this poem of Robert Frost's to memorize because...* Then, call on your audience to comment on what they liked about the poem that you shared.

Key Idea: Share the poetry of Robert Frost.

Math Exploration [S]

Choose **one** of the math options listed below.

★ *Singapore Primary Mathematics 4A/4B or 5A/5B* (see Appendix for schedules), or *Math with Confidence,* or *Apologia Math*

★ Your own math program

Key Idea: Use a step-by-step math program.

Science Exploration [I]

★ Read *Land Animals of the Sixth Day* p. 163 – top of p. 169. Now, skip to the "Experiment" on p. 170. Turn to the science experiment section in your science binder or sketchbook. At the top of a blank page, write: *Why does a giraffe need such high blood pressure?* Under the question, write: *'Guess'.* Write down your guess.

Follow the directions for the experiment in *Land Animals of the Sixth Day* p. 170. Next, on the paper write: *'Procedure'.* Draw a labeled picture of the experiment. At the bottom of the paper, write: *'Conclusion'.* Explain what you learned from the experiment.

Key Idea: For the giraffe to get the blood it needs to its brain, the heart must squeeze hard to increase the pressure and cause the blood to rise up the giraffe's very long neck.

Learning through History
Focus: The Reign of King Saul

Reading about History | I |

Read about history in the following resource:

⭐ *The Story of the Ancient World:*
Ch. LXVII-LXVIII p. 140 - middle of p. 143

In ancient times, slings were used as weapons. Where could you look to research more about a **sling**? Read about the Israelites' use of slings in 1 Samuel 17:40, 49; Judges 20:16; 2 Kings 3:25; 1 Chronicles 12:2; and 2 Chronicles 26:14. You may also wish to check another resource like www.wikipedia.org.

Answer one or more of the following questions from your research: *What did a sling look like? How was a sling used? Name some examples from the Bible of times when the Israelites used slings. Of what use was a sling to a shepherd? Which other ancient cultures used slings?*

Key Idea: The Israelites were using slings at the time of the Judges as noted in Scripture.

History Project | S |

In this unit you will be making a sling like those used by the ancient Israelites and by David when he killed Goliath. First, measure and cut 6 pieces of yarn that are each 25" long. Tie 3 of the pieces of yarn together with a knot at the top. Then, braid them and tie a knot at the bottom. Repeat the activity to make one more braid using the other 3 pieces of yarn. Save the braids for Day 2.

Key Idea: Samuel did as God told him and anointed Saul as king of Israel.

Storytime | T |

Choose one of the following read aloud options:

⭐ *Jashub's Journal: Sivan* p. 51-58

⭐ Read at least one historical fiction book for the next 12 days of plans.

After the reading, students will give a detailed oral narration. Select one paragraph from the story to read out loud to the students. This will be the starting point for the narration. Set a timer for 3-5 minutes. When the timer rings the narration is over, even if it isn't complete. A detailed, descriptive narration is the goal. See *Narration Tips* in the Appendix as needed.

Key Idea: Use oral narration to retell the story.

Bible Quiet Time | I |

Bible Reading: Choose one option below.

⭐ *The Illustrated Family Bible* p. 122-125

⭐ Your own Bible: 1 Samuel 8:1-9; 9:15-17; 13:1-14

Scripture Focus: Highlight 1 Samuel 8:5-7.

Prayer Focus: Pray a prayer of adoration to worship and honor God. Begin by reading the highlighted verses out loud as a prayer. End by praying, *You are King over all. Help me to treat you as King in my life by...*

Scripture Memory: Recite Philippians 2:10.
Music: *Philippians 2* CD: Track 2 (vs. 5-10)

Key Idea: The people asked Samuel for a king.

Independent History Study | I |

Open your *Student Notebook* to Unit 10. In Box 6, copy in cursive 1 Samuel 8:6-7.

Key Idea: When Samuel grew old, his sons became judges in Israel, but they were not honest and did not walk in God's ways. So, the Israelites asked Samuel for a king instead, like those that the pagan nations had around them. They were rejecting God as their king.

Learning the Basics
Focus: Language Arts, Math, Geography, Bible, and Science

Bible Study — T

Read aloud and discuss with the students the following page:

 The Radical Book for Kids p. 72-74

<u>Key Idea</u>: During Old Testament times, a person could walk about 20 miles per day. Walking was the most common mode of travel. By riding a donkey, a person could travel about 23 miles a day. In a horse-drawn chariot, a person could travel 45 miles a day. Use the provided charts to calculate the number of days various Biblical trips would have taken.

Language Arts — S

Have students complete one studied dictation exercise (see Appendix for directions and passages).

Help students complete one lesson from the following reading program:

 Drawn into the Heart of Reading

Work with the students to complete **one** of the English options listed below:

★ *Building with Diligence:* Lesson 18

★ *Following the Plan:* Lesson 16

★ Your own grammar program

<u>Key Idea</u>: Practice language arts skills.

Poetry — I

Open *Paint Like a Poet* to Lesson 8. Read aloud the poem *"Misgiving"*. On a 3 x 5 index card, neatly copy in black ink or in pencil the following highlighted lines from the poem:

All crying, 'We will go with you, O Wind!'
The foliage follow him, leaf and stem;
But a sleep oppresses them as they go,
And they end by bidding them as they go,
And they end by bidding him stay with
them.

-Robert Frost

Check your work to make sure it is correctly copied. Then, cut around your copywork. You may choose to outline the edge of the cut-out with an orange marker. Save it for Day 3.

<u>Key Idea</u>: Read and appreciate classic poetry.

Math Exploration — S

Choose **one** of the math options listed below.

★ *Singapore Primary Mathematics 4A/4B or 5A/5B* (see Appendix for schedules), or *Math with Confidence,* or *Apologia Math*

★ Your own math program

<u>Key Idea</u>: Use a step-by-step math program.

Science Exploration — I

★ Read *Land Animals of the Sixth Day* p. 171 – bottom of p. 175. Get your book about animal tracks that you began in Unit 2. At the top of the next page in your book of tracks, copy in cursive Genesis 3:14. Beneath the verse, draw and label lizard tracks and snake tracks as shown and described in the "Track It" section on p. 189-190.

Then, use a globe or a world map to find the locations of the animals listed in the **first column** of the "Map It" section on p. 189.

<u>Key Idea</u>: Lizards, turtles, and snakes are in the class Reptilia. They're cold-blooded and covered with thick, scaly skin. Reptiles molt or shed their skin as they grow. They also move by creeping or slithering.

Learning through History
Focus: The Reign of King Saul

Reading about History | I

Read about history in the following resource:

★ *The Story of the Ancient World:*
Ch. LXIX-LXX p. 143-146

You will be choosing a portion from today's reading that you found memorable or worthy of being reread to copy. Open your *Student Notebook* to Unit 10. In Box 4, carefully copy in cursive the portion from today's reading that you selected. Then, compare your written work to the original. Last, draw a small colorful picture in Box 4 to illustrate your sentences.

Key Idea: When Saul did not follow God's instructions, Samuel told Saul that God had left him. God instructed Samuel to anoint David.

Storytime | T

Choose one of the following read aloud options:

★ *Jashub's Journal: Tammuz* p. 59-70

★ Read aloud the next portion of the historical fiction book that you selected.

After reading, give each person 2 slips of paper. Each person must think of 2 questions to ask about the book and write one question on each slip of paper. Next, fold up the slips of paper and place them in a container. Each person must select at least one question from the container to answer.

Key Idea: Use questioning to share the story.

History Project | S

Today you will continue making your sling. To make the part of your sling which will hold the "stone", choose either a piece of cloth, felt, or a coffee filter. Then, measure and cut a 4" x 2" piece out of the material that you chose. Next, on each of the shorter sides of the material, cut a ¾" vertical slit inside the edge of each end. Now, take out the two pieces of yarn you braided on Day 1. Thread one braided piece of yarn through one slit in the material, and knot it back to the yarn itself. Repeat the threading and knotting for the other braided piece of yarn and the other slit. See the picture of the sling in your *Student Notebook* in Unit 10 to make sure that you have knotted the yarn correctly. Save your sling for Day 3.

Key Idea: With God's help, David used his sling to defeat the Philistine giant Goliath.

Bible Quiet Time | I

Reading: Choose one option below.

★ *The Illustrated Family Bible* p. 126-129

★ Your own Bible: 1 Samuel 16:1-13; ch. 17

Scripture Focus: Highlight 1 Samuel 16:7.

Prayer Focus: Pray a prayer of confession to admit or acknowledge your sins to God. Begin by reading the highlighted verse out loud as a prayer. End by praying, *I confess that my motives and thoughts are not always right. Help me to be a person with a pleasing heart.*

Scripture Memory: Recite Philippians 2:10.
Music: *Philippians 2* CD: Track 2 (vs. 5-10)

Key Idea: God chose David to be the next king, and He filled David with His Spirit. David was known as a man after God's own heart.

Independent History Study | I

Open your *Student Notebook* to "Prophecies About Christ". Under "Prophecy" write, *Isaiah 11:1-2*. Read the Scripture from your Bible to discover the prophecy. Under "Fulfillment" write, *Acts 13:22-23*. Read the fulfillment Scripture. Under "Description", write a few phrases to describe the prophecy about Jesus.

Key Idea: David was the son of Jesse from whose descendents would one day come the Savior, Jesus.

Learning the Basics
Focus: Language Arts, Math, Geography, Bible, and Science

Geography [T]

Read aloud to the students the following pages:

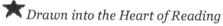 *A Child's Geography Vol. II* p. 64 (second column) – p. 66

Discuss with the students the **first two** "Field Notes" on p. 70.

Key Idea: The Great Rift Valley is a large crack in the earth's surface. The Jordan River runs through the Jordan Rift Valley, which is part of the Great Rift Valley. The Jordan River is the Biblical site of the healing of Naaman and the baptism of Jesus. This river gets its water from Mount Hermon, Israel's highest peak. The Jordan River feeds into Lake Kinneret, which in Bible times was called the Sea of Galilee.

Poetry [I]

Open *Paint Like a Poet* to Lesson 8. Read aloud the poem *"Misgiving"* by Robert Frost.

Today, you will be painting an autumn backdrop. You will need painting paper, a palette, water, a large flat paintbrush, plastic wrap, and yellow, red, and orange paint.

After gathering your supplies, turn to the "Step-by-Step Watercolor Tutorial" for Lesson 8 in *Paint Like a Poet*. Follow steps 1-3 to complete "Part One: Autumn Backdrop". Then, let your background dry. You will complete "Part Two" of the tutorial on Day 3.

Key Idea: Use painting to illustrate poetry.

Language Arts [S]

Help students complete one lesson from the following reading program:

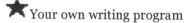 *Drawn into the Heart of Reading*

Work with the students to complete **one** of the writing options listed below:

 Writing & Rhetoric Book 1: Fable p. 59 – top of p. 63 (Note: Omit p. 57-58. Read the text aloud while the students follow along. Then, discuss.)

 Your own writing program

Key Idea: Practice language arts skills.

Math Exploration [S]

Choose **one** of the math options listed below.

 Singapore Primary Mathematics 4A/4B or *5A/5B* (see Appendix for schedules), or *Math with Confidence,* or *Apologia Math*

 Your own math program

Key Idea: Use a step-by-step math program.

Science Exploration [I]

 Read *Land Animals of the Sixth Day* bottom of p. 175 – bottom of p. 180. Orally retell or narrate to an adult the portion of text that you read today. Use the *Narration Tips* in the Appendix for help as needed.

Key Idea: Many snakes lay eggs. To hatch from their eggs, baby snakes have an egg tooth to tear open their shell. They lose their egg tooth when they molt. Snakes move by using their scales, called scutes, to grip the ground. Rattlesnakes, cottonmouths, and copperheads are poisonous pit vipers. The coral snake is also a poisonous snake. Colubrid snakes are the typical backyard snakes, such as garter snakes, king snakes, and grass snakes. Boas, pythons, and anacondas bite and constrict their prey.

Learning through History
Focus: The Reign of King Saul

Reading about History $\boxed{I}$

Read about history in the following resource:

★ *The Story of the Ancient World: Ch. LXXI-LXXII* p. 147 - middle of p. 150

You will be adding to your timeline in your *Student Notebook* today. In Unit 10 – Box 1, draw and color a crown. Label it, *Samuel anoints Saul as King (1095 B.C.)*. In Box 2, draw and color a horn with oil. Label it, *Samuel anoints David as King (1063 B.C.)*. In Box 3, draw and color 5 stones. Label it, *David slays Goliath (1063 B.C.)*.

Key Idea: Saul became jealous of David and tried to kill him with his spear.

Storytime $\boxed{T}$

Choose one of the following read aloud options:

★ *Jashub's Journal: Ab* p. 71-80

★ Read aloud the next portion of the historical fiction book that you selected.

After the reading, students will give a summary oral narration. The oral narration must be no longer than 5 sentences and should summarize the reading. As students narrate, have them hold up one finger for each sentence shared. Remind students that the focus should be on the big ideas, rather than on the details.

Key Idea: Summarize the story by narrating.

History Project $\boxed{S}$

Take out your sling that you made on Day 2. On paper, draw a red, bull's-eye target. Tape the target to the wall high up. (Remember, Goliath was 9 feet tall.) Use either a large marshmallow, a large cotton ball, a ping pong ball, or a tightly wadded and taped chunk of paper as your "stone". Follow the diagrams in your *Student Notebook* on Unit 10 to see how to use your sling. Practice trying to hit the bull's-eye with your stone.

Remember to never use a real stone unless you are outside all alone. Even then, you should only use a pebble or you could really hurt someone! Remember a stone from David's sling killed Goliath.

Key Idea: After David killed Goliath, he could have been prideful. Instead, he glorified God.

Bible Quiet Time $\boxed{I}$

Reading: Choose one option below.

★ *The Illustrated Family Bible* p. 130-131

★ Your own Bible: 1 Samuel 18

Scripture Focus: Highlight 1 Samuel 18:7-9.

Prayer Focus: Pray a prayer of thanksgiving to express gratitude for God's divine goodness. Begin by reading the highlighted verses out loud as a prayer. End by praying, *Help me to be thankful for any success that you may give me, Lord, and not to be jealous of others.*

Scripture Memory: Recite Philippians 2:10.
Music: *Philippians 2* CD: Track 2 (vs. 5-10)

Key Idea: Saul could see God was with David.

Independent History Study $\boxed{I}$

Open your *Student Notebook* to Unit 10. In Box 7, copy in cursive 1 Samuel 17:45.

Key Idea: After David used his sling to slay Goliath, Saul grew more and more jealous of David's fame. Yet, Saul's son Jonathan and David became good friends. Jonathan could see that David was God's choice to be the next king of Israel, even though Jonathan was next in line to be king. Jonathan accepted God's choice willingly.

Learning the Basics
Focus: Language Arts, Math, Geography, Bible, and Science

Bible Study | T |

Read aloud and discuss with the students the following pages:

 The Radical Book for Kids p. 75-79

Key Idea: It is important to consider what is at the center of your life. Only God is designed to fill the space at the center of your life. When you try to center your life around other things, these "things" will eventually fail you. Glorifying or magnifying God is to be central to all you do. When you enjoy something, be sure to thank God for it!

Language Arts | S |

Have students complete one studied dictation exercise (see Appendix for directions and passages).

Work with the students to complete **one** of the writing options listed below:

 Writing & Rhetoric Book 1: Fable p. 64-67 (Note: Omit "Writing Time" p. 63. Guide students through the lesson, so they are successful writing a summary.)

 Your own writing program

Key Idea: Practice language arts skills.

Poetry | I |

Open *Paint Like a Poet* to Lesson 8. Read aloud the poem *"Misgiving"* by Robert Frost.

Get the autumn backdrop that you painted on Day 2. Today, you will be adding falling leaves. You will need a palette, water, a small flat paintbrush, a pencil, 2 leaves (if possible), and red paint.

After gathering your supplies, turn to the "Step-by-Step Watercolor Tutorial" for Lesson 8 in *Paint Like a Poet*. Follow steps 4-6 to complete "Part Two: Falling Leaves". When your painting is dry, glue your poetry copywork from Day 1 to your painting. Store your completed artwork in the place you have chosen for it.

Key Idea: Explore poetry moods with painting.

Math Exploration | S |

Choose **one** of the math options listed below.

 Singapore Primary Mathematics 4A/4B or 5A/5B (see Appendix for schedules), or *Math with Confidence,* or *Apologia Math*

 Your own math program

Key Idea: Use a step-by-step math program.

Science Exploration | I |

 Read *Land Animals of the Sixth Day* bottom of p. 180 - 184. Write the answer to each numbered question on lined paper. You do not need to copy the question. Use the listed pages for reference.
1. Use a Venn diagram to compare lizards and snakes, as shown in "Notebook Activities" on p. 190.
2. What causes a chameleon to change colors? (p. 182)
3. Write the words *dewlap* and *setae* and give their definitions. (p. 183-184)
4. Use a globe or a world map to find the locations of the animals in the **second column** of the "Map It" section of p. 189.
5. What can we learn about the snake from Genesis 3:1?

Key Idea: Lizards often have four legs with five claws on each foot. They have ears, eyelids, and tails.

Unit 10 - Day 4

Reading about History [I]

Read about history in the following resource:

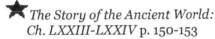 *The Story of the Ancient World:*
Ch. LXXIII-LXXIV p. 150-153

You will be writing a narration about *Chapter LXXIII: David's Generosity,* which is part of today's history reading.

To prepare for writing your narration, think about the questions below. If you do not know the answers, find them on p. 150-152 of *The Story of the Ancient World.* Ask yourself, *Where did God tell David to go fight? Who did David defeat in Keilah? When David left Keilah, where did he go? What did David do in the cave in Engedi? When David showed Saul the piece of his robe, what was Saul's response? How did David and his men support themselves? What did Nabal do? How did Abigail solve the problem Nabal created? When Nabal died, what did David do? Where was Michel, David's first wife?*

After you have thought about the answers to the questions, turn to Unit 10 in your *Student Notebook.* In Box 5, write a 5-8 sentence narration. When you have finished writing, read your sentences out loud to catch any mistakes. Check for the following things: *Did you include **who** the reading was mainly about? Did you include **what** important thing(s) happened? Did you include **how** it ended? If not, add those things.*

Then, underline or highlight the main idea sentence in the narration. Use the *Written Narration Skills* in the Appendix as a guide for editing the narration.

Key Idea: Saul began to pursue David to kill him. David fled and hid with men loyal to him.

Storytime [T]

Choose one of the following read aloud options:

★ *Jashub's Journal: Elul* p. 81-86

★ Read aloud your historical fiction book.

After the reading, have each person get a Bible and open it anywhere in Proverbs. Explain, *We will have 5 minutes to skim through the verses in Proverbs to find any connections to today's story. When a connection is found, read the verse out loud and quickly share the connection. At the end of 5 minutes, anyone who has not shared yet must read aloud one verse and make the best connection possible.*

Key Idea: Seek God's word for His guidance.

Bible Quiet Time [I]

Reading: Choose one option below.

★ *The Illustrated Family Bible* p. 132-135

★ Your own Bible: 1 Samuel chapters 25 and 28

Scripture Focus: Highlight 1 Samuel 25:28.

Prayer Focus: Pray a prayer of supplication to make a humble and earnest request of God. Begin by reading the highlighted verse out loud as a prayer. End by praying, *Please keep me from wrong, so my life may honor you. Help me to ask for forgiveness when I do sin.*

Scripture Memory: Copy Philippians 2:10 in your Common Place Book.
Music: *Philippians 2* CD: Track 2 (vs. 5-10)

Key Idea: Saul died just as Samuel had said.

Independent History Study [I]

Open your *Student Notebook* to "Prophecies About Christ". Under "Prophecy" write, *Psalm 40:7-8.* Read the Scripture from your Bible to discover the prophecy. Under "Fulfillment" write, *Hebrews 10:5-9.* Read the fulfillment Scripture. Under "Description", write a few phrases to describe the prophecy about Jesus.

Key Idea: David desired to do God's will. It was prophesied that Jesus would come to do God's will.

Learning the Basics
Focus: Language Arts, Math, Geography, Bible, and Science

Geography [T]

Read aloud to the students the following pages:

 A Child's Geography Vol. II p. 67-70
Discuss the **last two** "Field Notes" on p. 70.

Key Idea: Lake Kinneret provides fresh water to families and to crops all over Israel. Meanwhile, the Jordan River ends in the Dead Sea, which is the lowest place on earth. The Dead Sea is so salty that only brine shrimp can live in it.

Language Arts [S]

Have students complete one dictation exercise.

Guide students to complete one reading lesson.

 Drawn into the Heart of Reading

Help students complete **one** English lesson.

⭐ *Building with Diligence:* Lesson 19

⭐ *Following the Plan:* Lesson 17

⭐ Your own grammar program

Key Idea: Practice language arts skills.

Poetry [I]

Open *Paint Like a Poet* to Lesson 8. Today, you will be performing a poetry reading of *"Misgiving"*. Practice reading the poem aloud with expression that matches the mood of the poem. Then, read the poem aloud in front of your chosen audience. At the end of the reading, share the following, *When I read this poem by Robert Frost, it made me think of...* Call on your audience to share what thoughts the poem brought to their minds. Last, say, *Did you know that after the move to New Hampshire, Robert worked as a cobbler to help his mother pay the rent? He nailed heels to boots. He also went to a small village school in Salem. His mother was his teacher.*

Key Idea: Share the poetry of Robert Frost.

Math Exploration [S]

Choose **one** of the math options listed below.

⭐ *Singapore Primary Mathematics 4A/4B or 5A/5B* (see Appendix for schedules), or *Math with Confidence,* or *Apologia Math*

⭐ Your own math program

Key Idea: Use a step-by-step math program.

Science Exploration [I]

⭐ Read *Land Animals of the Sixth Day* p. 185 – middle of p. 189. Turn to the science experiment section in your science binder or sketchbook. At the top of a blank page, write: *How does a chameleon's skin change colors?* Under the question, write: *'Guess'*. Write down your guess. Cut out four 2" x 2" squares from a white paper towel or napkin. Each square will be one layer of the chameleon's skin. The bottom layer of a chameleon's skin is white. So, place one white square on a piece of waxed paper to represent the bottom layer of skin. The next layer of skin contains dark colors like blue and brown. So, on the next square, use watercolor markers to color it brown and blue. Lay this layer on top of the white layer. The next layer of skin contains yellows and reds. So, color the third white square with yellow and red watercolor markers. Lay this layer on top of the blue and brown layer. The fourth layer of skin is the epidermis, which is for protection. So, lay the fourth white square on top of the red and yellow square. Now, use a water dropper to drip water on the layers and see the colors of the chameleon's various layers of skin mix to produce one color that you can see through the top layer. Next, on the paper write: *'Procedure'*. Draw a picture of the experiment. Write: *'Conclusion'* and explain what you learned. Repeat the experiment with different colors. **Note:** The "Projects" on p. 190 are optional.

Key Idea: Chameleons are lizards that can change colors based on the light, time of day, mood, or mating.

Learning through History
Focus: King David's Reign

Unit 11 - Day 1

Reading about History I

Read about history in the following resource:

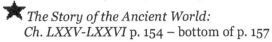 *The Story of the Ancient World:*
Ch. LXXV-LXXVI p. 154 – bottom of p. 157

When David became King of Israel, Hiram of Tyre was king of Phoenicia. Where could you look to research more about **Phoenicia**? Use a Bible, a reference book, or an online resource like www.wikipedia.org.

Answer one or more of the following questions from your research: *Where was Tyre located? Why did Hiram of Tyre make an alliance with King David? For what things were the ancient Phoenicians known? Where and how did they travel to trade? According to Ezekial 27:12-25, what things were traded in Tyre?*

Key Idea: David defeated the Amalekites.

History Project S

In this unit you will make an ancient board game that was played by the Phoenicians called *Twenty Squares*. First, measure and cut out a 1" x 1" square as a pattern. Next, on white paper trace around your square pattern to make the shape of the gameboard shown in Unit 11 of your *Student Notebook*. Then, cut your gameboard out and place it on a piece of waxed paper. Dip a tea bag in water and dab it on the board to make it look old. If you do not have a tea bag, use a paper towel to dab on cold coffee or watered down brown paint instead. Allow the board to dry until Day 2.

Key Idea: After David defeated the Philistines, the Phoenicians made an alliance with him.

Storytime T

Choose one of the following read aloud options:

 Jashub's Journal: Ethanim p. 87-92

 Read at least one historical fiction book for the next 8 days of plans.

After the reading, students will give a detailed oral narration. Select one paragraph from the story to read out loud to the students. This will be the starting point for the narration. Set a timer for 3-5 minutes. When the timer rings the narration is over, even if it isn't complete. A detailed, descriptive narration is the goal. See *Narration Tips* in the Appendix as needed.

Key Idea: Use oral narration to retell the story.

Bible Quiet Time I

Bible Reading: Choose one option below.

 The Illustrated Family Bible p. 136-139

 Your own Bible: 2 Samuel 2:1-7; 5:1-5; chapter 6

Scripture Focus: Highlight 2 Samuel 6:12.

Prayer Focus: Pray a prayer of adoration to worship and honor God. Begin by reading the highlighted verse out loud as a prayer. End by praying, *I rejoice and praise you for being Lord of all. Help me to give you the honor and reverence that you deserve by...*

Scripture Memory: Recite Philippians 2:11.
Music: *Philippians 2* CD: Track 2 (vs. 5-11)

Key Idea: David brought the Ark to Jersualem.

Independent History Study I

Open your *Student Notebook* to "Prophecies About Christ". Under "Prophecy" write, *2 Samuel 7:12-13*. Read the Scripture to discover the prophecy. Under "Fulfillment" write, *Luke 1:31-32*. Read the fulfillment Scripture. Under "Description", write a few phrases to describe the prophecy about Jesus.

Key Idea: God prophecied to David that his throne would be established forever, and through Jesus his kingdom would never end.

Learning the Basics
Focus: Language Arts, Math, Geography, Bible, and Science

Bible Study   [T]

Read aloud and discuss with the students the following pages:

 The Radical Book for Kids p. 80-81

Key Idea: Often our fears become too big in our minds. These fears make God seem small to us. The Bible says we are to fear the Lord, or be in awe of Him. Fearing God means remembering how big God is. When we remember how big God is, we also remember He is strong and able to help us. Then, we need not be afraid.

Language Arts   [S]

Have students complete one studied dictation exercise (see Appendix for directions and passages).

Help students complete one lesson from the following reading program:

 Drawn into the Heart of Reading

Work with the students to complete **one** of the English options listed below:

★ *Building with Diligence:* Lesson 20

★ *Following the Plan:* Lesson 18

★ Your own grammar program

Key Idea: Practice language arts skills.

Poetry   [I]

Open *Paint Like a Poet* to Lesson 9. Read aloud the poem *"Fragmentary Blue"*. On a 3 x 5 index card, neatly copy in black ink or in pencil the following highlighted lines from the poem:

Why make so much of fragmentary blue
In here and there a bird, or butterfly,
Or flower, or wearing-stone, or open eye,
When heaven presents in sheets the solid hue?

-Robert Frost

Check your work to make sure it is correctly copied. Then, cut around your copywork. You may choose to outline the edge of the cut-out with a blue marker. Save it for Day 3.

Key Idea: Read and appreciate a variety of classic poetry.

Math Exploration   [S]

Choose **one** of the math options listed below.

 ★ *Singapore Primary Mathematics 4A/4B* or *5A/5B* (see Appendix for schedules), or *Math with Confidence*, or *Apologia Math*

★ Your own math program

Key Idea: Use a step-by-step math program.

Science Exploration   [I]

★ Read *Land Animals of the Sixth Day* p. 191 – middle of p. 196. Get your book about animal tracks that you began in Unit 2. At the top of the next page in your book of tracks, copy in cursive Exodus 8:5-6. Beneath the verse, draw and label alligator or crocodile tracks and frog or toad tracks as shown and described in the "Track It" section on p. 209. You will read about these animals on Days 2-4.

Key Idea: Land species of turtles have a domed shell on their back, which keeps them safe from predators. Most turtles can pull their head and limbs into their shells. Side-necked turtles flatten their head against their shoulder to tuck it into their shell. Hidden-neck turtles pull their neck straight back into their shell. Turtles do not have ears, but they do have a good sense of smell. They have a horny beak instead of teeth and are often omnivores.

Unit 11 - Day 2

Reading about History | I |

Read about history in the following resource:

 The Story of the Ancient World: Ch. XXVII-LXXVIII p. 157 – top of p. 161

You will be choosing a portion from today's reading that you found memorable or worthy of being reread to copy. Open your *Student Notebook* to Unit 11. In Box 4, carefully copy in cursive the portion from today's reading that you selected. Then, compare your written work to the original. Last, draw a small colorful picture in Box 4 to illustrate your sentences.

<u>Key Idea</u>: When David sinned by having Uriah killed so he could take Bathsheba as his wife, God sent the prophet Nathan to confront him. David repented of his sin, but the consequences of the sin affected the rest of David's life.

History Project | S |

Today you will make the game pieces for *Twenty Squares*. Remove the crusts from 2 slices of bread. Tear the bread into very small pieces and put the pieces in a bowl with 2 Tablespoons of white glue. Stir the mixture. Add flour a little at at time to the mixture until it is no longer sticky. Then, knead it with your hands until it is a soft dough. Roll a very small ball of dough in between your hands. Place it on a piece of waxed paper. Dip the bottom of a glass in flour and use the glass bottom to flatten the ball of dough. It should be a flat disc the size of a dime. Make 9 other discs the same size. Paint 5 of the discs with black paint. Leave the other 5 discs white. Let them dry.

<u>Key Idea</u>: *Twenty Squares* is an ancient game.

Storytime | T |

Choose one of the following read aloud options:

 Jashub's Journal: Bul p. 93-100

 Read aloud the next portion of the historical fiction book that you selected.

After reading, work with the students to plan a 3 minute skit with simple props to act out part of today's reading. Set a timer for 3 minutes to quickly prepare for the skit. Make sure that you participate in the skit along with the students. When the timer rings, set it again for 3 minutes and perform the skit. You do not need an audience, as the goal is the retelling.

<u>Key Idea</u>: Use a skit to retell part of the story.

Bible Quiet Time | I |

Reading: Choose one option below.

 The Illustrated Family Bible p. 140-141

 Your own Bible: 2 Samuel 12:1-25

Scripture Focus: Highlight 2 Samuel 12:13.

Prayer Focus: Pray a prayer of confession to admit or acknowledge your sins to God. Begin by reading the highlighted verse out loud as a prayer. End by praying, *I confess my sins to you Lord, knowing that sin has consequences. Please forgive me for...*

Scripture Memory: Recite Philippians 2:11.
Music: *Philippians 2* CD: Track 2 (vs. 5-11)

<u>Key Idea</u>: In spite of David's sin, God forgave him. Later, Solomon was born to David and Bathsheba. The Bible says God loved Solomon.

Independent History Study | I |

 Listen to *What in the World?* Disc 2, Track 5: "Joshua Through David".

<u>Key Idea</u>: The first child of David and Bathsheba died as prophecied. Yet, God in His mercy allowed David and Bathsheba to have another son, Solomon, who would be God's choice to be king after David.

Learning the Basics

Focus: Language Arts, Math, Geography, Bible, and Science

Geography [T]

Have students get both the blank map and the labeled map of **Israel & Jordan** that they began in Unit 8.

Then, assign students the following page:

 A Child's Geography Vol. II p. 71

Note: Do only the "Map Notes" section.

Key Idea: Practice finding and recording the locations of various places on a map of Israel.

Language Arts [S]

Help students complete one lesson from the following reading program:

 Drawn into the Heart of Reading

Work with the students to complete **one** of the writing options listed below:

 Writing & Rhetoric Book 1: Fable p. 68-69 (Note: Reread the fable on p. 60 first. Then, brainstorm ideas with the students for today's lesson. You may read aloud the example in the Teacher's Guide p. 68 for help.)

 Your own writing program

Key Idea: Practice language arts skills.

Poetry [I]

Open *Paint Like a Poet* to Lesson 9. Read aloud the poem *"Fragmentary Blue"* by Robert Frost.

Today, you will be painting a fragmented sky. You will need painting paper, a palette, water, a large flat paintbrush, and light blue paint.

After gathering your supplies, turn to the "Step-by-Step Watercolor Tutorial" for Lesson 9 in *Paint Like a Poet*. Follow steps 1-3 to complete "Painting One: Fragmented Sky". Then, let your painting dry. Store your completed artwork in the place you have chosen for it.

Key Idea: Use painting to illustrate poetry.

Math Exploration [S]

Choose **one** of the math options listed below.

 Singapore Primary Mathematics 4A/4B or *5A/5B* (see Appendix for schedules), or *Math with Confidence,* or *Apologia Math*

 Your own math program

Key Idea: Use a step-by-step math program.

Science Exploration [I]

★ Read *Land Animals of the Sixth Day* middle of p. 196 – bottom of p. 200. Orally retell or narrate to an adult the portion of text that you read today. Use the *Narration Tips* in the Appendix for help as needed. Then, use a globe or a world map to find the locations of the animals in the **first column** of the "Map It" section of p. 209.

Key Idea: Alligators, gavials, crocodiles, and caimans are large reptiles in the order Crocodilia. Crocodiles or gavial's teeth can be seen even when their mouths are closed. They also have a V-shaped snout. Alligators or caimans have a U-shaped snout, and when their mouths are closed, you see very few teeth.

Reading about History | I |

Read about history in the following resource:

 ★ *The Story of the Ancient World: Ch. XXIX-LXXX* p. 161 – middle of p. 164

You will be adding to your timeline in your *Student Notebook* today. In Unit 11 – Box 1, draw and color a crown. Label it, *David is King of Judah and Israel (1048 B.C.)*. In Box 2, draw and color a tree. Label it, *Absalom Rebels (1023 B.C.)*. In Box 3, draw and color 4 stick figure giants. Label it, *Revolt against the Philistines (1018 B.C.)*.

Key Idea: David's children from his multiple wives quarreled among themselves. Absalom eventually killed Amnon and fled.

History Project | S |

Get the game board that you made on Day 1. Glue it on a black, light blue, or brown sheet of paper. Open your *Student Notebook* to the diagram of the gameboard in Unit 11. Follow the diagram to paint a light blue rosette on the square spaces on your gameboard that match the marked spaces in the diagram. While the gameboard is drying, get out 4 craft sticks to be throwing sticks. If you do not have craft sticks, you may use clothespins or toothpicks instead. Place your throwing sticks on a paper towel. Paint **one** side of each throwing stick black. Leave the other side unpainted. When your gameboard and throwing sticks are dry, use the pieces you made on Day 2 to play *Twenty Squares* according to the rules.

Key Idea: Israel and Phoenicia were neighbors.

Storytime | T |

Choose one of the following read aloud options:

★ *Jashub's Journal: Kislev* p. 101-106

★ Read aloud the next portion of the historical fiction book that you selected.

After the reading, students will give a summary oral narration. The oral narration must be no longer than 5 sentences and should summarize the reading. As students narrate, have them hold up one finger for each sentence shared. Remind students that the focus should be on the big ideas, rather than on the details.

Key Idea: Summarize the story by narrating.

Bible Quiet Time | I |

Reading: Choose one option below.

★ *The Illustrated Family Bible* p. 142-143 Optional Extension: p. 120

★ Your own Bible: 2 Samuel 15:1-17; 18:1-18

Scripture Focus: Highlight 2 Samuel 14:25.

Prayer Focus: Pray a prayer of thanksgiving to express gratitude for God's divine goodness. Begin by reading the highlighted verse out loud as a prayer. End by praying, *I am thankful that you look at the inside of a person rather than at the outside. Help me be pleasing to you...*

Scripture Memory: Recite Philippians 2:11.
Music: *Philippians 2* CD: Track 2 (vs. 5-11)

Key Idea: Absalom returned to Jerusalem to overthrow his father David as king.

Independent History Study | I |

Open your *Student Notebook* to Unit 11. Read the rules of the ancient Phoenician game *Twenty Squares*. This game was also played in ancient Egypt. When you have finished making your game board for your history project, play the game with a partner. You may wish to copy the rules to include with your board.

Key Idea: King David and Hiram of Tyre made an alliance between Israel and Phoenicia.

Learning the Basics
Focus: Language Arts, Math, Geography, Bible, and Science

Bible Study [T]

Read aloud and discuss with the students the following pages:

 The Radical Book for Kids p. 82-84

Key Idea: God gave you a mind to think and remember. By connecting facts to what you already know, you can remember better. Visualizing facts as pictures helps in recollection. Writing out facts or verses helps you memorize them. Reading a passage over and over aloud helps you memorize it. Answering questions about God's Word helps you recall what the Bible says.

Language Arts [S]

Have students complete one studied dictation exercise (see Appendix for directions and passages).

Work with the students to complete **one** of the writing options listed below:

 Writing & Rhetoric Book 1: Fable p. 70 – top of p. 74 (Note: Read aloud the text while the students follow along. Then, discuss.)

 Your own writing program

Key Idea: Practice language arts skills.

Poetry [I]

Open *Paint Like a Poet* to Lesson 9. Read aloud the poem *"Fragmentary Blue"* by Robert Frost.

Today, you will be painting a cloudy sky. You will need painting paper, a palette, water, a large flat paintbrush, a dropper, a paper towel, and blue paint.

After gathering your supplies, turn to the "Step-by-Step Watercolor Tutorial" for Lesson 9 in *Paint Like a Poet*. Follow steps 1-3 to complete "Painting Two: Cloudy Sky". When your painting is dry, glue your poetry copywork from Day 1 to your painting. Store your completed artwork in the place you have chosen for it.

Key Idea: Explore poetry moods with painting.

Math Exploration [S]

Choose **one** of the math options listed below.

 Singapore Primary Mathematics 4A/4B or 5A/5B (see Appendix for schedules), or *Math with Confidence,* or *Apologia Math*

 Your own math program

Key Idea: Use a step-by-step math program.

Science Exploration [I]

 Read *Land Animals of the Sixth Day* bottom of p. 200 – middle of p. 205. Write the answer to each numbered question on lined paper. You do not need to copy the question. Use the listed pages for help.
1. Describe one of the following: crocodiles, gavials, caimans, or alligators. (p. 201-202)
2. Write the words *endangered* and *extinct* and give their definitions. (p. 203)
3. What are the six stages that a typical frog goes through? (p. 203-204)
4. Use a globe or a world map to find the locations of the animals in the **second column** of the "Map It" section of p. 209.
5. Use a Venn diagram to compare reptiles and amphibians. See an example diagram on p. 190.

Key Idea: Amphibians begin life in water and then move to live on land. They have a unique life cycle.

Reading about History | I |

Read about history in the following resource:

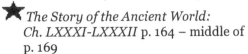 *The Story of the Ancient World: Ch. LXXXI-LXXXII p. 164 – middle of p. 169*

You will be writing a narration about *Chapter LXXXI: The Seafaring Phoenicians*, which is part of today's history reading.

To prepare for writing your narration, think about the questions below. If you do not know the answers, find them on p. 164-166 of *The Story of the Ancient World*. Ask yourself, *For what were the Phoenicians famous? From whom were the Phoenicians descended? How did the Phoenicians obtain their wealth? What other things were the Phoenicians known for? Who were their first customers? Which coasts did the Phoenicians visit to trade? What was the name of the most famous Phoenician colony. Describe a Phoenician trading expedition.*

After you have thought about the answers to the questions, turn to Unit 11 in your *Student Notebook*. In Box 5, write a 5-8 sentence narration. When you have finished writing, read your sentences out loud to catch any mistakes. Check for the following things: *Did you include **who** the reading was mainly about? Did you include **what** important thing(s) happened? Did you include **how** it ended? If not, add those things.*

Then, underline or highlight the main idea sentence in the narration. Use the *Written Narration Skills* in the Appendix as a guide for editing the narration.

Key Idea: The Phoenicians were descendents of Canaan. Their first city was at Sidon. They were best known for their purple dye.

Storytime | T |

Choose one of the following read aloud options:

 Jashub's Journal: Tebeth p. 107-111

Read aloud your historical fiction book.

After the reading, have each person get a Bible and open it anywhere in Proverbs. Explain, *We will have 5 minutes to skim through the verses in Proverbs to find any connections to today's story. When a connection is found, read the verse out loud and quickly share the connection. At the end of 5 minutes, anyone who has not shared yet must read aloud one verse and make the best connection possible.*

Key Idea: Seek God's word for His guidance.

Bible Quiet Time | I |

Reading: Choose one option below.

The Illustrated Family Bible p. 144-145 Optional extension: p. 121

Your own Bible: 2 Samuel 24; 1 Kings 1

Scripture Focus: Highlight 1 Kings 1:30.

Prayer Focus: Pray a prayer of supplication to make a humble and earnest request of God. Begin by reading the highlighted verse out loud as a prayer. End by praying, *Lord, please surround me with Christians whose counsel will help me walk in your ways and guide me to do your will.*

Scripture Memory: Copy Philippians 2:11 in your Common Place Book.
Music: *Philippians 2* CD: Track 2 (vs. 5-11)

Key Idea: Solomon was David's chosen heir.

Independent History Study | I |

Open your *Student Notebook* to Unit 11. In Box 6, copy in cursive 1 Kings 5:1, 12.

Key Idea: Hiram of Tyre made an alliance with David of Israel. Solomon continued the alliance.

Learning the Basics
Focus: Language Arts, Math, Geography, Bible, and Science

Geography · T

Go to the website link listed on p. 6 of *A Child's Geography Vol. II*. At the link, select "History & Geography". Then, under "Knowledge Quest" select ACG2-Extra Activities". Print the "Travel Log Template" of your choice from p. 39-42. Also at the link, for older students, print and assign the "Chapter Five Review" on p. 71. Assign all students the following page:

★ *A Child's Geography Vol. II* p. 71
Note: Do only the "Travel Notes" section. The "Books" and "Poetry" on p. 72 are optional.

<u>Key Idea:</u> Share three sights from Israel.

Language Arts · S

Have students complete one dictation exercise.

Guide students to complete one reading lesson.

★ *Drawn into the Heart of Reading*

Help students complete **one** English lesson.

★ *Building with Diligence:* Lesson 21

★ *Following the Plan:* Lesson 19

★ Your own grammar program

<u>Key Idea:</u> Practice language arts skills.

Poetry · I

Open *Paint Like a Poet* to Lesson 9. Today, you will be performing a poetry reading of *"Fragmentary Blue"*. Practice reading the poem aloud with expression that matches the mood of the poem. Then, read the poem aloud in front of your chosen audience.

At the end of the reading, share the following, *When I read this poem by Robert Frost, it made me think of...* Call on your audience to share what thoughts the poem brought to their minds. Last, say, *Did you know that Robert Frost's grandfather paid for the train fare so that Robert could attend high school in Lawrence? Robert became the top student in his class.*

<u>Key Idea:</u> Share the poetry of Robert Frost.

Math Exploration · S

Choose **one** of the math options listed below.

★ *Singapore Primary Mathematics 4A/4B* or *5A/5B* (see Appendix for schedules), or *Math with Confidence,* or *Apologia Math*

★ Your own math program

<u>Key Idea:</u> Use a step-by-step math program.

Science Exploration · I

★ Read *Land Animals of the Sixth Day* middle of p. 205 – top of p. 209. Turn to the science experiment section in your science binder or sketchbook. At the top of a blank page, write: *How do frogs breathe when they are in mud or underwater?* Under the question, write: *'Guess'*. Write down your guess. In the summer heat, frogs often bury themselves under mud or in the water to keep themselves cool and wet. Use an uncooked egg as your frog. Gently place the egg in the bottom of a glass bowl or glass pan to be your pond. Fill your container partway full of water so that it covers the top of your egg. After 10 minutes, what do you notice forming around the egg? Why do tiny air bubbles form around the egg? An egg has a semi-permeable membrane through which oxygen can pass. Frogs can absorb oxygen through their skin too, even in mud or water. Now, gently move the glass container, while watching the egg through the side of the container. What do you notice rising from the bottom of the egg to the surface of the water? Next, on the paper write: *'Procedure'*. Draw a picture of the experiment. Write: *'Conclusion'* and explain what you learned. **Note:** The "Project" on p. 210 is optional.

<u>Key Idea:</u> When frogs bury themselves in mud or water, they continue to breathe by absorbing oxygen through their skin. Frogs also have lungs for breathing on land.

Learning through History
Focus: From Solomon to a Divided Kingdom

Unit 12 - Day 1

Reading about History   [I]

Read about history in the following resource:

 ★ *The Story of the Ancient World: Ch. LXXXIII-LXXXIV* p. 169 - bottom of p. 173

God gave Solomon the job of building His Temple. Where could you look to research more about **Solomon's Temple**? Use a Bible, an online resource like www.wikipedia.org, or take a virtual tour at museumbibletours.com.

Answer one or more of the following questions from your research: *Where was the Temple built? How long did it take for the Temple to be built? What were some of the materials used in building the Temple? Describe the outside of the Temple. Describe the inside of the Temple. When the Temple was complete, what did Solomon do? How do we know that the Lord was pleased with His Temple?*

Key Idea: Solomon was 19 when he became God's anointed leader as Israel's next king.

History Project   [S]

In this unit you will make a project to show the division of the 12 tribes of Israel. Get one sheet of white paper and one sheet of pastel paper. Measure and cut out twelve 3" x 2" rectangles, ten white and two pastel. Fold each rectangle in half to make twelve 1 ½" x 2" pockets. Staple each pocket on the sides leaving the top open. Next, measure and cut out two 5" x 3" rectangles, one white and one pastel. Fold and staple them into pockets and save them.

Key Idea: Solomon ruled all 12 of the tribes.

Storytime   [T]

Choose one of the following read aloud options:

★ *God King* p. ix-xi and p. 1-13

★ Read at least one historical fiction book for the next 4 days of plans.

After the reading, students will give a detailed oral narration. Select one paragraph from the story to read out loud to the students. This will be the starting point for the narration. Set a timer for 3-5 minutes. When the timer rings the narration is over, even if it isn't complete. A detailed, descriptive narration is the goal. See *Narration Tips* in the Appendix as needed.

Key Idea: Use oral narration to retell the story.

Bible Quiet Time   [I]

Bible Reading: Choose one option below.

★ *The Illustrated Family Bible* p. 146-149

★ Your own Bible: 1 Kings 3; 5:1-12; 9:1-9

Scripture Focus: Highlight 1 Kings 3:5, 9.

Prayer Focus: Pray a prayer of adoration to worship and honor God. Begin by reading the highlighted verses out loud as a prayer. End by praying, *Lord, you are exalted above all things. Help me to have the wisdom and discernment that only you can give.*

Scripture Review: Philippians 2:1-11.
Music: *Philippians 2* CD: Tracks 1-2 (all)

Key Idea: At Gibeon, God spoke to Solomon. God was pleased with Solomon's request.

Independent History Study   [I]

Open your *Student Notebook* to "Prophecies About Christ". Under "Prophecy" write, *Psalm 45:1-7*. Read the Scripture to discover the prophecy. Under "Fulfillment" write, *Hebrews 1:8-9*. Read the fulfillment Scripture. Under "Description", write a few phrases to describe the prophecy about Jesus.

Key Idea: This Psalm, written for Solomon's wedding, also describes Christ as the righteous anointed one.

Learning the Basics
Focus: Language Arts, Math, Geography, Bible, and Science

Bible Study [T]

Read aloud and discuss the following pages:

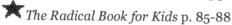 *The Radical Book for Kids* p. 85-88

Key Idea: God designed man in His image. We were created to glorify God. When sin entered the world, we not only displayed God's image but also our own sinful image. When Jesus was born, He was the perfect reflection of God. He fulfilled God's mission by living a sinless life and dying the death we should have had. Because of Jesus' resurrection, all followers of Christ can now reflect His glory!

Language Arts [S]

Have students complete one studied dictation exercise (see Appendix for directions and passages).

Help students complete one lesson from the following reading program:

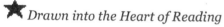 *Drawn into the Heart of Reading*

Work with the students to complete **one** of the English options listed below:

★ *Building with Diligence:* Lesson 22

★ *Following the Plan:* Lesson 20

★ Your own grammar program

Key Idea: Practice language arts skills.

Poetry [I]

Open *Paint Like a Poet* to Lesson 10. Read aloud the poem *"Going for Water"*. On a 3 x 5 index card, neatly copy in black ink or in pencil the following highlighted lines from the poem:

We ran as if to meet the moon
That slowly dawned behind the trees,
The barren boughs without the leaves,
Without the birds, without the breeze.
                    -Robert Frost

Check your work to make sure it is correctly copied. Then, cut around your copywork. You may choose to outline the edge of the cut-out with a purple marker. Save it for Day 3.

Key Idea: Read and appreciate a variety of classic poetry.

Math Exploration [S]

Choose **one** of the math options listed below.

★ *Singapore Primary Mathematics 4A/4B or 5A/5B* (see Appendix for schedules), or *Math with Confidence,* or *Apologia Math*

★ Your own math program

Key Idea: Use a step-by-step math program.

Science Exploration [I]

★ Read *Land Animals of the Sixth Day* p. 211 – middle of p. 216. Get your book about animal tracks that you began in Unit 2. At the top of the next page in your book of tracks, copy in cursive Job 40:15-17. Beneath the verse, draw and label the dinosaur track shown and described in the "Track It" section on p. 227.

Key Idea: At one time, enormous animals roamed the earth. Giant-sized dinosaurs, wombats, sloths, kangaroos, and crocodiles once existed. "Dinosaur" is a fairly new term, which means it isn't found in the Bible or in other ancient writings. However, the Bible does describe very large animals that resemble dinosaurs. Petroglyphs that resemble dinosaurs have also been found. Fossilized dinosaur bones are studied to learn about dinosaurs. This leaves paleontologists guessing as to the type of skin dinosaurs had.

Learning through History
Focus: From Solomon to a Divided Kingdom

Unit 12 - Day 2

Reading about History [I]

Read about history in the following resource:

★ *The Story of the Ancient World:*
   Ch. LXXXV p. 173 - middle of p. 176

You will be choosing a portion from today's reading that you found memorable or worthy of being reread to copy. Open your *Student Notebook* to Unit 12. In Box 5, carefully copy in cursive the portion from today's reading that you selected. Then, compare your written work to the original. Last, draw a small colorful picture in Box 5 to illustrate your sentences.

Key Idea: Solomon married 700 different foreign women, and his wives turned his heart away from God. So, God allowed Hadad, prince of Edom to raid Solomon's borders.

Storytime [T]

Choose one of the following read aloud options:

★ *God King* p. 14-30

★ Read aloud your historical fiction book.

After reading, give students a few minutes to prepare a short advertisement speech for the book. During the speech, students should hold up the book and say the book title and the name of the author. The wording of the advertisement should provide a peek into the book without giving away the ending. The goal should be for listeners to feel like they've "Got to Have This Book"!

Key Idea: Use an ad speech to share the story.

History Project [S]

Get out the 14 pockets that you made on Day 1. Label each of the 10 small white pockets with one of the following tribe names: Reuben, Simeon, Gad, Dan, Asher, Zebulun, Naphtali, Issachar, Ephraim, and Manasseh. Label each of the small pastel colored pockets with one of the following tribe names: Judah and Benjamin. Label the large white pocket *Israel* and the large pastel pocket *Judah*. Open your *Student Notebook* to Unit 12. On the page with the heading "The Divided Kingdom", glue each pocket into a matching white space. Leave the *Student Notebook* open to dry until Day 3.

Key Idea: The Lord warned Solomon that worshipping other gods would result in punishment. Ahijah prophecied God would tear Israel into pieces and give ten tribes to Jeroboam.

Bible Quiet Time [I]

Reading: Choose one option below.

★ *The Illustrated Family Bible* p. 150-153

★ Your own Bible: 1 Kings 10:1-13; 11:1-13

Scripture Focus: Highlight 1 Kings 11:4

Prayer Focus: Pray a prayer of confession to admit or acknowledge your sins to God. Begin by reading the highlighted verse out loud as a prayer. End by praying, *Lord, I confess that sometimes my heart is not as fully devoted to you as it should be. Help me be more devoted to you.*

Scripture Review: Philippians 2:1-11.
Music: *Philippians 2* CD: Tracks 1-2 (all)

Key Idea: The Queen of Sheba tested Solomon.

Independent History Study [I]

Open your *Student Notebook* to "Prophecies About Christ". Under "Prophecy" write, *Psalm 72:10-11*. Read the Scripture to discover the prophecy. Under "Fulfillment" write, *Matthew 2:1-11*. Read the fulfillment Scripture. Under "Description", write a few phrases to describe the prophecy about Jesus.

Key Idea: This Psalm prophecied that Christ, like Solomon, would have kings bow down and bring gifts.

Learning the Basics
Focus: Language Arts, Math, Geography, Bible, and Science

Geography [T]

Read aloud to the students the following pages:

 A Child's Geography Vol. II p. 73-75

Discuss with the students the **first** "Field Note" on p. 80.

Key Idea: Many people go on a pilgrimage each year to visit the Holy places where Jesus walked. Bethlehem was the birthplace of Jesus. In Bethlehem, the Church of the Nativity was built upon the spot thought to be the place of Jesus' birth. Bethlehem is mainly populated with Muslims today.

Language Arts [S]

Help students complete one lesson from the following reading program:

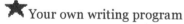 *Drawn into the Heart of Reading*

Work with the students to complete **one** of the writing options listed below:

★ *Writing & Rhetoric Book 1: Fable* p. 75 – top of p. 78 (Note: Omit p. 74. Guide students through the lesson, so they are successful writing an amplification.)

★ Your own writing program

Key Idea: Practice language arts skills.

Poetry [I]

Open *Paint Like a Poet* to Lesson 10. Read aloud the poem *"Going for Water"* by Robert Frost.

Today, you will be painting a night backdrop. You will need painting paper, a palette, water, a large flat paintbrush, masking tape, a paper towel, and purple and dark blue paint.

After gathering your supplies, turn to the "Step-by-Step Watercolor Tutorial" for Lesson 10 in *Paint Like a Poet*. Follow steps 1-3 to complete "Part One: Night Backdrop". Then, let your background dry. You will complete "Part Two" of the tutorial on Day 3.

Key Idea: Use painting to illustrate poetry.

Math Exploration [S]

Choose **one** of the math options listed below.

★ *Singapore Primary Mathematics 4A/4B* or *5A/5B* (see Appendix for schedules), or *Math with Confidence*, or *Apologia Math*

★ Your own math program

Key Idea: Use a step-by-step math program.

Science Exploration [I]

★ Read *Land Animals of the Sixth Day* middle of p. 216 – top of p. 219. Orally retell or narrate to an adult the portion of text that you read today. Use the *Narration Tips* in the Appendix for help as needed. "Try This" at the top of p. 219 is an optional extra.

Key Idea: Dinosaur names often come from a feature on the dinosaur, from the place where it was discovered, or from the name of the person who discovered it. Lizard-hipped dinosaurs are separated into theropods and sauropods. Sauropods walked on four legs, while theropods walked on two legs. Sauropods were herbivores, and theropods were carnivores.

Reading about History | I |

Read about history in the following resource:

 The Story of the Ancient World: Ch. LXXXVI-LXXXVII p. 176-179

You will be adding to your timeline in your *Student Notebook* today. In Unit 12 – Box 1, draw and color 2 rings. Label it, *Solomon marries Pharaoh's daughter (1014 B.C.).* In Box 2, draw and color the Temple. Label it, *Temple completed (1004 B.C.).* In Box 3, write *Judah / Israel.* Label it, *Divided kingdom (975 B.C.).* In Box 4, draw and color a pyramid. Label it, *Pharaoh Shishak invades Judah (971 B.C.).*

Key Idea: After Solomon's death, Jeroboam ruled Israel, and Rehoboam ruled Judah.

Storytime | T |

Choose one of the following read aloud options:

⭐ *God King* p. 31-45

⭐ Read aloud the next portion of the historical fiction book that you selected.

After the reading, students will give a summary oral narration. The oral narration must be no longer than 5 sentences and should summarize the reading. As students narrate, have them hold up one finger for each sentence shared. Remind students that the focus should be on the big ideas, rather than on the details.

Key Idea: Summarize the story by narrating.

History Project | S |

Choose a cloth rag for today's activity to go with the Bible reading 1 Kings 11:26-43. Tear the rag into 12 very small pieces. Open your *Student Notebook* to Unit 12. Place one piece of cloth inside each of the 12 small pockets to signify the rending of the cloak, representing the 12 tribes of Israel. Then, take the cloth out of the 10 white pockets and place those pieces into the large *Israel* pocket. Last, take the cloth out of the 2 pastel colored pockets and place those pieces in the large *Judah* pocket to show the fulfillment of the prophecy.

Key Idea: The prophet Ahijah tore his cloak into 12 pieces and handed 10 to Jeroboam, who was one of Solomon's officials. This prophecy showed that God would punish Solomon's disobedience by tearing 10 tribes from the hand of his son and giving them to Jeroboam.

Bible Quiet Time | I |

Reading: Choose one option below.

⭐ *The Illustrated Family Bible* p. 156-157

⭐ Your own Bible: 1 Kings 11:26-43

Scripture Focus: Highlight 1 Kings 12:8.

Prayer Focus: Pray a prayer of thanksgiving to express gratitude for God's divine goodness. Begin by reading the highlighted verse out loud as a prayer. End by praying, *Thank you for providing me with wise adults who walk in your ways. Help me listen to their wise counsel, rather than listening to counsel from those my own age.*

Scripture Review: Philippians 2:1-11.
Music: *Philippians 2* CD: Tracks 1-2 (all)

Key Idea: Rehoboam took the wrong advice.

Independent History Study | I |

⭐ Listen to *What in the World?* Disc 2, Track 6: "Solomon Through Jeroboam".

Key Idea: Solomon's son Rehoboam continued taxing the people heavily and was left only with the tribes of Judah and Benjamin. Jeroboam ruled the other 10 tribes of Israel, and he built idols to worship.

Learning the Basics
Focus: Language Arts, Math, Geography, Bible, and Science

Bible Study [T]

Read aloud and discuss with the students the following pages:

 The Radical Book for Kids p. 89-94

Key Idea: Amy Charmichael and Lottie Moon were both women who gave their lives for Christ. In spite of physical trials and hardship, Amy became a missionary in India for most of her life. She bravely rescued young girls from slavery in the Hindu temples and taught them the love of Jesus. Lottie was a tireless missionary to China for almost 40 years. Her articles and letters encouraged many other men and women to become missionaries.

Language Arts [S]

Have students complete one studied dictation exercise (see Appendix for directions and passages).

Work with the students to complete **one** of the writing options listed below:

 Writing & Rhetoric Book 1: Fable p. 78 (Note: Reread the fable on p. 71 first. Then, brainstorm ideas with students for today's lesson.)

 Your own writing program

Key Idea: Practice language arts skills.

Poetry [I]

Open *Paint Like a Poet* to Lesson 10. Read aloud the poem *"Going for Water"* by Robert Frost.

Get the night backdrop that you painted on Day 2. Today, you will be adding the moon and some trees. You will need a palette, water, a small round paintbrush, a toothpick, and grey, white, and black paint.

After gathering your supplies, turn to the "Step-by-Step Watercolor Tutorial" for Lesson 10 in *Paint Like a Poet*. Follow steps 4-6 to complete "Part Two: Moon and Trees". When your painting is dry, glue your poetry copywork from Day 1 to your painting. Store your completed artwork in the place you have chosen for it.

Key Idea: Explore poetry moods with painting.

Math Exploration [S]

Choose **one** of the math options listed below.

 Singapore Primary Mathematics 4A/4B or 5A/5B (see Appendix for schedules), or *Math with Confidence*, or *Apologia Math*

 Your own math program

Key Idea: Use a step-by-step math program.

Science Exploration [I]

 Read *Land Animals of the Sixth Day* top of p. 219 - 223. Write the answer to each numbered question on lined paper. You do not need to copy the question. Use the listed page to help you answer each question.
1. What are the names of some of the common sauropod fossils that have been found? (p. 219)
2. Who are some of the common theropods that have been discovered? (p. 220-221)
3. Write the words *sauropod* and *theropod* and give their definitions. (p. 217)
4. Give some examples of the bird-hipped dinosaurs. (p. 222-223)
5. Use a globe or a world map to find the locations of the animals in the "Map It" section of p. 227.

Key Idea: Sauropods and theropods are saurischians, or lizard-hipped. Ornithischia are bird-hipped.

Reading about History · I

Read about history in the following resource:

 *The Story of the Ancient World:
Ch. LXXXVIII-LXXXIX* p. 180 – top of p. 184

You will be writing a narration about *Chapter LXXXVIII: Two Kings of Judah,* which is part of today's history reading.

To prepare for writing your narration, think about the questions below. If you do not know the answers, find them on p. 180-181 of *The Story of the Ancient World.* Ask yourself, *Who was King of Judah after Solomon? How did Rehoboam's reign start out? When Judah turned to idol worship, how did God punish them? Who came against Jerusalem? What did Rehoboam do when Pharaoh Shishak arrived in Jerusalem? When Rehoboam died, who was Judah's next king? What did Abijah say to Israel and to Jeroboam? Even though Jeroboam had Abijah surrounded, what happened? Why did God punish Israel? Who became Judah's next king after Abijah?*

After you have thought about the answers to the questions, turn to Unit 12 in your *Student Notebook.* In Box 6, write a 5-8 sentence narration. When you have finished writing, read your sentences out loud to catch any mistakes. Check for the following things: *Did you include **who** the reading was mainly about? Did you include **what** important thing(s) happened? Did you include **how** it ended? If not, add those things.*

Then, underline or highlight the main idea sentence in the narration. Use the *Written Narration Skills* in the Appendix as a guide for editing the narration.

Key Idea: God punished Judah's idol worship by allowing Pharaoh Shishak to invade them.

Storytime · T

Choose one of the following read aloud options:

 God King p. 46-59

Read aloud the next portion of the historical fiction book that you selected.

After the reading, have each person get a Bible and open it anywhere in Proverbs. Explain, *We will have 5 minutes to skim through the verses in Proverbs to find any connections to today's story. When a connection is found, read the verse out loud and quickly share the connection. At the end of 5 minutes, anyone who has not shared yet must read aloud one verse and make the best connection possible.*

Key Idea: Seek God's word for His guidance.

Bible Quiet Time · I

Reading: Choose one option below.

The Illustrated Family Bible p. 154

Your own Bible: 1 Kings 14:21-31; 15:1-24

Scripture Focus: Highlight 1 Kings 15:3.

Prayer Focus: Pray a prayer of supplication to make a humble and earnest request of God. Begin by reading the highlighted verse out loud as a prayer. End by praying, *Knowing my own children will follow my example, help me not to fall into a pattern of sinning but instead to be fully devoted to you Lord, like David.*

Scripture Review: Philippians 2:1-11.
Music: *Philippians 2* CD: Tracks 1-2 (all)

Key Idea: The sons of both Jeroboam and Rehoboam did mostly evil in the eyes of God.

Independent History Study · I

Open your *Student* Notebook to Unit 12. In Box 7, copy in cursive 1 Kings 11:11-12.

Key Idea: God's people turned to idol worship, and God punished them so that they would repent.

Learning the Basics

Focus: Language Arts, Math, Geography, Bible, and Science

Geography [T]

Read aloud to the students the following pages:

⭐ *A Child's Geography Vol. II* p. 76 – first paragraph in the second column of p. 80

Discuss with the students the last **three** "Field Notes" on p. 80.

Key Idea: Nazareth was Jesus' hometown. Today, half of the people in Nazareth are Christians, and the other half are Muslims. Jerusalem is claimed as the capital city of Israel by Israelis and also as the future capital of Palestine by the Palestinians. Conflict continues over Jerusalem.

Language Arts [S]

Have students complete one dictation exercise.

Guide students to complete one reading lesson.

⭐ *Drawn into the Heart of Reading*

Help students complete **one** English lesson.

⭐ *Building with Diligence:* Lesson 23

⭐ *Following the Plan:* Lesson 21 (Half)

⭐ Your own grammar program

Key Idea: Practice language arts skills.

Poetry [I]

Open *Paint Like a Poet* to Lesson 10. Today, you will be performing a poetry reading of *"Going for Water"*. Practice reading the poem aloud with expression that matches the mood of the poem. Then, read the poem aloud in front of your chosen audience.

At the end of the reading, share the following, *When I read this poem by Robert Frost, it made me think of...* Call on your audience to share what thoughts the poem brought to their minds. Last, say, *Did you know that when Robert Frost graduated from high school in 1892, he shared the top honors in his class with his future wife, Elinor White? By this time Robert was already writing poetry, leaving little time for studying at Dartmouth (as his grandfather wished for him to do).*

Key Idea: Share the poetry of Robert Frost.

Math Exploration [S]

Choose **one** of the math options listed below.

⭐ *Singapore Primary Mathematics 4A/4B or 5A/5B* (see Appendix for schedules), or *Math with Confidence*, or *Apologia Math*

⭐ Your own math program

Key Idea: Use a step-by-step math program.

Science Exploration [I]

⭐ Read *Land Animals of the Sixth Day* p. 224-226. Now, skip to the "Experiment" on the bottom of p. 227-228. Turn to the science experiment section in your science binder or sketchbook. At the top of a blank page, write: *How did a dinosaur's stance affect the way it moved?* Under the question, write: *'Guess'*. Write down your guess. Follow the directions for the experiment in *Land Animals of the Sixth Day* p. 227-228. You may wish to substitute tinker toys for the coat hangers. If you do not have the supplies to do the experiment, you can still complete steps 5-9 on p. 228.

Next, on the paper write: *'Procedure'*. Draw a labeled picture of the experiment. At the bottom of the paper, write: *'Conclusion'*. Explain what you learned from the experiment.

Key Idea: A lizard's legs are positioned outside its body, giving it a sprawling stance. A dinosaur's legs were positioned beneath its body, giving it the ability to run more easily.

Learning through History
Focus: Israel and Judah at the Time of Elijah and Elisha

Reading about History | I

Read about history in the following resource:

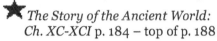 *The Story of the Ancient World:*
Ch. XC-XCI p. 184 – top of p. 188

Ten of the twelve tribes of Israel formed the Northern Kingdom. Where could you look to research more about the **Northern Kingdom of Israel**? Use the Bible, a reference book, or an online resource like www.wikipedia.org.

Answer one or more of the following questions from your research: *Name the various capital cities of the northern kingdom in the order in which each was the capital. Which king made Samaria his capital city? What did Ahab hope to gain by marrying the king of Phoenicia's daughter? What worship did Jezebel bring to the northern kingdom? During what years did the northern kingdom exist? What caused the end of the northern kingdom?*

Key Idea: Ahab was the son of Omri.

History Project | S

In this unit you will make a clay or dough map of Israel, Judah, and the neighbors that surrounded them in ancient times. Make paper labels with the names of these locations: Israel, Judah, Syria, Phoenicia, Philistia, Ammon, Moab, Edom, Egypt, The Great Sea (Mediterranean Sea), and The Salt Sea. Attach the labels to toothpicks to make flags. Store the flags in a baggie until Day 3.

Key Idea: After Jeroboam died, Israel was reigned by a succession of kings including Nadab, Baasha, Elah, Zimri, Omri, and Ahab. As the seventh king of Israel, Ahab was the mightiest and the most wicked king.

Storytime | T

Choose one of the following read aloud options:

 God King p. 60-76

★ Read at least one fantasy for the next 16 days of plans (see Appendix for suggestions).

After the reading, students will give a detailed oral narration. Select one paragraph from the story to read out loud to the students. This will be the starting point for the narration. Set a timer for 3-5 minutes. When the timer rings the narration is over, even if it isn't complete. A detailed, descriptive narration is the goal. See *Narration Tips* in the Appendix as needed.

Key Idea: Use oral narration to retell the story.

Bible Quiet Time | I

Bible Reading: Choose one option below.

★ *The Illustrated Family Bible* p. 158-159

★ Your own Bible: 1 Kings 16:29-34; 17

Scripture Focus: Highlight 1 Kings 17:1.

Prayer Focus: Pray a prayer of adoration to worship and honor God. Begin by reading the highlighted verse out loud as a prayer. End by praying, *I give you praise and adoration for the rain and dew that we often take for granted. Although Baal was supposed to be a weather god, only you can bring the rain.*

Scripture Memory: Recite Philippians 2:12.
Music: *Philippians 2* CD: Track 3 (verse 12)

Key Idea: Ahab sinned by marrying Jezebel, the daughter of the Phoenician king of Sidon.

Independent History Study | I

★ Open your *Student Notebook* to Unit 13. In box 6, copy in cursive Psalm 2:1-2.

Key Idea: Jezebel encouraged Ahab to worship Baal and persecuted the prophets of God in Israel.

Learning the Basics
Focus: Language Arts, Math, Geography, Bible, and Science

Bible Study [T]

Read aloud and discuss with the students the following pages:

 The Radical Book for Kids p. 95-97

Key Idea: Latin words and phrases are a common part of the English language. Approximately 60% of English words have Latin origins. Latin was the language spoken in Ancient Rome 2,500 years ago by the Caesars.

Language Arts [S]

Have students complete one studied dictation exercise (see Appendix for directions and passages).

Help students complete one lesson from the following reading program:

 Drawn into the Heart of Reading

Work with the students to complete **one** of the English options listed below:

⭐ *Building with Diligence:* Lesson 24

⭐ *Following the Plan:* Lesson 21 (Last half)

⭐ Your own grammar program

Key Idea: Practice language arts skills.

Poetry [I]

Open *Paint Like a Poet* to Lesson 11. Read aloud the poem *"Range-Finding"*. On a 3 x 5 index card, neatly copy in black ink or in pencil the following highlighted lines from the poem:

On the bare upland pasture there had spread
O'ernight 'twixt mullein stalks a wheel of thread
And straining cables wet with silver dew.
A sudden passing bullet shook it dry.
The indwelling spider ran to greet the fly,
But finding nothing, sullenly withdrew.
                    -Robert Frost

Check your work to make sure it is correctly copied. Then, cut around your copywork. You may choose to outline the edge of the cut-out with a green marker. Save it for Day 3.

Key Idea: Read and appreciate classic poetry.

Math Exploration [S]

Choose **one** of the math options listed below.

 Singapore Primary Mathematics 4A/4B or 5A/5B (see Appendix for schedules), or *Math with Confidence*, or *Apologia Math*

⭐ Your own math program

Key Idea: Use a step-by-step math program.

Science Exploration [I]

⭐ Read *Land Animals of the Sixth Day* p. 229 – top of p. 232. Today you will add to your science notebook. At the top of an unlined paper, copy Job 8:13-15 in cursive. Beneath the verse, draw and color the spider from p. 229 of *Land Animals of the Sixth Day*. Label each part of the spider with the correct name. Beneath the diagram of the spider, write the following heading: *Two spiders to watch out for in the United States*. Then, draw and color a picture of the brown recluse from p. 231 and the black widow from p. 232. Write the name of the spider beneath each drawing.

Key Idea: Spiders, ticks, mites, scorpions, and harvestmen are arachnids. They have eight legs and two pedipalps used for handling food and for defending themselves. Arachnids have multiple eyes and can sense things by using the hairs on their legs, which are called setae. They also have fangs and venom.

Learning through History
Focus: Israel and Judah at the Time of Elijah and Elisha

Reading about History   I

Read about history in the following resource:

★ *The Story of the Ancient World:*
Ch. XCII-XCIII p. 188-191

You will be choosing a portion from today's reading that you found memorable or worthy of being reread to copy. Open your *Student Notebook* to Unit 13. In Box 4, carefully copy in cursive the portion from today's reading that you selected. Then, compare your written work to the original. Last, draw a small colorful picture in Box 3 to illustrate your sentences.

Key Idea: God judged the weather god Baal by sending a drought that no amount of prayers to Baal could change. God showed that there is only one true God.

Storytime   T

Choose one of the following read aloud options:

★ *God King* p. 77-88

★ Read aloud the next portion of the fantasy that you selected.

After reading, give each person a white piece of paper or a markerboard and a marker. Set a timer for 3-5 minutes and instruct each person to do a quick outline sketch about the story. Ideas for sketches include settings, characters, actions, important objects, or symbols. When the timer rings, briefly share the sketches.

Key Idea: Use sketching to share the story.

History Project   S

Today you will use colored clay or playdough to make the shape of the map shown in your *Student Notebook* on Unit 13. Place a piece of waxed paper on top of your work surface. Flatten the playdough or clay on the waxed paper in the shape of the various countries shown on the map. Alternate different colors of clay or playdough to better show each individual region. When you have completed forming the map, leave the map on the waxed paper and place it inside a lidded container to store for Day 3.

Key Idea: In Phoenicia, Baal was worshipped as a weather god. Jezebel brought the worship of Baal to Israel when she married Ahab. She persecuted the prophets of God.

Bible Quiet Time   I

Reading: Choose one option below.

★ *The Illustrated Family Bible* p. 160-161

★ Your own Bible: 1 Kings 18

Scripture Focus: Highlight 1 Kings 18:17-18.

Prayer Focus: Pray a prayer of confession to admit or acknowledge your sins to God. Begin by reading the highlighted verses out loud as a prayer. End by praying, *I confess that I too blame others for my sins just as Ahab did. Forgive me for my sinful nature when I...*

Scripture Memory: Recite Philippians 2:12.
Music: *Philippians 2* CD: Track 3 (verse 12)

Key Idea: After three years of drought, God sent Elijah to Ahab to summon the people of Israel and the prophets of Baal to Mt. Carmel.

Independent History Study   I

Open your *Student Notebook* to the map in Unit 13. Jezebel was the daughter of the king of Phoenicia. She came from the city of Sidon. Find Phoenicia on the map. Ahab was king of the Northern Kingdom of Israel. His capital city was Samaria. Find Israel and the city of Samaria on the map.

Key Idea: Ahab's father, Omri, had made Samaria the capital of the Northern Kingdom of Israel.

Geography   T

Read aloud to the students the following pages:

 A Child's Geography Vol. II p. 80 (second paragraph in the second column) – p. 83

Discuss with the students "Field Notes" p. 83.

<u>Key Idea</u>: The Mosque of Omar, or the Dome of the Rock, is a holy shrine in Jerusalem for Muslims. Muslims think it houses the rock from which Mohammed ascended up to Allah. The Dome of the Rock is also the site of Mount Moriah, where Abraham was ready to sacrifice Isaac, and the site where the Jewish Temple's Holy of Holies once stood! The Church of the Holy Sepulchre is thought to stand where Jesus was nailed to the cross and over His tomb.

Language Arts   S

Complete one lesson from the program below.

★ *Drawn into the Heart of Reading*

Work with the students to complete **one** of the writing options listed below:

★ *Writing & Rhetoric Book 1: Fable* p. 79-87 (Note: Have students choose **either** the part of the fisherman **or** his wife. You will read all other parts. You will only do one reading of the fairy tale.)

★ Your own writing program

<u>Key Idea</u>: Practice language arts skills.

Poetry   I

Open *Paint Like a Poet* to Lesson 11. Read aloud the poem *"Range-Finding"* by Robert Frost.

Today, you will be painting a grassy backdrop. You will need painting paper, a palette, water, a large flat paintbrush, a paper towel, and green paint.

After gathering your supplies, turn to the "Step-by-Step Watercolor Tutorial" for Lesson 11 in *Paint Like a Poet*. Follow steps 1-3 to complete "Part One: Grassy Backdrop". Then, let your background dry. You will complete "Part Two" of the tutorial on Day 3.

<u>Key Idea</u>: Use painting to illustrate poetry.

Math Exploration   S

Choose **one** of the math options listed below.

★ *Singapore Primary Mathematics 4A/4B* or *5A/5B* (see Appendix for schedules), or *Math with Confidence,* or *Apologia Math*

★ Your own math program

<u>Key Idea</u>: Use a step-by-step math program.

Science Exploration   I

★ Read *Land Animals of the Sixth Day* p. 232-237. Orally retell or narrate to an adult the portion of text that you read today. Use the *Narration Tips* in the Appendix for help as needed. **Note:** Wait to do "Try This" on p. 234 until Day 4. If you have access to the internet, you may wish to learn about arthropods through the Virtual Insect Collection Lab at the following site: https://arthropods.nmsu.edu/making-an-insect-collection/virtual-insect-collection-lab.html

<u>Key Idea</u>: Spiders produce silk using their spinnerets. They produce different kinds of silk for different purposes. Dragline silk makes a strong safety line for spiders. Capture silk is used to catch prey. Egg-case silk is wrapped around the spider's eggs for protection. Orb webs, funnel webs, tangle webs (or cobwebs), and sheet webs are four of the most common kinds of webs that spiders weave.

Reading about History | I |

Read about history in the following resource:

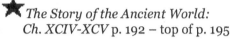 ★ *The Story of the Ancient World:*
Ch. XCIV-XCV p. 192 – top of p. 195

You will be adding to your timeline in your *Student Notebook* today. In Unit 13 – Box 1, draw a blue star. Label it, *Samaria becomes Israel's capitol (924 B.C.).* In Box 2, draw and color an altar on fire. Label it, *Elijah at Mt. Carmel (906 B.C.).* In Box 3, draw a black music note. Label it, *God fights for Jehoshaphat and Judah (897 B.C.).*

Key Idea: Jehoshaphat was king in Judah when Ahab was king in Israel. Even though Jehoshaphat was a good king, he encouraged his son to marry the daughter of Ahab and Jezebel. This marriage would bring much heartache to Judah.

History Project | S |

Get the clay or playdough map in the container that you saved from Day 2 and the flags that you saved from Day 1. Refer to the map on Unit 13 in your *Student Notebook* as you add the flags to label the corresponding places on your clay or playdough map. After labeling your map, study it for a few minutes and then remove the flags. Next, close your *Student Notebook* and try to replace each flag in its correct position on your clay or playdough map. Then, open your *Student Notebook* and check to see how many flags you placed correctly.

Key Idea: Micaiah prophecied that Ahab would lose his life in the war with the king of Damascus. The prophecy came true.

Storytime | T |

Choose one of the following read aloud options:

★ *God King* p. 89-103

★ Read aloud the next portion of the fantasy that you selected.

After the reading, students will give a summary oral narration. The oral narration must be no longer than 5 sentences and should summarize the reading. As students narrate, have them hold up one finger for each sentence shared. Remind students that the focus should be on the big ideas, rather than on the details.

Key Idea: Summarize the story by narrating.

Bible Quiet Time | I |

Reading: Choose one option below.

★ *The Illustrated Family Bible* p. 162-163

★ Your own Bible: 1 Kings 21

Scripture Focus: Highlight 1 Kings 21:29.

Prayer Focus: Pray a prayer of thanksgiving to express gratitude for God's divine goodness. Begin by reading the highlighted verse out loud as a prayer. End by praying, *Thank you Lord for the mercy that you show me when I humble myself before you and am sorry. Show me my sins so I may ask for forgiveness.*

Scripture Memory: Recite Philippians 2:12.
Music: *Philippians 2* CD: Track 3 (verse 12)

Key Idea: Although Ahab had sinned against God greatly, God took pity on him when Ahab repented and humbled himself before God.

Independent History Study | I |

Ahab was killed in a war with the king of Damascus. Damascus is the capital of Syria. Find Syria on the map in your *Student Notebook* – Unit 13. Ahab was buried in Samaria, Israel's capital city at the time.

Key Idea: Even though Ahab tried to disguise himself to avoid death, he was killed anyway as prophecied.

Learning the Basics
Focus: Language Arts, Math, Geography, Bible, and Science

Bible Study | T |

Read aloud and discuss with the students the following pages:

 The Radical Book for Kids p. 98-100

Key Idea: In the Bible, the high priest's breastplate had twelve gemstones to represent the twelve tribes of Israel. As God's people, we are His special treasure. We are like jewels to our heavenly King, and he treasures us!

Language Arts | S |

Have students complete one studied dictation exercise (see Appendix for directions and passages).

Work with the students to complete **one** of the writing options listed below:

 Writing & Rhetoric Book 1: Fable p. 88-91 (Note: Read the text aloud while the students follow along. Guide students as needed to discover the moral for each example.)

 Your own writing program

Key Idea: Practice language arts skills.

Poetry | I |

Open *Paint Like a Poet* to Lesson 11. Read aloud the poem *"Range-Finding"* by Robert Frost.

Get the grassy backdrop that you painted on Day 2. Today, you will be adding grass, blooms, and a web. You will need a palette, water, a small round paintbrush, a toothpick, and green, yellow, and white paint.

After gathering your supplies, turn to the "Step-by-Step Watercolor Tutorial" for Lesson 11 in *Paint Like a Poet*. Follow steps 4-6 to complete "Part Two: Grass, Blooms, and Web". When your painting is dry, glue your poetry copywork from Day 1 to your painting. Store your completed artwork in the place you have chosen for it.

Key Idea: Explore poetry moods with painting.

Math Exploration | S |

Choose **one** of the math options listed below.

 Singapore Primary Mathematics 4A/4B or *5A/5B* (see Appendix for schedules), or *Math with Confidence,* or *Apologia Math*

 Your own math program

Key Idea: Use a step-by-step math program.

Science Exploration | I |

 Read *Land Animals of the Sixth Day* bottom of p. 238 – middle of p. 243. Write the answer to each numbered question on lined paper. You do not need to copy the question. Use the listed pages for help.
1. Why aren't daddy longlegs considered to be spiders? (p. 238-239)
2. Draw and label the parts of a scorpion. (p. 239)
3. Write the words *parasite* and *mange* and give their definitions. (p. 241-242)
4. Why is it important to wash your sheets and to vacuum and sweep? (p. 242)
5. What should you do if you find a tick on you? (p. 243)

Key Idea: Harvestmen are spider-like arachnids who are not really spiders. Scorpions are arachnids with a venomous stinger. Mites and ticks are arachnids called acarina. They are very plentiful parasites.

Reading about History [I]

Read about history in the following resource:

⭐ *The Story of the Ancient World:*
   Ch. XCVI-XCVII p. 195 – middle of p. 198

You will be writing a narration about *Chapter XCVI: The Chariot of Fire,* which is part of today's history reading.

To prepare for writing your narration, think about the questions below. If you do not know the answers, find them on p. 195-196 of *The Story of the Ancient World.* Ask yourself, *Who was the new king of Israel in today's story? What was the name of Joram's mother? Where have you heard about Jezebel before? At this time, what had God commanded Elijah to do? How did Elijah test Elisha? Where did Elijah and Elisha travel together? What happened when Elijah reached the banks of the Jordan River? What did Elisha ask of Elijah? How was Elijah taken to heaven? What sign was given to Elisha that God had granted his request?*

After you have thought about the answers to the questions, turn to Unit 13 in your *Student Notebook.* In Box 5, write a 5-8 sentence narration. When you have finished writing, read your sentences out loud to catch any mistakes. Check for the following things: *Did you include **who** the reading was mainly about? Did you include **what** important thing(s) happened? Did you include **how** it ended? If not, add those things.*

Then, underline or highlight the main idea sentence in the narration. Use the *Written Narration Skills* in the Appendix as a guide for editing the narration.

Key Idea: Joram was King Ahab's son.

Storytime [T]

Choose one of the following read aloud options:

⭐ *God King* p. 104-115

⭐ Read aloud the next portion of the fantasy.

After the reading, have each person get a Bible and open it anywhere in Proverbs. Explain, *We will have 5 minutes to skim through the verses in Proverbs to find any connections to today's story. When a connection is found, read the verse out loud and quickly share the connection. At the end of 5 minutes, anyone who has not shared yet must read aloud one verse and make the best connection possible.*

Key Idea: Seek God's word for His guidance.

Bible Quiet Time [I]

Reading: Choose one option below.

⭐ *The Illustrated Family Bible* p. 164-165

⭐ Your own Bible: 2 Kings 2:1-18; 4:8-37

Scripture Focus: Highlight 2 Kings 2:9.

Prayer Focus: Pray a prayer of supplication to make a humble and earnest request of God. Begin by reading the highlighted verse out loud as a prayer. End by praying, *Lord, I ask to do your work on earth and to follow in the footsteps of those you call into your service. Help me be led by your Spirit to do your will.*

Scripture Memory: Copy Philippians 2:12 in your Common Place Book.
Music: *Philippians 2* CD: Track 3 (verse 12)

Key Idea: God took Elijah to heaven.

Independent History Study [I]

Elisha traveled with Elijah to Bethel and then to Jericho. The Jordan River that Elijah crossed is near Jericho. In your *Student Notebook* – Unit 13, find Bethel, Jericho, and the place where Elijah was taken.

Key Idea: Elisha asked God to give him a double portion of Elijah's spirit. God granted Elisha's request.

Learning the Basics
Focus: Language Arts, Math, Geography, Bible, and Science

Geography [T]

Have students get both the blank map and the labeled map of **Israel & Jordan** that they began in Unit 8.

Then, assign students the following page:

 ⭐ *A Child's Geography Vol. II* p. 84
Note: Do only the "Map Notes" section. Then, save both the labeled map and the blank map to use when you read about Jordan.

<u>Key Idea</u>: Practice finding and recording the locations of various places on a map of Israel.

Language Arts [S]

Have students complete one dictation exercise.

Guide students to complete one reading lesson.

⭐ *Drawn into the Heart of Reading*

Help students complete **one** English lesson.

⭐ *Building with Diligence:* Lesson 25
⭐ *Following the Plan:* Lesson 22
⭐ Your own grammar program

<u>Key Idea</u>: Practice language arts skills.

Poetry [I]

Open *Paint Like a Poet* to Lesson 11. Today, you will be performing a poetry reading of *"Range-Finding"*. Practice reading the poem aloud with expression that matches the mood of the poem. Then, read the poem aloud in front of your chosen audience. At the end of the reading, share the following, *When I read this poem by Robert Frost, it made me think of...* Call on your audience to share what thoughts the poem brought to their minds.

Last, say, *Did you know that Robert Frost left Dartmouth College after only a few months and returned home to work in a textile mill and write poetry? His poem "My Butterfly" was published in a magazine when he was 19.*

<u>Key Idea</u>: Share the poetry of Robert Frost.

Math Exploration [S]

Choose **one** of the math options listed below.

⭐ *Singapore Primary Mathematics 4A/4B* or *5A/5B* (see Appendix for schedules), or *Math with Confidence*, or *Apologia Math*
⭐ Your own math program

<u>Key Idea</u>: Use a step-by-step math program.

Science Exploration [I]

⭐ Read *Land Animals of the Sixth Day* bottom of p. 243 – top of p. 247. Turn to the science experiment section in your science binder or sketchbook. At the top of a blank page, write: *How does a spider form its web?* Under the question, write: *'Guess'*. Write down your guess. Follow the steps to make the web on *Land Animals of the Sixth Day* p. 234. You may wish to make your web on paper instead, using liquid glue to attach your yarn to the paper. When you get to "Step 5" and are adding the extra circles, use a different colored yarn or string to signify that part of the web is made with capture silk, which is sticky. When the web is complete, rinse out and dry a milk cap or a juice cap. Then, place sugar in the cap and place the cap on your web. The capful of sugar represents an insect. You are the spider, carrying a dropper of water, which represents venom. As the spider, use your fingers to step on only the non-sticky parts of the web to get to your prey. When you get to the insect, pour your venom into the insect to liquefy it. Then, use your dropper to suck up the liquid for your meal. Next, on the paper write: *'Procedure'*. Draw a labeled picture of the steps in making a web. At the bottom of the paper, write: *'Conclusion'*. Explain what you learned from the experiment. **Note:** The "Experiment" on p. 247-248 is optional.

<u>Key Idea</u>: Spiders build their orb web between two "posts", following a general pattern as they weave.

Learning through History
Focus: The Assyrian Conquests

Reading about History | I |

Read about history in the following resource:

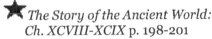 *The Story of the Ancient World: Ch. XCVIII-XCIX p. 198-201*

At the time when Elisha was a prophet in Israel, Aram (or Syria) often waged war on Israel. Where could you look to research more about **Aram** (or Syria)? Read 2 Kings 5:1-18 for more information on Aram. You may also wish to use a reference book or an online resource like www.wikipedia.org.

Answer one or more of the following questions from your research: *Where was Aram or Syria located? What was the capital city of Aram? What two rivers flowed near Damascus? Who was the ruler of Aram when Naaman was the captain of the Syrian army? Who was king in Israel at the time Ben-Hadad II was king in Aram? Who was the principle god worshiped in Aram?*

<u>Key Idea</u>: Naaman, the captain of the Syrian army, had leprosy. Elisha healed him.

History Project | S |

In this unit you will be making a mosaic like those found within Assyrian palaces. On white paper, measure and cut out a 4" x 4" box. In the box, draw a large picture of a horse and a chariot, like the one shown on p. 209 or on the wall on p. 211 of *The Story of the Ancient World*. You may choose whether to include a chariot driver. Save the sketch for Day 2.

<u>Key Idea</u>: When the Syrians came to fight Israel, the Lord caused them to hear horses and chariots in their camp. The Syrians fled for home, leaving behind all of their provisions.

Storytime | T |

Choose one of the following read aloud options:

 God King p. 116-127

Read at least one fantasy for the next 12 days of plans.

After the reading, students will give a detailed oral narration. Select one paragraph from the story to read out loud to the students. This will be the starting point for the narration. Set a timer for 3-5 minutes. When the timer rings the narration is over, even if it isn't complete. A detailed, descriptive narration is the goal. See *Narration Tips* in the Appendix as needed.

<u>Key Idea</u>: Use oral narration to retell the story.

Bible Quiet Time | I |

Bible Reading: Choose one option below.

⭐ *The Illustrated Family Bible* p. 166-167 and 2 Kings 7:1-19

⭐ Your own Bible: 2 Kings 5:1-19; 7:1-19

Scripture Focus: Highlight 2 Kings 5:14.

Prayer Focus: Pray a prayer of adoration to worship and honor God. Begin by reading the highlighted verse out loud as a prayer. End by praying, *I worship you for your healing power and praise you for your wondrous works. I know all healing comes from your mighty hand. Thank you for healing me when...*

Scripture Memory: Recite Philippians 2:13.
Music: *Philippians 2* CD: Track 3 (vs. 12-13)

<u>Key Idea</u>: Elisha was God's prophet in Israel. God protected Elisha from the Syrian army.

Independent History Study | I |

Open your *Student Notebook* to Unit 14. In Box 7, copy in cursive 2 Kings 7:5-7.

<u>Key Idea</u>: The Syrians (Arameans) thought that Israel had hired the Egyptians and Hittites to attack them.

Learning the Basics

Focus: Language Arts, Math, Geography, Bible, and Science

Bible Study   [T]

Read aloud and discuss with the students the following pages:

⭐ *The Radical Book for Kids* p. 101-103

Key Idea: When making decisions, it is important to consider what the Bible says. Next, weigh what is good about the choice you are making. Ask whether you can thank God for that choice, and whether He would be glorified by it. Weigh whether the choice is wise, or whether it makes sin look acceptable. Last, ask whether the choice makes something more important to you than God.

Language Arts   [S]

Have students complete one dictation exercise (see Appendix for directions and passages).

Help students complete one lesson from the following reading program:

⭐ *Drawn into the Heart of Reading*

Work with the students to complete **one** of the English options listed below:

⭐ *Building with Diligence:* Lesson 26 (Half)

⭐ *Following the Plan:* Lesson 23

⭐ Your own grammar program

Key Idea: Practice language arts skills.

Poetry   [I]

Open *Paint Like a Poet* to Lesson 12. Read aloud the poem *"The Road Not Taken"*. On a 3 x 5 index card, neatly copy in black ink or in pencil the following highlighted lines from the poem:

I shall be telling this with a sigh
Somewhere ages and ages hence:
Two roads diverged in a wood, and I –
I took the one less traveled by,
And that has made all the difference.
                              -Robert Frost

Check your work to make sure it is correctly copied. Then, cut around your copywork. You may choose to outline the edge of the cut-out with a yellow marker. Save it for Day 3.

Key Idea: Read and appreciate a variety of classic poetry.

Math Exploration   [S]

Choose **one** of the math options listed below.

⭐ *Singapore Primary Mathematics 4A/4B* or *5A/5B* (see Appendix for schedules), or *Math with Confidence,* or *Apologia Math*

⭐ Your own math program

Key Idea: Use a step-by-step math program.

Science Exploration   [I]

⭐ Read *Land Animals of the Sixth Day* p. 249 – middle of p. 253. "Try This" on p. 251 is optional.

Today you will add to your science notebook. At the top of an unlined paper, copy Genesis 8:19 in cursive. Beneath the verse, write the heading "Gastropod Anatomy". Beneath the heading, draw and color the gastropod illustrated on p. 251 of *Land Animals of the Sixth Day*. Label each part of the gastropod with the correct name.

Key Idea: Snails and slugs are in the class Gastropoda, which is a part of the phylum Mollusca. These animals move by using their belly like a foot. Snails and slugs produce mucus as they slide along. The mucus can be used as a defense too. Snails and slugs also have two optic tentacles with eyes.

Reading about History   I

Read about history in the following resource:

 The Story of the Ancient World: Ch. C-CI p. 202 – bottom of p. 205

You will be choosing a portion from today's reading that you found memorable or worthy of being reread to copy. Open your *Student Notebook* to Unit 14. In Box 4, carefully copy in cursive the portion from today's reading that you selected. Then, compare your written work to the original. Last, draw a small colorful picture in Box 4 to illustrate your sentences.

Key Idea: Jezebel encouraged idol worship in Israel, and her daughter Athaliah encouraged idol worship in Judah. God eventually judged these two wicked queens as evidenced by their very untimely deaths.

History Project   S

Take out the drawing of the horse and chariot that you made on Day 1. Use crayons to brightly color your drawing. Make sure to color the entire 4" x 4" square so that no white space is left anywhere on the paper. Save the colored drawing for Day 3.

Key Idea: According to God's command, Jehu was anointed as the next king of Israel after Joram. As captain of Israel's armies, Jehu killed all of Ahab's family including Jezebel and King Ahaziah of Judah (who was the son of Athaliah, daughter of Jezebel and Ahab).

Storytime   T

Choose one of the following read aloud options:

 God King p. 128-138

★ Read aloud the next portion of the fantasy that you selected.

After reading, give each person 2 slips of paper. Each person must think of 2 questions to ask about the book and write one question on each slip of paper. Next, fold up the slips of paper and place them in a container. Each person must select at least one question from the container to answer.

Key Idea: Use questioning to share the story.

Bible Quiet Time   I

Reading: Choose one option below.

★ *The Illustrated Family Bible* p. 10-13 and 2 Kings 12:1-5

★ Your own Bible: 2 Kings 11; 12:1-5

Scripture Focus: Highlight 2 Kings 12:2.

Prayer Focus: Pray a prayer of confession to admit or acknowledge your sins to God. Begin by reading the highlighted verse out loud as a prayer. End by praying, *Lord, I confess that I need Godly people in my life to give me a good example of how to live for you. Surround me with Godly companions like...*

Scripture Memory: Recite Philippians 2:13.
Music: *Philippians 2* CD: Track 3 (vs. 12-13)

Key Idea: Joash became king of Judah as a boy. He repaired God's temple.

Independent History Study   I

★ Look on the timeline on p. 260 of *A Story of the Ancient World.* Who became king in Assyria right after Jehu killed Jehoram king of Israel and Ahaziah king of Judah? After Athaliah was killed and Joash became king in Judah, who became king in Assyria? What did these two kings do for Assyria?

Key Idea: God used Jehu to cut off Ahab's descendents due to their idolatry. Athaliah was killed later too.

Learning the Basics

Focus: Language Arts, Math, Geography, Bible, and Science

Geography [T]

Go to the website link listed on p. 6 of *A Child's Geography Vol. II*. At the link, select "History & Geography". Then, under "Knowledge Quest" select ACG2-Extra Activities". Print the "Travel Log Template" of your choice from p. 39-42. Also at the link, for older students, print and assign the "Chapter Six Review" on p. 72-73.

Assign all students the following page:

 A Child's Geography Vol. II p. 84
Note: Do only the "Travel Notes" section.

Key Idea: Share three sights from Israel.

Language Arts [S]

Help students complete one lesson from the following reading program:

 Drawn into the Heart of Reading

Work with the students to complete **one** of the writing options listed below:

 Writing & Rhetoric Book 1: Fable
p. 92 – middle of p. 95 (Note: Read aloud the text while the students follow along. Then, discuss the assigned pages. Save "Go Deeper" for Day 3.)

⭐ Your own writing program

Key Idea: Practice language arts skills.

Poetry [I]

Open *Paint Like a Poet* to Lesson 12. Read aloud the poem *"The Road Not Taken"* by Robert Frost.

Today, you will be painting a branching road. You will need painting paper, a palette, water, a large flat paintbrush, a pencil, a dropper (optional), a paper towel, and brown and yellow paint.

After gathering your supplies, turn to the "Step-by-Step Watercolor Tutorial" for Lesson 12 in *Paint Like a Poet*. Follow steps 1-3 to complete "Part One: Branching Road". Then, let your background dry. You will complete "Part Two" of the tutorial on Day 3.

Key Idea: Use painting to illustrate poetry.

Math Exploration [S]

Choose **one** of the math options listed below.

 Singapore Primary Mathematics 4A/4B or *5A/5B* (see Appendix for schedules), or *Math with Confidence,* or *Apologia Math*

 Your own math program

Key Idea: Use a step-by-step math program.

Science Exploration [I]

⭐ Read *Land Animals of the Sixth Day* middle of p. 253 – bottom of p. 257. "Try This" on p. 256-257 is optional. Orally retell or narrate to an adult the portion of text that you read today. Use the *Narration Tips* in the Appendix for help as needed.

Key Idea: Flatworms, segmented worms, and roundworms are annelids. Flatworms are flat and can live as parasites in people and animals. This is why it's important to have safety regulations on meat products and to cook meat until it is well-done. Roundworms are very abundant and can truly live anywhere. Two common parasitic roundworms are ascaris and whipworms.

Learning through History
Focus: The Assyrian Conquests

Reading about History   I

Read about history in the following resource:

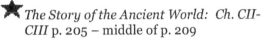 *The Story of the Ancient World:* Ch. CII-CIII p. 205 – middle of p. 209

You will be adding to your timeline in your *Student Notebook* today. In Unit 14 – Box 1, draw and color a crown. Label it, *Shalmaneser, King of Assyria (858 B.C.).* In Box 2, draw and color a round stone. Label it, *Death of Elisha (839 B.C.).* In Box 3, draw and color a broken wall. Label it, *Judah defeated by Israel (826 B.C.).*

Key Idea: Assyria began military campaigns against Israel's neighbors. All of them submitted and paid tribute to Assyria.

Storytime   T

Choose one of the following read aloud options:

★ *God King* p. 139-157 (violent content)

★ Read aloud the next portion of the fantasy that you selected.

After the reading, students will give a summary oral narration. The oral narration must be no longer than 5 sentences and should summarize the reading. As students narrate, have them hold up one finger for each sentence shared. Remind students that the focus should be on the big ideas, rather than on the details.

Key Idea: Summarize the story by narrating.

History Project   S

Get the colored drawing you saved from Day 2. Turn the drawing over, so the blank side of the paper is facing up. Make sure that the horse and chariot are not upside down when you turn it over. Have an adult help you measure and make pencil lines to form 8 rows of 8 squares, with each square measuring ½" x ½". Number the squares in the top row, starting on the **right** and moving across to the **left** from 1-8. Number the squares in the second row going from **right** to **left** from 9-16. Number the squares in the third row going from **right** to **left** from 17-24. Continue numbering in this manner through 64. Then, carefully cut the squares apart on the pencil lines. Open your *Student Notebook* to Unit 14. In Box 8, glue square number 1 in box 1, square 2 in box 2, and so on until all of the squares are glued in.

Key Idea: Assyria and Babylon fought often.

Bible Quiet Time   I

Reading: Choose one option below.

★ *The Illustrated Family Bible* p. 16-17 and 2 Chronicles 25

★ Your own Bible: 2 Chronicles 25

Scripture Focus: Highlight 2 Chron. 25:2.

Prayer Focus: Pray a prayer of thanksgiving to express gratitude for God's divine goodness. Begin by reading the highlighted verse out loud as a prayer. End by praying, *Thank you for the times in my life when you help me do what is right in your eyes. Help me honor you more by serving you with my whole heart.*

Scripture Memory: Recite Philippians 2:13.
Music: *Philippians 2* CD: Track 3 (vs. 12-13)

Key Idea: Joash's son, Amaziah, became king in Judah. At times, Amaziah listened to God, but he worshipped idols too.

Independent History Study   I

Open your *Student Notebook* to Unit 14. In Box 6, copy in cursive Jonah 1:1-3.

Key Idea: Asshur founded Assyria and built Nineveh. Asshur was worshipped as a god by the Assyrians.

Learning the Basics

Focus: Language Arts, Math, Geography, Bible, and Science

Bible Study   T

Read aloud and discuss with the students the following pages:

 The Radical Book for Kids p. 104-107

Key Idea: As Christians, we need to rely on Jesus and His wisdom as our example for how to live. Jesus shows us how to relate to God, to others, to the world, and to life's situations. To grow in wisdom, we should ask God for wisdom through prayer and reading His Word. We should also listen to the teaching of wise Christian parents. As we grow in wisdom, we should fear the Lord and take the good paths in life even when they are diffficult.

Language Arts   S

Have students complete one studied dictation exercise (see Appendix for directions and passages).

Work with the students to complete **one** of the writing options listed below:

 Writing & Rhetoric Book 1: Fable middle of p. 95-97 (Note: Guide the students as needed to complete the lesson.)

 Your own writing program

Key Idea: Practice language arts skills.

Poetry   I

Open *Paint Like a Poet* to Lesson 12. Read aloud the poem *"The Road Not Taken"* by Robert Frost.

Get the branching road backdrop that you painted on Day 2. Today, you will be adding bushes and trees. You will need a palette, water, a small flat paintbrush, a paper towel, and green, blue, yellow, and brown paint.

After gathering your supplies, turn to the "Step-by-Step Watercolor Tutorial" for Lesson 12 in *Paint Like a Poet*. Follow steps 4-6 to complete "Part Two: Bushes and Trees". When your painting is dry, glue your poetry copywork from Day 1 to your painting. Store your completed artwork in the place you have chosen for it.

Key Idea: Explore poetry moods with painting.

Math Exploration   S

Choose **one** of the math options listed below.

 Singapore Primary Mathematics 4A/4B or 5A/5B (see Appendix for schedules), or *Math with Confidence,* or *Apologia Math*

 Your own math program

Key Idea: Use a step-by-step math program.

Science Exploration   I

 Read *Land Animals of the Sixth Day* bottom of p. 257 – middle of p. 261. Write the answer to each numbered question on lined paper. You do not need to copy the question. Use the listed page to help you answer each question.

1. How can wearing shoes outside help prevent you from getting a hookworm infection? (p. 258)
2. Why is it important to have clean drinking water? (p. 258)
3. Write the words *stylet* and *lymph node* and give their definitions. (p. 259)
4. List 3 kinds of roundworms that cause diseases in developed countries. (p. 260-261)
5. Why is it a good idea to wash your hands before eating when you're at the park? (p. 261)

Key Idea: Roundworms can be parasitic. Infections are most common in countries without clean water.

Reading about History $\boxed{\text{I}}$

Read about history in the following resource:

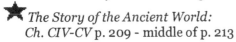 *The Story of the Ancient World:
Ch. CIV-CV p. 209 - middle of p. 213*

You will be writing a narration about *Chapter CV: The Prophets' Warning,* which is part of today's history reading.

To prepare for writing your narration, think about the questions below. If you do not know the answers, find them on p. 211-213 of *The Story of the Ancient World.* Ask yourself, *For what were the Assyrians known? Who was the son of Asshurnazirpal? Where did Shalmaneser build his palaces? Where did Assyria get her wealth? Who were some of the prophets that prophecied in Israel and Judah during this time? What messages from God did the prophets give the people? How was Judah different from the countries surrounding it at this time?*

After you have thought about the answers to the questions, turn to Unit 14 in your *Student Notebook.* In Box 5, write a 5-8 sentence narration. When you have finished writing, read your sentences out loud to catch any mistakes. Check for the following things: *Did you include **who** the reading was mainly about? Did you include **what** important thing(s) happened? Did you include **how** it ended? If not, add those things.*

Then, underline or highlight the main idea sentence in the narration. Use the *Written Narration Skills* in the Appendix as a guide for editing the narration.

Key Idea: As king of Assyria, Asshurnazirpal was known for his military conquests. His son, Shalmaneser, continued the Assyrian conquests to even further lands.

Storytime $\boxed{\text{T}}$

Choose one of the following read aloud options:

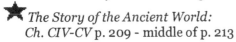 *God King* p. 158-177

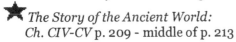 Read aloud the next part of the fantasy.

After the reading, have each person get a Bible and open it anywhere in Proverbs. Explain, *We will have 5 minutes to skim through the verses in Proverbs to find any connections to today's story. When a connection is found, read the verse out loud and quickly share the connection. At the end of 5 minutes, anyone who has not shared yet must read aloud one verse and make the best connection possible.*

Key Idea: Seek God's word for His guidance.

Bible Quiet Time $\boxed{\text{I}}$

Reading: Choose one option below.

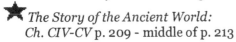 *The Illustrated Family Bible* p. 18-19

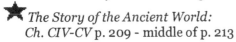 Your own Bible: 2 Kings 13:10-25; 14:23-29

Scripture Focus: Highlight 2 Kings 13:11.

Prayer Focus: Pray a prayer of supplication to make a humble and earnest request of God. Begin by reading the highlighted verse out loud as a prayer. End by praying, *Help me turn away from my sins so that I do not continue to do them. Help me with the sin of...*

Scripture Memory: Copy Philippians 2:13 in your Common Place Book.
Music: *Philippians 2* CD: Track 3 (vs. 12-13)

Key Idea: The kings in Israel and Judah often did not do what was right in God's eyes.

Independent History Study $\boxed{\text{I}}$

 Listen to *What in the World?* Disc 2, Track 7: "Jonah Goes to Nineveh".

Key Idea: God sent the prophet Jonah to the Assyrian city of Nineveh to preach repentence. Since the Assyrians were known to be very wicked and to be cruel conquerors, Jonah ran from God and his task.

Learning the Basics
Focus: Language Arts, Math, Geography, Bible, and Science

Geography |T|

Have bagels with cream cheese (or lox) with the students following the directions in the "Food" section of p. 85.

While having your bagels, read aloud the prayer with the students on the following page:

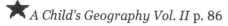 ★ *A Child's Geography Vol. II* p. 86

Note: Wait to make Hamentaschen, as it is an upcoming history project.

Key Idea: It's important to pray for those in other countries who need to know the Lord.

Language Arts |S|

Have students complete one dictation exercise.

Guide students to complete one reading lesson.

★ *Drawn into the Heart of Reading*

Help students complete **one** English lesson.

★ *Building with Diligence:* Lesson 26 (Half)

★ *Following the Plan:* Lesson 24

★ Your own grammar program

Key Idea: Practice language arts skills.

Poetry |I|

Open *Paint Like a Poet* to Lesson 12. Today, you will be performing a poetry reading of *"The Road Not Taken"*. Practice reading the poem aloud with expression that matches the mood of the poem. Then, read the poem aloud in front of your chosen audience.

At the end of the reading, share the following, *When I read this poem by Robert Frost, it made me think of...* Call on your audience to share what thoughts the poem brought to their minds. Last, say, *Did you know that after Robert's poem was published, he knew that he wanted to be a poet? Yet, he needed an income, so he tried writing for a weekly newspaper called "The Sentinel". He liked to write but didn't like prying into people's lives.*

Key Idea: Share the poetry of Robert Frost.

Math Exploration |S|

Choose **one** of the math options listed below.

★ *Singapore Primary Mathematics 4A/4B* or *5A/5B* (see Appendix for schedules), or *Math with Confidence,* or *Apologia Math*

★ Your own math program

Key Idea: Use a step-by-step math program.

Science Exploration |I|

★ Read *Land Animals of the Sixth Day* middle of p. 261 - 264. "Try This" on p. 262 and p. 265 are optional. Now, skip to the "Experiment" on the bottom of p. 266. Turn to the science experiment section in your science binder or sketchbook. At the top of a blank page, write: *Do worms prefer cold or warm temperatures?* Under the question, write: *'Guess'*. Write down your guess. Follow the directions for the experiment in *Land Animals of the Sixth Day* p. 266. Note: If you do not have earthworms, and you have access to the internet, then go to the following link to complete an earthworm observation lab instead: https://www.youtube.com/watch?v=BUx5leb3RKE

Next, on the paper write: *'Procedure'*. Draw a labeled picture of the experiment. At the bottom of the paper, write: *'Conclusion'*. Explain what you learned from the experiment.

Key Idea: Earthworms are annelids with a cuticle that must stay wet for them to breathe through it. Cool, moist conditions are best for earthworms.

Reading about History | I

Read about history in the following resource:

★ *The Story of the Ancient World:*
Ch. CVI-CVII p. 213 - middle of p. 216

Nineveh was the ancient capital city of the Assyrian Empire. Where could you look to research more about **Nineveh**? Use a Bible, a reference book, or an online resource like www.wikipedia.org.

Answer one or more of the following questions from your research: *In Genesis 10:11, who does it say built Nineveh? Where was the ancient city of Nineveh located? What was used to build most of the buildings in the city? Describe Nineveh. Which Assyrian rulers made Nineveh into a great city? Why didn't Jonah want to go to Nineveh? Who eventually conquered Nineveh? What happened to the city according to God's judgment in Nahum 1:7-8 and 2:6-11?*

Key Idea: God sent Jonah to warn Nineveh.

History Project | S

In this unit you will make an oragami prayer box. Get two 8 ½" x 11" sheets of colored paper. Cut off the bottoms of both papers to make two 8 ½" x 8 ½" squares. Next, open your *Student Notebook* to Unit 15. Follow the included directions using one of the paper squares to make the bottom of the prayer box. Then, repeat the directions using the second square to make the top of the prayer box. Last, slide one box over top of the other box like a lid. Save the box for Day 2.

Key Idea: Jonah knew God would save Nineveh if the people prayed and repented.

Storytime | T

Choose one of the following read aloud options:

★ *God King* p. 178-194

★ Read at least one fantasy for the next 8 days of plans.

After the reading, students will give a detailed oral narration. Select one paragraph from the story to read out loud to the students. This will be the starting point for the narration. Set a timer for 3-5 minutes. When the timer rings the narration is over, even if it isn't complete. A detailed, descriptive narration is the goal. See *Narration Tips* in the Appendix as needed.

Key Idea: Use oral narration to retell the story.

Bible Quiet Time | I

Bible Reading: Choose one option below.

★ *The Illustrated Family Bible* p. 168-169

★ Your own Bible: Jonah chapters 1 and 3

Scripture Focus: Highlight Jonah 1:15-16.

Prayer Focus: Pray a prayer of adoration to worship and honor God. Begin by reading the highlighted verses out loud as a prayer. End by praying, *I worship you for being in control of all things. You are to be feared and praised. Help me to treat you with the reverence that you deserve.*

Scripture Memory: Recite Philippians 2:14.
Music: *Philippians 2* CD: Track 4 (verse 14)

Key Idea: Jonah ran from God, but God used a big fish to save Jonah. Then, Jonah repented and went to Nineveh.

Independent History Study | I

Open your *Student Notebook* to Unit 15. In Box 6, copy in cursive Jonah 3:1-2, 10.

Key Idea: Jonah didn't want the people of Nineveh to be saved, because the Assyrians were their enemies.

Learning the Basics
Focus: Language Arts, Math, Geography, Bible, and Science

Bible Study   T

Read and discuss the following pages:

 The Radical Book for Kids p. 108-111

<u>Key Idea</u>: The book of Job mentions untamed animals like the lion and wild ox. It also describes monster-like creatures like the Behemoth and Leviathan. These creatures are all under God's rule. He controls all things. As King of the universe and Creator of all, no situation is out of God's control.

Language Arts   S

Have students complete one studied dictation exercise (see Appendix).

Help students complete one lesson from the following reading program:

 Drawn into the Heart of Reading

Work with the students to complete **one** of the English options listed below:

★ *Building with Diligence:* Lesson 27

★ *Following the Plan:* Lesson 25

★ Your own grammar program

<u>Key Idea</u>: Practice language arts skills.

Poetry   I

Open *Paint Like a Poet* to Lesson 13. Read aloud the poem *"Once by the Pacific"*. On a 3 x 5 index card, neatly copy in black ink or in pencil the following highlighted lines from the poem:

The shattered water made a misty din.
Great waves looked over others coming in,
And thought of doing something to the shore
That water never did to land before.
           -Robert Frost

Check your work to make sure it is correctly copied. Then, cut around your copywork. You may choose to outline the edge of the cut-out with a blue marker. Save it for Day 3.

<u>Key Idea</u>: Read and appreciate a variety of classic poetry.

Math Exploration   S

Choose **one** of the math options listed below.

★ *Singapore Primary Mathematics 4A/4B or 5A/5B* (see Appendix for schedules), or *Math with Confidence,* or *Apologia Math*

★ Your own math program

<u>Key Idea</u>: Use a step-by-step math program.

Science Exploration   I

★ Read *Birds of the Air* p. 1-3. Today, you will begin a book that is about birds in your area. You will add to this book for the next 4 units. You may make your book either by adding a "Birds" section to your hardcover "Tracks" book, or you may make a paper book for "Birds" similar to the one described in Unit 2 – Day 1. At the top of a clean page in your book, copy Song of Solomon 2:12 in cursive. Beneath the verse, sketch 1-3 birds that are common to your area. You can do this by using a pocket field guide and sketching birds from your area, or if you have internet access you may refer to https://ebird.org/home. If you choose the internet option, click on "Explore." Then, under "Explore Regions," enter your state, or enter your country. After that a list of birds sighted in your area will come up. Choose 1-3 birds to click on and sketch that are not water birds. Color the birds and label them.

<u>Key Idea</u>: When learning to recognize birds, look at the body, tail, beak, color, size, and any special marks.

Learning through History
Focus: Israel Falls to Assyria and Judah Is Saved

Reading about History I

Read about history in the following resource:

⭐ *The Story of the Ancient World:*
Ch. CVIII-CIX p. 216 – top of p. 220

You will be choosing a portion from today's reading that you found memorable or worthy of being reread to copy. Open your *Student Notebook* to Unit 15. In Box 4, carefully copy in cursive the portion from today's reading that you selected. Then, compare your written work to the original. Last, draw a small colorful picture in Box 4 to illustrate your sentences.

Key Idea: Pul, the king of Assyria and Babylon died. Nabonassar became the new king of Babylon by force, and Tiglathpileser seized the throne of Assyria at Nineveh. At the same time in Judah, Ahaz stripped the temple to pay Tiglathpileser to relieve him of his enemies Israel and Syria.

History Project S

Get the prayer box that you made on Day 1. On the lid of the prayer box, copy the following 4 parts of prayer to guide you as you pray:
A = **A**doration
C = **C**onfession
T = **T**hanksgiving
S = **S**upplication

What word do you notice that the first letter of the 4 parts of prayer make? Why would it be important to begin your prayers with adoration? Why is it important to note that there is more to prayer than supplication?

Key Idea: The Israelites often prayed to idols.

Storytime T

Choose one of the following read aloud options:

⭐ *God King* p. 195-206 and *Author's Note*

⭐ Read aloud the next portion of the fantasy that you selected.

After reading, work with the students to plan a 3 minute skit with simple props to act out part of today's reading. Set a timer for 3 minutes to quickly prepare for the skit. Make sure that you participate in the skit along with the students. When the timer rings, set it again for 3 minutes and perform the skit. You do not need an audience, as the goal is the retelling.

Key Idea: Use a skit to retell part of the story.

Bible Quiet Time I

Reading: Choose one option below.

⭐ *The Illustrated Family Bible* p. 170-173

⭐ Your own Bible: 2 Chronicles 26; 28

Scripture Focus: Highlight 2 Chron. 28:24.

Prayer Focus: Pray a prayer of confession to admit or acknowledge your sins to God. Begin by reading the highlighted verse out loud as a prayer. End by praying, *I confess that I often forget what a blessing it is to worship you in your temple, the church. Help me rejoice in your house and be thankful its doors are open.*

Scripture Memory: Recite Philippians 2:14.
Music: *Philippians 2* CD: Track 4 (verse 14)

Key Idea: Assyria conquered Israel.

Independent History Study I

Open your *Student Notebook* to "Prophecies About Christ". Under "Prophecy" write, *Isaiah 9:1-2*. Read the Scripture to discover the prophecy. Under "Fulfillment" write, *Matthew 4:12-16*. Read the fulfillment Scripture. Under "Description", write a few phrases to describe the prophecy about Jesus.

Key Idea: Christ will come out of Galilee and be a light to Zebulun and Naphtali who were conquered.

Learning the Basics
Focus: Language Arts, Math, Geography, Bible, and Science

Geography [T]

Read aloud to the students the following pages:

 A Child's Geography Vol. II p. 87-91

Discuss with the students "Field Notes" p. 92.

Key Idea: Egypt is considered to be part of the Middle East, however much of it is in the continent of Africa. The Sinai Peninsula is where Moses led the twelve tribes of Israel out of Egypt. The mountain of Jubal Musa is thought to be the Mt. Sinai of the Bible. St. Catherine's Monastery is built around what is thought to be Moses' burning bush.

Language Arts [S]

Help students complete one lesson from the following reading program:

 Drawn into the Heart of Reading

Work with the students to complete **one** of the writing options listed below:

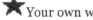 *Writing & Rhetoric Book 1: Fable* p. 99 – top of p. 101 (Note: Omit p. 98. Guide students through the lesson as needed.)

★ Your own writing program

Key Idea: Practice language arts skills.

Poetry [I]

Open *Paint Like a Poet* to Lesson 13. Read aloud the poem *"Once by the Pacific"* by Robert Frost.

Today, you will be painting an ocean backdrop. You will need painting paper, a palette, water, a large flat paintbrush, a paper towel, and dark blue and dark green paint.

After gathering your supplies, turn to the "Step-by-Step Watercolor Tutorial" for Lesson 13 in *Paint Like a Poet*. Follow steps 1-3 to complete "Part One: Ocean Backdrop". Then, let your background dry. You will complete "Part Two" of the tutorial on Day 3.

Key Idea: Use painting to illustrate poetry.

Math Exploration [S]

Choose **one** of the math options listed below.

 Singapore Primary Mathematics 4A/4B or 5A/5B (see Appendix for schedules), or *Math with Confidence,* or *Apologia Math*

 Your own math program

Key Idea: Use a step-by-step math program.

Science Exploration [I]

★ Read *Birds of the Air* p. 4-7. Orally retell or narrate to an adult the portion of text that you read today. Use the *Narration Tips* in the Appendix for help as needed.

Key Idea: Birds sing to reflect moods, just as people do. Their throats swell and quiver as they work their vocal chords to make notes and sing. In the spring, the father bird sings to the mother bird while she is building the nest and sitting on the eggs. After the baby birds have hatched, the father bird teaches the baby birds his song.

Reading about History [I]

Read about history in the following resource:

★ *The Story of the Ancient World:*
Ch. CX-CXI p. 220-223

You will be adding to your timeline in your *Student Notebook* today. In Unit 15 – Box 1, draw and color a fish. Label it, *Jonah prophecies in Nineveh (approx. 771 B.C.).* In Box 2, draw and color chains. Label it, *Sargon of Assyria conquers Israel (721 B.C.).* In Box 3, draw and color an angel. Label it, *Hezekiah, Destruction of Sennacherib (710 B.C.).*

Key Idea: The Assyrian king Sennacherib attacked and subdued Egypt. On his return march to Assyria, Sennacherib attacked the cities of Judah. He sent a letter to terrify Hezekiah, king of Judah, into resuming tribute to Assyria. But, God answered Hezekiah's prayer and saved Jerusalem from Sennacherib.

History Project [S]

Get your prayer box . On a small strip of paper, list some things you wish to remind yourself to pray about. Fold the slip of paper and place it inside your prayer box. Then, find a quiet place where you can be alone with God. Use the 4 parts of prayer listed on the lid of your prayer box as a guide as you pray. Remember to pray for the items that you listed on your slip of paper. Keep your prayer box in a special place. As your prayers are answered remove the slip of paper and replace it with a new one. You may have many slips of paper in your prayer box to remind you of prayers to be said.

Key Idea: God heard Hezekiah's prayer and granted him 15 more years upon the earth.

Storytime [T]

Choose one of the following read aloud options:

★ Your own Bible: Jonah chapter 1

★ Read aloud the next portion of the fantasy that you selected.

After the reading, students will give a summary oral narration. The oral narration must be no longer than 5 sentences and should summarize the reading. As students narrate, have them hold up one finger for each sentence shared. Remind students that the focus should be on the big ideas, rather than on the details.

Key Idea: Summarize the story by narrating.

Bible Quiet Time [I]

Reading: Choose one option below.

★ *The Illustrated Family Bible* p. 174-175

★ Your own Bible: 2 Chronicles 29:1-11; 32

Scripture Focus: Highlight 2 Kings 20:3.

Prayer Focus: Pray a prayer of thanksgiving to express gratitude for God's divine goodness. Begin by reading the highlighted verse out loud as a prayer. End by praying, *I thank you for Hezekiah's faith in you and his wholehearted devotion. Help the same to be true of me.*

Scripture Memory: Recite Philippians 2:14.
Music: *Philippians 2* CD: Track 4 (verse 14)

Key Idea: Hezekiah served the Lord with wholehearted devotion, and God answered his prayers to deliver him from Sennacherib.

Independent History Study [I]

★ Listen to *What in the World?* Disc 3, Track 1: "Assyria".

Key Idea: When Israel did not listen to the warnings of God's prophets, He allowed Northern Israel and Samaria to be conquered by Assyria. Then, Samaria was resettled with captured people from many lands.

Learning the Basics
Focus: Language Arts, Math, Geography, Bible, and Science

Bible Study [T]

Read aloud and discuss with the students the following pages:

 The Radical Book for Kids p. 112-115

Key Idea: Manners are not specifically listed in the Bible, yet having good manners helps you serve others and enjoy people. God's love for you does not have anything to do with your manners, but your manners can show love to others.

Language Arts [S]

Have students complete one studied dictation exercise (see Appendix for directions and passages).

Work with the students to complete **one** of the writing options listed below:

 Writing & Rhetoric Book 1: Fable top of p. 101-103 (Note: Guide students through the lesson, so they are successful writing a summary.)

 Your own writing program

Key Idea: Practice language arts skills.

Poetry [I]

Open *Paint Like a Poet* to Lesson 13. Read aloud the poem *"Once by the Pacific"* by Robert Frost.

Get the ocean backdrop that you painted on Day 2. Today, you will be adding ocean waves. You will need a palette, water, a small flat paintbrush, and dark blue, dark green, and white paint.

After gathering your supplies, turn to the "Step-by-Step Watercolor Tutorial" for Lesson 13 in *Paint Like a Poet*. Follow steps 4-5 to complete "Part Two: Ocean Waves". When your painting is dry, glue your poetry copywork from Day 1 to your painting. Store your completed artwork in the place you have chosen for it.

Key Idea: Explore poetry moods with painting.

Math Exploration [S]

Choose **one** of the math options listed below.

 Singapore Primary Mathematics 4A/4B or 5A/5B (see Appendix for schedules), or *Math with Confidence,* or *Apologia Math*

 Your own math program

Key Idea: Use a step-by-step math program.

Science Exploration [I]

 Read *Birds of the Air* p. 8-12. Write the answer to each numbered question on lined paper. You do not need to copy the question. Use the listed page to help you answer each question.
1. Describe a Chaffinch's cup-nest. (p. 8)
2. What do Thrushes and Rooks use to plaster their nests? (p. 8-9)
3. Where do Larks and Plovers build their nests? Why must their young run about as soon as they hatch? (p. 9)
4. What is the difference between a Swallow's nest and a Martin's nest? (p. 9) What does Psalm 104:12 say about the birds' dwelling place?
5. Tell about the nest of one of the following birds: Woodpecker, Pigeon, Reed-warbler, or Wren. (p. 10-11)

Key Idea: Birds make different types of nests. Some are cup-like. Others are mud-lined or roughly woven.

Learning through History
Focus: Israel Falls to Assyria and Judah Is Saved

Reading about History   I

Read about history in the following resource:

★ *The Story of the Ancient World: Ch. CXII-CXIII* p. 224 - top of p. 228

You will be writing a narration about *Chapter CXII: Manasseh, King of Judah,* which is part of today's history reading.

To prepare for writing your narration, think about the questions below. If you do not know the answers, find them on p. 224-226 of *The Story of the Ancient World.* Ask yourself, *Who was the king of Babylon that tried to throw off Assyrian rule? What did Sennacherib do in response? After Sennacherib was killed, who ruled in Assyria? What did Esarhaddon do first? Meanwhile in Judah, when Hezekiah died who became king? What wicked things did Manasseh do? How did God punish him? When Manasseh humbled himself before God, what happened? How did Manasseh show that he had changed?*

After you have thought about the answers to the questions, turn to Unit 15 in your *Student Notebook.* In Box 5, write a 5-8 sentence narration. When you have finished writing, read your sentences out loud to catch any mistakes. Check for the following things: *Did you include **who** the reading was mainly about? Did you include **what** important thing(s) happened? Did you include **how** it ended? If not, add those things.*

Then, underline or highlight the main idea sentence in the narration. Use the *Written Narration Skills* in the Appendix as a guide for editing the narration.

<u>Key Idea</u>: Sennacherib destroyed Babylon.

Storytime   T

Choose one of the following read aloud options:

★ Your own Bible: Jonah chapter 2

★ Read aloud the next part of the fantasy.

After the reading, have each person get a Bible and open it anywhere in Proverbs. Explain, *We will have 5 minutes to skim through the verses in Proverbs to find any connections to today's story. When a connection is found, read the verse out loud and quickly share the connection. At the end of 5 minutes, anyone who has not shared yet must read aloud one verse and make the best connection possible.*

<u>Key Idea</u>: Seek God's word for His guidance.

Bible Quiet Time   I

Reading: Choose one option below.

★ *The Illustrated Family Bible* p. 176-177

★ Your own Bible: 2 Chronicles 33 and 34

Scripture Focus: Highlight 2 Chronicles 34:30-31

Prayer Focus: Pray a prayer of supplication to make a humble and earnest request of God. Begin by reading the highlighted verse out loud as a prayer. End by praying, *Please put a love for your word in my heart and help me keep your commands with all my heart and soul.*

Scripture Memory: Copy Philippians 2:14 in your Common Place Book.
Music: *Philippians 2* CD: Track 4 (verse 14)

<u>Key Idea</u>: Josiah dedicated himself to God.

Independent History Study   I

Open your *Student Notebook* to Unit 16 – Box 6. Follow the directions from *Draw and Write Through History* p. 6-8 to draw the hanging gardens of Babylon. You will color your drawing on Unit 16-Day 1.

<u>Key Idea</u>: After Sennacherib destroyed Babylon, his son Esarhaddon rebuilt it in all its magnificence after Sennacherib's death.

Geography [T]

Read aloud to the students the following pages:

 A Child's Geography Vol. II – Read p. 92 (second column) – p. 96. Discuss with the students "Field Notes" p. 96.

<u>Key Idea</u>: The Suez Canal in Egypt saves ships from having to sail all the way around Africa. Egyptian pharaohs, Ptolemy, Cleopatra, and Napoleon all worked at finishing the project, but could not. It is a modern-day engineering feat! Meanwhile, in the Arabian Desert, the oil rigs pump 750,000 barrels of oil a day.

Language Arts [S]

Have students complete one dictation exercise.

Guide students to complete one reading lesson.

⭐ *Drawn into the Heart of Reading*

Help students complete **one** English lesson.

⭐ *Building with Diligence:* Lesson 28

⭐ *Following the Plan:* Lesson 26

⭐ Your own grammar program

<u>Key Idea</u>: Practice language arts skills.

Poetry [I]

Open *Paint Like a Poet* to Lesson 13. Today, you will be performing a poetry reading of *"Once by the Pacific"*. Practice reading the poem aloud with expression that matches the mood of the poem. Then, read the poem aloud in front of your chosen audience.

At the end of the reading, share the following, *When I read this poem by Robert Frost, it made me think of...* Call on your audience to share what thoughts the poem brought to their minds. Last, say, *Did you know that after Robert Frost stopped writing for "The Sentinel" he taught Latin at a school with his mother? He also was engaged to his high school classmate, Elinor White.*

<u>Key Idea</u>: Share the poetry of Robert Frost.

Math Exploration [S]

Choose **one** of the math options listed below.

⭐ *Singapore Primary Mathematics 4A/4B* or *5A/5B* (see Appendix for schedules), or *Math with Confidence*, or *Apologia Math*

⭐ Your own math program

<u>Key Idea</u>: Use a step-by-step math program.

Science Exploration [I]

⭐ Read *Birds of the Air* p. 13-18. Turn to the science experiment section in your science binder or sketchbook. At the top of a blank page, write: *How does a baby chick breathe inside its egg?* Under the question, write: *'Guess'*. Write down your guess. Then, place a raw egg in a glass. Add white vinegar until the egg is completely covered. You will see bubbles form on the egg's surface. Allow the egg to sit in the vinegar for 3 days. Then, take the egg out and discard the vinegar. Rinse the egg under water, being careful not to break it. The vinegar should have dissolved most of the egg's shell, which is made of calcium carbonate. Since the shell is no longer there, how does the egg keep its egg-shape? Notice the covering beneath the eggshell, which is called the membrane. The water in the vinegar passed through the membrane causing the egg to swell. What else could pass through the membrane that the chick needs to breathe? Now, place the egg in a different glass. Add corn syrup until the egg is covered. Allow the egg to sit in the corn syrup for 3 days. Then, take the egg out and discard the corn syrup. Where did the water that was inside the egg go? How did it move out of the egg? Next, on the paper write: *'Procedure'*. Draw a picture of both experiments. At the bottom of the paper, write: *'Conclusion'*. Explain what you learned.

<u>Key Idea</u>: The egg allows air to pass through its membrane, just like the water in the vinegar and the water in the egg did. This allows the baby chick to breathe while it's inside the egg.

Learning through History
Focus: Judah Falls to the Babylonians

Reading about History   I

Read about history in the following resource:

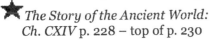 *The Story of the Ancient World:*
Ch. CXIV p. 228 – top of p. 230

The Babylonians and the Medians attacked Nineveh and destroyed it. Then, the Babylonians became the next world empire. Where could you look to research more about **Babylon**? Use a Bible, an online resource like www.wikipedia.org, or a reference book.

Answer one or more of the following questions from your research: *Where was the city of Babylon located? Near what modern-day city are the ruins of Babylon found? What was the Code of Hammurabi? Which Assyrian king completely destroyed Babylon? Which Assyrian king rebuilt it? Who made Babylon the capital of his empire? For what wonders in Babylon is Nebuchadnezzar known? How did Cyrus, king of Persia, enter Babylon?*

Key Idea: God judged the city of Nineveh.

History Project   S

In this unit you will make a cookie model of the statue in Nebuchadnezzar's dream. In a bowl, mix 1½ cups powdered sugar, 1 cup margarine or butter (softened), 1 egg, 1 tsp. vanilla, and ½ tsp. almond extract. Then, mix in 2½ cups flour, 1 tsp. baking soda, and 1 tsp. cream of tartar. Divide the dough into 5 parts. Add food coloring to make the following colors of dough: gold (or yellow), grey (or light blue), brown (or light orange), black, and natural colored dough. Cover the dough and refrigerate it overnight.

Key Idea: Babylon would soon conquer Judah.

Storytime   T

Choose one of the following read aloud options:

 Your own Bible: Jonah chapters 3-4

Read at least one fantasy for the next 4 days of plans.

After the reading, students will give a detailed oral narration. Select one paragraph from the story to read out loud to the students. This will be the starting point for the narration. Set a timer for 3-5 minutes. When the timer rings the narration is over, even if it isn't complete. A detailed, descriptive narration is the goal. See *Narration Tips* in the Appendix as needed.

Key Idea: Use oral narration to retell the story.

Bible Quiet Time   I

Bible Reading: Choose the option below.

Your own Bible: Nahum 1; 3:18-19

Scripture Focus: Highlight Nahum 1:3.

Prayer Focus: Pray a prayer of adoration to worship and honor God. Begin by reading the highlighted verse out loud as a prayer. End by praying, *I am so thankful Lord that you are slow to anger, for in your great power you hold each of us in your hands. You control all things.*

Scripture Memory: Recite Philippians 2:15.
Music: *Philippians 2* CD: Track 4 (vs. 14-15)

Key Idea: The destruction of Nineveh was foretold by the prophet Nahum.

Independent History Study   I

Open your *Student Notebook* to Unit 16 – Box 6. Use *Draw and Write Through History* p. 5 as a guide to color your sketch of the hanging gardens of Babylon. You may finish coloring on Day 2, if needed.

Key Idea: After the fall of Nineveh, the Assyrian empire was taken over by the Babylonians.

Learning the Basics
Focus: Language Arts, Math, Geography, Bible, and Science

Bible Study [T]

Read aloud and discuss with the students the following pages:

 The Radical Book for Kids p. 116-118

<u>Key Idea</u>: John Bunyan was a British author who lived 300 years ago. While he was in prison for many years, he wrote *Pilgrim's Progress*. Bunyan's *Pilgrim's Progress* is an allegory about a man named Christian and his journey to the Celestial City. Bunyan also wrote *Holy War,* another allegory where the city of Mansoul is under attack by Satan.

Language Arts [S]

Have students complete one studied dictation exercise (see Appendix for directions and passages).

Help students complete one lesson from the following reading program:

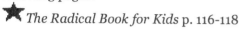 *Drawn into the Heart of Reading*

Work with the students to complete **one** of the English options listed below:

★ *Building with Diligence:* Lesson 29

★ *Following the Plan:* Lesson 27

★ Your own grammar program

<u>Key Idea</u>: Practice language arts skills.

Poetry [I]

Open *Paint Like a Poet* to Lesson 14. Read aloud the poem *"Dust of Snow"*. On a 3 x 5 index card, neatly copy in black ink or in pencil the following highlighted lines from the poem:

The way a crow
Shook down on me
The durst of snow
From a hemlock tree

Has given my heart
A change of mood
And saved some part
Of a day I had rued.
             - Robert Frost

Check your work to make sure it is correctly copied. Then, cut around your copywork. You may choose to outline the edge of the cut-out with a blue marker. Save it for Day 3.

<u>Key Idea</u>: Read and appreciate classic poetry.

Math Exploration [S]

Choose **one** of the math options listed below.

★ *Singapore Primary Mathematics 4A/4B* or *5A/5B* (see Appendix for schedules), or *Math with Confidence*, or *Apologia Math*

★ Your own math program

<u>Key Idea</u>: Use a step-by-step math program.

Science Exploration [I]

★ Read *Birds of the Air* p. 19-23. Get your book about birds that you began last unit. At the top of the next page in your book, copy in cursive Luke 12:24. Beneath the verse, sketch a Pigeon that is common to your area. You can do this by using a pocket field guide and sketching birds from your area, or if you have internet access you may refer to https://ebird.org/home. If you choose the internet option, click on "Explore." Then, under "Explore Regions," enter your state, or enter your country. After that a list of birds sighted in your area will come up. Scroll through the list to find any Pigeons sighted in your area. Then, click on the Pigeon in the list and a picture and description will come up. Draw and color the Pigeon and label it. Note: If there are no Pigeons in your area, select a different bird common to your area to sketch instead.

<u>Key Idea</u>: Baby Pigeons are born naked with closed eyes and jointed wings. Their feathers grow over time.

Learning through History
Focus: Judah Falls to the Babylonians

Unit 16 - Day 2

Reading about History | I |

Read about history in the following resource:

★ *The Story of the Ancient World:*
 Ch. CXV-CXVI p. 230 – top of p. 234

You will be choosing a portion from today's reading that you found memorable or worthy of being reread to copy. Open your *Student Notebook* to Unit 16. In Box 4, carefully copy in cursive the portion from today's reading that you selected. Then, compare your written work to the original. Last, draw a small colorful picture in Box 4 to illustrate your sentences.

Key Idea: Jeremiah prophecied in Judah that Babylon would soon invade Jerusalem and destroy the city and the Temple.

Storytime | T |

Choose one of the following read aloud options:

★ Your own Bible: Esther chapter 1

★ Read aloud the next portion of the fantasy.

After reading, give students a few minutes to prepare a short advertisement speech for the book. During the speech, students should hold up the book and say the book title and the name of the author. The wording of the advertisement should provide a peek into the book without giving away the ending. The goal should be for listeners to feel like they've "Got to Have This Book"!

Key Idea: Use an ad speech to share the story.

History Project | S |

Get the dough from Day 1 out of the refrigerator. Open your *Student Notebook* to Unit 16. Use the diagram of the statue to guide you as you make a large cookie in the shape of the statue. Begin by rolling the gold dough 3/16" thick on a lightly floured surface. Cut the dough into the shape of the statue's head. It should be about the size of your fist. Then, place the cut out near the top of a lightly greased cookie sheet. Use a toothpick to etch the details of the head on the cookie. Repeat the process using the silver (or light blue) dough to make the chest and arms, the brown (or light orange) dough to make the belly and thighs, the black dough to make the legs, and the black and natural dough to make the feet. Heat the oven to 375 degrees. Bake the cookie until the edges are light brown (7-8 minutes).

Key Idea: Nebuchadnezzar ruled Babylon.

Bible Quiet Time | I |

Reading: Choose one option below.

★ *The Illustrated Family Bible* p. 178-179
 Optional extension: p. 155

★ Your own Bible: 2 Chronicles 36:1-21

Scripture Focus: Highlight 2 Chronicles 36:15-16.

Prayer Focus: Pray a prayer of confession to admit or acknowledge your sins to God. Begin by reading the highlighted verses out loud as a prayer. End by praying, *I confess that I don't always listen carefully to your word or always listen to your messengers, like my pastor or my parents. Help me to develop the habit of attention, so I may listen better.*

Scripture Memory: Recite Philippians 2:15.
Music: *Philippians 2* CD: Track 4 (vs. 14-15)

Key Idea: God judged Judah with destruction.

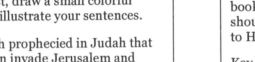

Independent History Study | I |

★ Open your *Student Notebook* to Unit 16 - Box 7. Finish coloring your drawing from Day 1, if needed. Then, in Box 7, copy in cursive the text of *Draw and Write Through History* p. 9.

Key Idea: When the Babylonians destroyed Jerusalem, many Jews were taken to Babylon as captives.

Learning the Basics
Focus: Language Arts, Math, Geography, Bible, and Science

Geography   [T]

Go to the website link listed under "Bringing It Home" on p. 6 of *A Child's Geography Vol. II*. At the link, select "History & Geography". Then, under "Knowledge Quest" select ACG2-Extra Activities". Print a copy of the labeled map of **Egypt, Iraq & Saudi Arabia** on p. 47 and the blank map of **Egypt, Iraq & Saudi Arabia** on p. 48 for each student.

Then, assign students the following page:

 A Child's Geography Vol. II p. 97

Note: Do only the "Map Notes" section. If desired, play "Music" from the links on p. 98.

<u>Key Idea</u>: Practice finding and recording the locations of various places on a map of Egypt.

Language Arts   [S]

Help students complete one lesson from the following reading program:

 Drawn into the Heart of Reading

Work with the students to complete **one** of the writing options listed below:

 Writing & Rhetoric Book 1: Fable p. 104-107 (Note: Read aloud the text while the students follow along. Then, discuss.)

 Your own writing program

<u>Key Idea</u>: Practice language arts skills.

Poetry   [I]

Open *Paint Like a Poet* to Lesson 14. Read aloud the poem *"Dust of Snow"* by Robert Frost.

Today, you will be painting a snowy hill. You will need painting paper, a palette, water, a large flat paintbrush, salt, and white, light blue, and purple paint.

After gathering your supplies, turn to the "Step-by-Step Watercolor Tutorial" for Lesson 14 in *Paint Like a Poet*. Follow steps 1-3 to complete "Part One: Snowy Hill". Then, let your background dry. You will complete "Part Two" of the tutorial on Day 3.

<u>Key Idea</u>: Use painting to illustrate poetry.

Math Exploration   [S]

Choose **one** of the math options listed below.

 Singapore Primary Mathematics 4A/4B or *5A/5B* (see Appendix for schedules), or *Math with Confidence,* or *Apologia Math*

 Your own math program

<u>Key Idea</u>: Use a step-by-step math program.

Science Exploration   [I]

 Read *Birds of the Air* p. 24-29. Orally retell or narrate to an adult the portion of text that you read today. Use the *Narration Tips* in the Appendix for help as needed.

<u>Key Idea</u>: Some birds are born naked, and others are born downy-feathered. Some birds are born blind, and others are born seeing. There are many different kinds of baby birds. Usually, mother birds must work very hard to keep their young fed and their nest clean. Sometimes the father birds help with feeding and caring for the young. Often, parent birds continue feeding their young for awhile, even after the young birds can fly.

Learning through History
Focus: Judah Falls to the Babylonians

Reading about History [I]

Read about history in the following resource:

★ *The Story of the Ancient World:*
Ch. CXVII-CXVIII p. 234-237

You will be adding to your timeline in your *Student Notebook* today. In Unit 16 – Box 1, draw and color a broken wall. Label it, *Fall of Nineveh to Babylon and Media (625 B.C.).* In Box 2, draw and color a statue. Label it, *Nebuchadnezzar dreams of a statue (604 B.C.).* In Box 3, draw and color a fire. Label it, *Jerusalem destroyed by Nebuchadnezzar (588 B.C.).*

Key Idea: God used Nebuchadnezzar as His instrument of destruction, and He prophecied to Nebuchadnezzar through dreams.

Storytime [T]

Choose one of the following read aloud options:

★ Your own Bible: Esther chapter 2

★ Read aloud the next portion of the fantasy that you selected.

After the reading, students will give a summary oral narration. The oral narration must be no longer than 5 sentences and should summarize the reading. As students narrate, have them hold up one finger for each sentence shared. Remind students that the focus should be on the big ideas, rather than on the details.

Key Idea: Summarize the story by narrating.

History Project [S]

Get the cookie statue that you made on Day 2. Read Daniel 2:32-45. Then, open your *Student Notebook* to the picture of the statue on Unit 16. With the help of your *Student Notebook,* point to each part of your cookie statue and name the kingdom that it most likely represents. Next, get a rock from outside. Clean the rock by washing it in soap and water and drying it. Then, use the rock to smash the feet of iron and clay. Make sure not to break or dent the cookie sheet! Remember, Christ is the rock of the kingdom that will endure forever. Last, start with the top of your statue and break off and eat a piece of each color naming the kingdom it represents.

Key Idea: The Lord revealed the meaning of Nebuchadnezzar's dream to Daniel. The statue represented the various kingdoms to come.

Bible Quiet Time [I]

Reading: Choose one option below.

★ *The Illustrated Family Bible* p. 180-181

★ Your own Bible: Daniel chapters 1-2

Scripture Focus: Highlight Daniel 1:17.

Prayer Focus: Pray a prayer of thanksgiving to express gratitude for God's divine goodness. Begin by reading the highlighted verse out loud as a prayer. End by praying, *Thank you for giving each person the skills needed to do what you call that person to do. I pray that I will use my skills for your glory.*

Scripture Memory: Recite Philippians 2:15.
Music: *Philippians 2* CD: Track 4 (vs. 14-15)

Key Idea: Even in captivity, God did not forsake His people. He answered their prayers.

Independent History Study [I]

★ Listen to *What in the World?* Disc 3, Half of Track 2: "Babylon".

Key Idea: Nebuchadnezzar made a golden image of himself for all of his people to worship. God used a miracle to save Shadrach, Meshach, and Abednego from death when they refused to worship the image.

Bible Study | T |

Read aloud and discuss with the students the following pages:

 The Radical Book for Kids p. 119-122

Key Idea: C.S. Lewis was a British professor and author. After his conversion to Christianity, Lewis wrote his famous book *Mere Christianity*. Lewis is also remembered for his tales of adventure. He has captivated children and grown-ups for years with *The Chronicles of Narnia* series. Lewis's Narnia series is filled with Christian symbolism.

Language Arts | S |

Have students complete one studied dictation exercise (see Appendix for directions and passages).

Work with the students to complete **one** of the writing options listed below:

 Writing & Rhetoric Book 1: Fable p. 109 – top of p. 112 (Note: Omit p. 108. Guide students through the lesson, so they are successful writing an amplification. "Speak It" on p. 112-113 is optional.)

 Your own writing program

Key Idea: Practice language arts skills.

Poetry | I |

Open *Paint Like a Poet* to Lesson 14. Read aloud the poem *"Dust of Snow"* by Robert Frost.

Get the snowy hill backdrop that you painted on Day 2. Today, you will be adding a snowy tree. You will need a palette, water, a small flat paintbrush, a small round paintbrush, a toothpick, and brown, dark green, and white paint.

After gathering your supplies, turn to the "Step-by-Step Watercolor Tutorial" for Lesson 14 in *Paint Like a Poet*. Follow steps 4-6 to complete "Part Two: Snowy Tree". When your painting is dry, glue your poetry copywork from Day 1 to your painting. Store your completed artwork in the place you have chosen for it.

Key Idea: Explore poetry moods with painting.

Math Exploration | S |

Choose **one** of the math options listed below.

 Singapore Primary Mathematics 4A/4B or *5A/5B* (see Appendix for schedules), or *Math with Confidence,* or *Apologia Math*

 Your own math program

Key Idea: Use a step-by-step math program.

Science Exploration | I |

 Read *Birds of the Air* p. 30-34. Write the answer to each numbered question on lined paper. You do not need to copy the question. Use the listed page to help you answer each question.
1. How do birds that sleep in hedges keep from falling off their branches as they sleep? (p. 31)
2. When a bird roosts, what does it do to keep warm in the cold air? (p. 31)
3. Write the words *plumage* and *roost* and give their definitions. (p. 31-32)
4. Where do birds sleep in bad weather? (p. 31-32)
5. Where do seashore birds roost? (p. 32-34) In Psalm 104:17, where does the stork make its nest?

Key Idea: At night, smaller birds roost in hedges. Swallows and Swifts perch in barn rafters in the summer and migrate in the winter. Wood-pigeons and Pheasants roost in tree branches. Partridges sleep in fields on the ground. Jackdaws sleep in holes, and Cormorants and Gulls sleep on cliff ledges.

Learning through History
Focus: Judah Falls to the Babylonians

Reading about History [I]

Read about history in the following resource:

★ *The Story of the Ancient World:*
   Ch. CXIX-CXX p. 238 – middle of p. 241

You will be writing a narration about *Chapter CXIX: The Coming of the Persians,* which is part of today's history reading.

To prepare for writing your narration, think about the questions below. If you do not know the answers, find them on p. 238-239 of *The Story of the Ancient World.* Ask yourself, *Which two nations helped Babylon overthrow Assyria? From whom did the Medians and Persians descend? When Nebuchadnezzar was king of Babylon, who made an alliance? Which king of Israel, from whom one day would come the Messiah, did Nebuchadnezzar take captive to Babylon? What did Cyrus learn as a prince on his visit to his grandfather in Media? Who was Cyrus' uncle? When Cyrus returned home to Persia, what did he learn? Why was Cyrus punished by his teacher?*

After you have thought about the answers to the questions, turn to Unit 16 in your *Student Notebook.* In Box 5, write a 5-8 sentence narration. When you have finished writing, read your sentences out loud to catch any mistakes. Check for the following things: *Did you include **who** the reading was mainly about? Did you include **what** important thing(s) happened? Did you include **how** it ended? If not, add those things.*

Then, underline or highlight the main idea sentence in the narration. Use the *Written Narration Skills* in the Appendix as a guide for editing the narration.

<u>Key Idea</u>: Cyrus and Darius grew up together.

Storytime [T]

Choose one of the following read aloud options:

★ Your own Bible: Esther chapter 3

★ Read aloud the next portion of the fantasy that you selected.

After the reading, have each person get a Bible and open it anywhere in Proverbs. Explain, *We will have 5 minutes to skim through the verses in Proverbs to find any connections to today's story. When a connection is found, read the verse out loud and quickly share the connection. At the end of 5 minutes, anyone who has not shared yet must read aloud one verse and make the best connection possible.*

<u>Key Idea</u>: Seek God's word for His guidance.

Bible Quiet Time [I]

Reading: Choose one option below.

★ *The Illustrated Family Bible* p. 182

★ Your own Bible: Daniel chapter 3

Scripture Focus: Highlight Daniel 3:16-18.

Prayer Focus: Pray a prayer of supplication to make a humble and earnest request of God. Begin by reading the highlighted verse out loud as a prayer. End by praying, *Help me stand firm in my faith no matter what happens. Guide me to trust you and to know that you are with me especially in times of trial.*

Scripture Memory: Copy Philippians 2:15 in your Common Place Book.
Music: *Philippians 2* CD: Track 4 (vs. 14-15)

<u>Key Idea</u>: The Hebrews had faith in God.

Independent History Study [I]

★ Listen to *What in the World?* Disc 3, Last Half of Track 2: "Babylon".

<u>Key Idea</u>: Cyrus was prince of Persia when his Uncle Darius was prince of Media. They were close in age.

Learning the Basics
Focus: Language Arts, Math, Geography, Bible, and Science

Geography [T]

Go to the website link listed on p. 6 of *A Child's Geography Vol. II*. At the link, select "History & Geography". Then, under "Knowledge Quest" select ACG2-Extra Activities". Print the "Travel Log Template" of your choice from p. 39-42. Also at the link, for older students, print and assign the "Chapter Seven Review" on p. 74. Assign all students the following page:

★ *A Child's Geography Vol. II* p. 97
Note: Do only the "Travel Notes" section. The "Art" section of p. 98 is an optional extra.

Key Idea: Share three sights from Egypt.

Language Arts [S]

Have students complete one dictation exercise.

Guide students to complete one reading lesson.

★ *Drawn into the Heart of Reading*

Help students complete **one** English lesson.

★ *Building with Diligence:* Lesson 30

★ *Following the Plan:* Lesson 28

★ Your own grammar program

Key Idea: Practice language arts skills.

Poetry [I]

Open *Paint Like a Poet* to Lesson 14. Today, you will be performing a poetry reading of *"Dust of Snow"*. Practice reading the poem aloud with expression that matches the mood of the poem. Then, read the poem aloud in front of your chosen audience.

At the end of the reading, share the following, *When I read this poem by Robert Frost, it made me think of...* Call on your audience to share what thoughts the poem brought to their minds.

Last, say, *Did you know that Robert Frost married Elinor White in 1895? His first son, Elliot, was born in 1896. Sadly, Elliot died of cholera when he was only 3. Elinor and Robert eventually had 5 more children.*

Key Idea: Share the poetry of Robert Frost.

Math Exploration [S]

Choose **one** of the math options listed below.

★ *Singapore Primary Mathematics 4A/4B* or *5A/5B* (see Appendix for schedules), or *Math with Confidence*, or *Apologia Math*

★ Your own math program

Key Idea: Use a step-by-step math program.

Science Exploration [I]

★ Read *Birds of the Air* p. 35-40. Turn to the science experiment section in your science binder or sketchbook. At the top of a blank page, write: *What adaptations do Swallows, Swifts, and Martins have to help them catch flies and gnats?* Under the question, write: *'Guess'*. Write down your guess. You will need 10 pieces of popped popcorn or 'O' shaped dry cereal to be flying insects. You will also need a small envelope, a tweezers, and a pair of tongs to be three different types of bird beaks. Get 10 pieces of popped popcorn or dry cereal to be flying insects. Have a helper gently toss in the air all 10 pieces at one time. Your job is to capture as many insects as possible with one type of beak. Repeat the trial 10 times for each beak, keeping a record of how many insects you caught each time. The insects must be caught while they are in the air. Make sure to open the envelope like a mouth to test that particular beak. Next, on the paper write: *'Procedure'*. Make a table to show the results of the experiment. At the bottom of the paper, write: *'Conclusion'*. Explain what you learned from the experiment.

Key Idea: Swallows, Swifts, and Martins have short, sharp beaks and mouths that open wide.

Reading about History I

Read about history in the following resource:

 The Story of the Ancient World:
Ch. CXXI-CXXII p. 241 – middle of p. 245

The Jewish people celebrate God's deliverence of His people from Haman, as told in the book of Esther. This holiday is called Purim. Where could you look to research more about **Purim**? Use a Bible, an online resource like www.wikipedia.org, or a reference book.

Answer one or more of the following questions from your research: *Why is Purim celebrated by the Jewish people? When is it celebrated? Where is the Purim story told? How is Purim celebrated? Why are food gifts given as part of Purim? What is charity? Why is charity an important part of Purim? Which foods are traditionally eaten during Purim? What are some new words you have learned from your research today?*

Key Idea: At the time of Cyrus and Belshazzar, the Jews were still captives in Babylon.

History Project S

In this unit you will make a gragger, which is a Jewish noisemaker used in the celebration of Purim. You will need a small empty box (i.e. a gelatin, pudding, rice, or small cereal box). Place small rocks, buttons, rice, dry beans, or macaroni noodles inside the box. Tape the ends of the box tightly closed. Shake the box to make sure it makes a loud noise. Neatly wrap the box in colored paper and decorate it. Save your gragger for Day 3.

Key Idea: God was with His people in Babylon.

Storytime T

Choose one of the following read aloud options:

 Your own Bible: Esther chapter 4

Read at least one mystery for the next 16 days of plans (see Appendix for suggestions).

After the reading, students will give a detailed oral narration. Select one paragraph from the story to read out loud to the students. This will be the starting point for the narration. Set a timer for 3-5 minutes. When the timer rings the narration is over, even if it isn't complete. A detailed, descriptive narration is the goal. See *Narration Tips* in the Appendix as needed.

Key Idea: Use oral narration to retell the story.

Bible Quiet Time I

Bible Reading: Choose one option below.

★ *The Illustrated Family Bible* p. 183-185

★ Your own Bible: Daniel chapters 5-6

Scripture Focus: Highlight Daniel 6:19-22.

Prayer Focus: Pray a prayer of adoration to worship and honor God. Begin by reading the highlighted verses out loud as a prayer. End by praying, *I give you praise and adoration for your power to save Daniel by shutting the lions' mouths. I know your will is always done.*

Scripture Memory: Recite Philippians 2:16.
Music: *Philippians 2* CD: Track 4 (vs. 14-16)

Key Idea: King Darius was tricked into putting Daniel in the lions' den, but God saved Daniel.

Independent History Study I

Open your *Student Notebook* to Unit 17. In Box 6, copy Daniel 6:26-28.

Key Idea: Even though Daniel was a captive in Babylon, God used him to change the lives of the kings that he advised. These kings included Nebuchadnezzar, Belshazzar, Darius the Mede, and Cyrus the Great.

Learning the Basics
Focus: Language Arts, Math, Geography, Bible, and Science

Bible Study · T

Read aloud and discuss with the students the following pages:

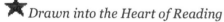 *The Radical Book for Kids* p. 123 – top of p. 126

<u>Key Idea</u>: As Christians, it is important to get to know God. When you believe on the Lord Jesus Christ and ask Him to forgive your sins, He sends His Spirit to live inside you. The Holy Spirit helps you know God through His Word. God is our Father, our judge, our source of life, our shelter, and our refuge.

Language Arts · S

Have students complete one studied dictation exercise (see Appendix for directions and passages).

Help students complete one lesson from the following reading program:

 Drawn into the Heart of Reading

Work with the students to complete **one** of the English options listed below:

★ *Building with Diligence:* Lesson 31

★ *Following the Plan:* Lesson 29 (Half)

★ Your own grammar program

<u>Key Idea</u>: Practice language arts skills.

Poetry · I

Choose one of Robert Frost's poems from Lessons 10-16 in *Paint Like a Poet* to memorize.

You will have 2 weeks (units) to memorize the entire poem. So, you should have half of your chosen poem memorized by Day 4 of this unit.

After you have chosen your poem to memorize, read it three times, adding actions to help you remember the words.

<u>Key Idea</u>: Read and appreciate a variety of classic poetry.

Math Exploration · S

Choose **one** of the math options listed below.

★ *Singapore Primary Mathematics 4A/4B or 5A/5B* (see Appendix for schedules), or *Math with Confidence*, or *Apologia Math*

★ Your own math program

<u>Key Idea</u>: Use a step-by-step math program.

Science Exploration · I

★ Read *Birds of the Air* p. 41-45. Get your book about birds that you began in unit 15. At the top of the next page in your book, copy in cursive Jeremiah 8:7. Beneath the verse, sketch 1-3 birds that migrate to or from your area. You can do this by using a pocket field guide and sketching the migratory birds from your area, or if you have internet access you may refer to https://www.allaboutbirds.org. If you choose the internet option, once you get to the website click on "Search" in the top toolbar. Next, in the "Search" type "migratory birds" followed by the name of your state. If you live outside the U.S., type in your region. Images of migratory birds in your area will come up. Choose 1-3 birds to click on, sketch, color, and label. Pay attention to the "Migration" path shown on the map that comes up when you click on a bird. Beneath each sketch, copy a portion of the text from the website under "Find This Bird" or "Cool Facts."

<u>Key Idea</u>: As summer ends, there is less food for the birds, so some of them migrate.

Learning through History
Focus: The Persian Empire

Reading about History   I

Read about history in the following resource:

★ *The Story of the Ancient World: Ch. CXXIII-CXXIV* p. 245 – middle of p. 248

You will be choosing a portion from today's reading that you found memorable or worthy of being reread to copy. Open your *Student Notebook* to Unit 17. In Box 4, carefully copy in cursive the portion from today's reading that you selected. Then, compare your written work to the original. Last, draw a small colorful picture in Box 4 to illustrate your sentences.

<u>Key Idea</u>: After 70 years of captivity in Babylon, the Jews were allowed to go home.

Storytime   T

Choose one of the following read aloud options:

★ Your own Bible: Esther chapter 5

★ Read aloud the next portion of the mystery that you selected.

After reading, give each person a white piece of paper or a markerboard and a marker. Set a timer for 3-5 minutes and instruct each person to do a quick outline sketch about the story. Ideas for sketches include settings, characters, actions, important objects, or symbols. When the timer rings, briefly share the sketches.

<u>Key Idea</u>: Use sketching to share the story.

History Project   S

Today you will make Hamantashen, which is a traditional Jewish cookie served to celebrate Purim. Mix 2 cups flour, 2 eggs, 3/8 cup sugar, 1 cup butter or margarine (softened), 2 tsp. baking power, 1 tsp. vanilla extract, and 1 Tbsp. orange juice (optional). Have an adult help you beat the mixture on high speed. Add more flour if needed. Roll dough into a ball and divide into 2 parts. Roll out each part to about 1/8" thickness. Use the open end of a glass to cut out 3-inch circles. Put a ½ tsp. of preserves in the center of the circle. Then, fold three sides of the circle in to form a triangular shaped cookie, leaving space in the center for the filling to poke through. Pinch the 3 corners of the triangle to seal each cookie. Place on a greased sheet and bake 20 min. at 350 degrees. Cool and store.

<u>Key Idea</u>: Not all Jews returned home. Some remained in Babylon at the time of Esther.

Bible Quiet Time   I

Reading: Choose one option below.

★ *The Illustrated Family Bible* p. 186-187

★ Your own Bible: Ezra 1:1-8; 5:7-17; 6:1-12

Scripture Focus: Highlight Ezra 1:1-2.

Prayer Focus: Pray a prayer of confession to admit or acknowledge your sins to God. Begin by reading the highlighted verses out loud as a prayer. End by praying, *I confess that I don't always do what I know in my heart is right. Please help me listen to the Holy Spirit and do what is right in your eyes.*

Scripture Memory: Recite Philippians 2:16.
Music: *Philippians 2* CD: Track 4 (vs. 14-16)

<u>Key Idea</u>: Cyrus fulfilled the word of the Lord.

Independent History Study   I

★ Listen to *What in the World?* Disc 3, Track 3: "Cyrus the Great". Then, read Isaiah 44:28 through 45:6 to see Isaiah's prophecy that Cyrus fulfilled.

<u>Key Idea</u>: In Isaiah's prophecy, God called Cyrus by name 150 years before he actually ruled. Isaiah also prophecied the fall of the Temple in Jerusalem 100 years before it happened. God is the author of history.

Geography [T]

Read aloud to the students the following pages:

 A Child's Geography Vol. II p. 99 – bottom of p. 101

Discuss with the students the **first** "Field Note" on p. 105.

Key Idea: The northern region in Egypt is called Lower Egypt; and the southern region is called Upper Egypt. This is because the Nile River flows north from the mountains of Africa, making northern Egypt downstream on the Nile River. The Nile has been a famous river throughout history and continues to be the source of much of life in Egypt today.

Poetry [I]

Today, you will copy half of the Robert Frost poem from *Paint Like a Poet* that you chose to memorize this week.

At the top of a clean page in your *Common Place Book,* copy the title and the author of the poem. Then, copy half of the poem in cursive, leaving the rest of the page blank.

You will copy the remaining half of the poem during the next unit.

Practice the portion of the poem that you copied today by reading it aloud.

Key Idea: Copy and memorize classic poetry.

Language Arts [S]

Help students complete one lesson from the following reading program:

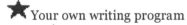 *Drawn into the Heart of Reading*

Work with the students to complete **one** of the writing options listed below:

★ *Writing & Rhetoric Book 1: Fable* p. 114 – bottom of p. 117 (Note: Read aloud the text while the students follow along. Then, discuss.)

★ Your own writing program

Key Idea: Practice language arts skills.

Math Exploration [S]

Choose **one** of the math options listed below.

★ *Singapore Primary Mathematics 4A/4B* or *5A/5B* (see Appendix for schedules), or *Math with Confidence,* or *Apologia Math*

★ Your own math program

Key Idea: Use a step-by-step math program.

Science Exploration [I]

★ Read *Birds of the Air* p. 46-50. Orally retell or narrate to an adult the portion of text that you read today. Use the *Narration Tips* in the Appendix for help as needed.

Key Idea: Birds are able to stay warm in the winter, but it is hard for them to find enough food. Sometimes they even starve. It is a good idea to share your leftover food with the birds in the winter. Make sure to cut it up into small pieces and add a little hot water. They will soon be coming to your door for their meal. If you live in town, you may need to choose a different place to put the food than by your front door.

Learning through History
Focus: The Persian Empire

Reading about History | I |

Read about history in the following resource:

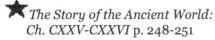
★ *The Story of the Ancient World:*
Ch. CXXV-CXXVI p. 248-251

You will be adding to your timeline in your *Student Notebook* today. In Unit 17 – Box 1, draw and color a hand writing on the wall. Label it, *Belshazzar's Feast/Babylon conquered by Medes and Persians (538 B.C.)*. In Box 2, draw and color a lion. Label it, *Daniel in the lions' den (538 B.C.)*. In Box 3, draw and color two gold pillars. Label it, *Jews rebuild Temple/Esther is Queen of Persia (515 B.C.)*.

Key Idea: After the death of Darius the Mede and Cyrus the Great, Cyrus' two sons divided the Persian Empire between them. After their deaths, Darius the Great became the next king of Persia.

History Project | S |

Get the gragger that you made on Day 1 and the Hamantashens (meaning "Haman's pockets) that you made on Day 2. On Purim the Jews read aloud from the book of Esther called the *Megilla*. As your parent reads aloud from the book of Esther for storytime today, you will use your gragger just like the Jews do during the reading of the Megilla at Purim. Each time Haman's name is mentioned during the reading, you will shake your gragger loudly to blot out the name of evil. At the end of the reading, you may eat your Hamantashens. Make sure to share with the rest of your family!

Key Idea: Haman hated the Jews. He served in King Ahasuerus' (Darius the Great's) court.

Storytime | T |

Choose one of the following read aloud options:

★ Your own Bible: Esther chapters 6-7

★ Read aloud the next portion of the mystery that you selected.

After the reading, students will give a summary oral narration. The oral narration must be no longer than 5 sentences and should summarize the reading. As students narrate, have them hold up one finger for each sentence shared. Remind students that the focus should be on the big ideas, rather than on the details.

Key Idea: Summarize the story by narrating.

Bible Quiet Time | I |

Reading: Choose one option below.

★ *The Illustrated Family Bible* p. 188-191

★ Your own Bible: Esther chapters 4-7

Scripture Focus: Highlight Esther 7:3.

Prayer Focus: Pray a prayer of thanksgiving to express gratitude for God's divine goodness. Begin by reading the highlighted verse out loud as a prayer. End by praying, *Thank you for never forgetting about your people even in times of trouble. I am so glad that I can always come before you and pray for your help and guidance. Guide me to…*

Scripture Memory: Recite Philippians 2:16.
Music: *Philippians 2* CD: Track 4 (vs. 14-16)

Key Idea: God used Esther to save His people.

Independent History Study | I |

Open your *Student Notebook* to Unit 17 – Box 7. On the map of Ancient Jerusalem find the walls at the time of David and Solomon. Then, find the walls that Nehemiah rebuilt. Last, note the third wall.

Key Idea: Cyrus allowed Jerusalem's Temple to be rebuilt. Darius the Great allowed the wall rebuilding.

Bible Study | T

Read aloud and discuss with the students the following pages:

Poetry | I

Practice reading aloud half of the poem that you chose to memorize from *Paint Like a Poet*, using the actions that you added to help you remember the words. Do this 2 times.

⭐ *The Radical Book for Kids* top of p. 126-129

Then, recite half of the poem without looking at the words.

<u>Key Idea</u>: Jesus is the Lamb of God, offered as a perfect sacrafice for our sin. He is the Lion of Judah, the conquering King. Jesus is the vine, and we are the branches. He is our source of life. The Holy Spirit is the "breath" of God quietly working within us. The Holy Spirit is like a bird hovering and bringing life. The Spirit is our Helper who teaches, strengthens, and encourages. The Spirit is like an anointing oil, giving Christians the power to do God's will.

You have 2 weeks (units) to memorize the entire poem. So, you should have half of your chosen poem memorized by Day 4 of this unit.

<u>Key Idea</u>: Memorize classic poetry.

Language Arts | S

Have students complete one dictation exercise.

Work with the students to complete **one** of the writing options listed below:

⭐ *Writing & Rhetoric Book 1: Fable* p. 119-120 (Note: Omit bottom of p. 117 and p. 118. Reread the fable on p. 115 first. Then, guide students through the lesson, so they are successful writing a fable.)

⭐ Your own writing program

<u>Key Idea</u>: Practice language arts skills.

Math Exploration | S

Choose **one** of the math options listed below.

⭐ *Singapore Primary Mathematics 4A/4B or 5A/5B* (see Appendix for schedules), or *Math with Confidence,* or *Apologia Math*

⭐ Your own math program

<u>Key Idea</u>: Use a step-by-step math program.

Science Exploration | I

⭐ Read *Birds of the Air* p. 51-54. Write the answer to each numbered question on lined paper. You do not need to copy the question. Use the listed page to help you answer each question.
1. How is a Goldfinch useful to us? (p. 51)
2. How does a Nuthatch open the nuts it eats? (p. 52)
3. Write the words *moult* (or *molt*) and *gorse* and give their definitions. (p. 51-52)
4. Choose one of the following birds to describe: Blackcap, Whitethroat, Stonechat, or Little Dipper. (p. 52-54)
5. What does Psalm 50:11 tell you about God?

<u>Key Idea</u>: It is interesting to study the small birds that live in your neighborhood. Each one was created by God and belongs to Him.

Learning through History
Focus: The Persian Empire

Reading about History | I |

Read about history in the following resource:

⭐ *The Story of the Ancient World:*
Ch. CXXVII p. 252 top of p. 254

You will be writing a narration about *Chapter CXXVII: Revival in Jerusalem,* which is part of today's history reading.

To prepare for writing your narration, think about the questions below. If you do not know the answers, find them on p. 252-254 of *The Story of the Ancient World.* Ask yourself, *Who became king after Darius the Great? When was the Temple in Jerusalem completed? Whom did the Lord call to return to Jerusalem after the Temple was completed? What did Ezra take with him on his journey? When Ezra arrived, why did he weep? What was the purpose of the synagogue? Why did Nehemiah come to Jerusalem? During the time of Nehemiah, what did Malachi prophecy?*

After you have thought about the answers to the questions, turn to Unit 17 in your *Student Notebook.* In Box 5, write a 5-8 sentence narration. When you have finished writing, read your sentences out loud to catch any mistakes. Check for the following things: *Did you include **who** the reading was mainly about? Did you include **what** important thing(s) happened? Did you include **how** it ended? If not, add those things.*

Then, underline or highlight the main idea sentence in the narration. Use the *Written Narration Skills* in the Appendix as a guide for editing the narration.

Key Idea: After the Temple was completed, God called Ezra and then Nehemiah to return.

Storytime | T |

Choose one of the following read aloud options:

⭐ Your own Bible: Esther chapter 8

⭐ Read aloud the next part of your mystery.

After the reading, have each person get a Bible and open it anywhere in Proverbs. Explain, *We will have 5 minutes to skim through the verses in Proverbs to find any connections to today's story. When a connection is found, read the verse out loud and quickly share the connection. At the end of 5 minutes, anyone who has not shared yet must read aloud one verse and make the best connection possible.*

Key Idea: Seek God's word for His guidance.

Bible Quiet Time | I |

Reading: Choose one option below.

⭐ *The Illustrated Family Bible* p. 192-195

⭐ Your own Bible: Nehemiah chapters 1-2

Scripture Focus: Highlight Nehemiah 1:4.

Prayer Focus: Pray a prayer of supplication to make a humble and earnest request of God. Begin by reading the highlighted verse out loud as a prayer. End by praying, *Guide me to do those hard tasks which honor you, knowing nothing is too difficult for you. Help me to ask for your success when I am doing a hard task.*

Scripture Memory: Copy Philippians 2:16 in your Common Place Book.
Music: *Philippians 2* CD: Track 4 (vs. 14-16)

Key Idea: Nehemiah prayed for God's success.

Independent History Study | I |

Open your *Student Notebook* to "Prophecies About Christ". Under "Prophecy" write, *Malachi 3:1.* Read the Scripture from the Bible to discover the prophecy. Under "Fulfillment" write, *Matthew 11:10-11.* Read the fulfillment Scripture. Under "Description", write a few phrases to describe the prophecy about Jesus.

Key Idea: Malachi prophecied that God would send a messenger to prepare the way for the Savior.

Learning the Basics

Focus: Language Arts, Math, Geography, Bible, and Science

Geography　[T]

Read aloud to the students the following pages:

★ *A Child's Geography Vol. II* bottom of p. 101 – middle of p. 105

Discuss with the students the **last three** "Field Notes" on p. 105.

Key Idea: The Egyptians built the Aswan Dam to create a reservoir, or man-made lake, on the Nile River. The water from the dam generates electricity, and the reservoir releases water throughout the year. In Egypt, tourism is an important industry.

Poetry　[I]

Practice reading aloud half of the poem that you chose to memorize from *Paint Like a Poet*, using the actions that you added to help you remember the words. Do this 2 times.

Then, recite half of the poem without looking at the words.

You have 2 weeks (units) to memorize the entire poem. So, you should have half of your chosen poem memorized by today.

Key Idea: Memorize classic poetry.

Language Arts　[S]

Have students complete one dictation exercise.

Guide students to complete one reading lesson.

★ *Drawn into the Heart of Reading*

Help students complete **one** English lesson.

★ *Building with Diligence:* Lesson 32

★ *Following the Plan:* Lesson 29 (Last half)

★ Your own grammar program

Key Idea: Practice language arts skills.

Math Exploration　[S]

Choose **one** of the math options listed below.

★ *Singapore Primary Mathematics 4A/4B* or *5A/5B* (see Appendix for schedules), or *Math with Confidence*, or *Apologia Math*

★ Your own math program

Key Idea: Use a step-by-step math program.

Science Exploration　[I]

★ Read *Birds of the Air* p. 55-60. Turn to the science experiment section in your science binder or sketchbook. At the top of a blank page, write: *Why are birds of prey at the top of the food chain?* Under the question, write: *'Guess'.* Write down your guess. You will need popcorn, raisins, or any small objects to represent seeds. You will need 2 Ziploc bags to be birds' stomachs. You will be a small seed-eating bird, so you will need a clothespin to be your bird beak. Scatter the seeds across the floor of a large area. Have a partner time you for 15 seconds. Use your beak to gather as many seeds as possible in that time. Place each gathered seed in your Ziploc bag. At the end of 15 seconds, count and record the number of seeds you gathered. Repeat the activity, but this time have the helper be a Hawk circling the area three times as you gather seeds, and then swooping in to tag you. Once you've been tagged, place your bag inside the Hawk's bag to show that you've been eaten by the Hawk. Then, count to see how many seeds you gathered before being eaten. What was different? Describe the food chain in this activity. Who were the consumers and the producer(s) in the food chain? Are there fewer or more consumers as you move up the food chain? Explain. What would happen if there were no birds of prey? Next, on the paper write: *'Procedure'.* Show the results of the experiment. At the bottom of the paper, write: *'Conclusion'.* Explain what you learned.

Key Idea: Owls, Hawks, Eagles, and Falcons are birds of prey. These birds prey upon small animals.

Unit 18 - Day 1

Reading about History [I]

Read about history in the following resource:

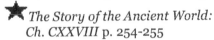 *The Story of the Ancient World:*
  Ch. CXXVIII p. 254-255

Alexander the Greek came from Macedonia. Where could you look to research more about the **Ancient Kingdom of Macedonia**? Use an online resource like www.wikipedia.org or a reference book.

Answer one or more of the following questions from your research: *According to the map in your Student Notebook-Unit 18, where was Macedonia located? What kingdoms bordered ancient Macedonia? Describe the topography of the land in Macedonia. What rivers flowed through Macedonia? Who were some of the famous kings of Macedonia? Which king of Persia ruled Macedonia for a time? What did Philip II do for Macedonia? Who was Philip II's famous son? Why was he famous?*

Key Idea: Macedonia was located north of Greece. Alexander the Great was Macedonian. He was the son of Philip II.

History Project [S]

In this unit you will do a project to study the geography of Greece and its city-states. Find Greece on a globe or a world map. On which continent is Greece located? Find the seas that surround Greece and give their names. Greece is a peninsula. What is a peninsula? Which countries border Greece today?

Key Idea: Greece is surrounded by water on three sides. It became an important kingdom.

Storytime [T]

Choose one of the following read aloud options:

 Your own Bible: Esther chapters 9-10

★ Read at least one mystery for the next 12 days of plans.

After the reading, students will give a detailed oral narration. Select one paragraph from the story to read out loud to the students. This will be the starting point for the narration. Set a timer for 3-5 minutes. When the timer rings the narration is over, even if it isn't complete. A detailed, descriptive narration is the goal. See *Narration Tips* in the Appendix as needed.

Key Idea: Use oral narration to retell the story.

Bible Quiet Time [I]

Bible Reading: Choose the option below.
★ Your own Bible: Daniel 10; 11:1-4

Scripture Focus: Highlight Daniel 11:2-4.

Prayer Focus: Pray a prayer of adoration to worship and honor God. Begin by reading the highlighted verses out loud as a prayer. End by praying, *Lord, you alone know the future. You set up kings and decide their reign. You prophecied about things to come, knowing what the future holds. I am in awe of you!*

Scripture Review: Recite Philippians 2:1-16.
Music: *Philippians 2* CD: Tracks 1-4 (all)

Key Idea: God revealed future kingdoms.

Independent History Study [I]

Open your *Student Notebook* to Unit 18. On the map in Box 6, use colored pencils to **lightly** shade Macedonia. Then, lightly shade each of the kingdoms bordering Macedonia in a different color.

Key Idea: Macedonia was an ancient Greek kingdom bordered by Epirus to the west, Thessaly to the south, Thrace to the east, and Paionia to the north.

Learning the Basics
Focus: Language Arts, Math, Geography, Bible, and Science

Bible Study [T]

Read aloud and discuss with the students the following pages:

 The Radical Book for Kids p. 130-134

Key Idea: The main characters in many books, plays, and movies often resemble the roles that Jesus fuflfills. Jesus is our King, our friend, our rescuer, and Savior. Many cultures have creation stories and flood stories that resemble the Bible. Many different people groups around the world believe in one divine Creator and speak of a divine lost book.

Language Arts [S]

Have students complete one dictation exercise

Help students complete one lesson from the following reading program:

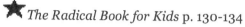 *Drawn into the Heart of Reading*

Work with the students to complete **one** of the English options listed below:

Building with Diligence: Lesson 33

Following the Plan: Lesson 30 (Half)

Your own grammar program

Key Idea: Practice language arts skills.

Poetry [I]

Continue memorizing the Robert Frost poem that you chose from *Paint Like a Poet* in Unit 17. You should have half of your chosen poem memorized already.

You should memorize the rest of the poem by Day 4 of this unit.

Today, read the entire poem 3 times, adding actions to the last half of the poem to help you memorize the words more easily.

Key Idea: Read and appreciate a variety of classic poetry.

Math Exploration [S]

Choose **one** of the math options listed below.

 Singapore Primary Mathematics 4A/4B or 5A/5B (see Appendix for schedules), or *Math with Confidence,* or *Apologia Math*

 Your own math program

Key Idea: Use a step-by-step math program.

Science Exploration [I]

Read *Birds of the Air* p. 61-65. Get your book about birds that you began in unit 15. At the top of the next page in your book, copy in cursive Psalm 104:12. Beneath the verse, sketch one or more birds that you have seen in your backyard. If time and weather allow, go outside and sit quietly, watching for any birds. Then, to determine which bird you saw, use either a pocket field guide or if you have internet access refer to https://www.allaboutbirds.org. If you choose the internet option, once you get to the website click on "Birds" in the top toolbar. Next, when the "Bird Guide" comes up, **under** the "Search" bar, select "Browse Bird Guide by Shape" to search by bird shape. Once you identify the bird you saw by shape, click on that bird outline. Pictures of those types of birds will come up. Once you've found the bird that you saw, sketch, color, and label it. This is your last assigned entry in your bird book; however, you may wish to continue adding sketches to your book whenever you see a new type of bird in your yard.

Key Idea: Rooks eat insects and seeds. Starlings, Jackdaws, and Fieldfares often feed with the Rooks.

Learning through History
Focus: The Geography and Beginning of Greece

Reading about History　[I]

Read about history in the following resource:

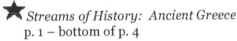 *Streams of History: Ancient Greece* p. 1 – bottom of p. 4

You will be choosing a portion from today's reading that you found memorable or worthy of being reread to copy. Open your *Student Notebook* to Unit 18. In Box 4, carefully copy in cursive the portion from today's reading that you selected. Then, compare your written work to the original. Last, draw a small colorful picture in Box 4 to illustrate your sentences.

Key Idea: The geography of Greece made it difficult for the various city-states to join together. The land was very mountainous.

Storytime　[T]

Choose one of the following read aloud options:

★ *Archimedes and the Door of Science* p. 1-8

★ Read aloud the next portion of the mystery that you selected.

After reading, give each person 2 slips of paper. Each person must think of 2 questions to ask about the book and write one question on each slip of paper. Next, fold up the slips of paper and place them in a container. Each person must select at least one question from the container to answer.

Key Idea: Use questioning to share the story.

History Project　[S]

Open your *Student Notebook* to Unit 18. Use your colored pencils to lightly color the islands surrounding Greece on the map in Box 6. Notice how they look like stepping stones.

Next, use a light blue pencil to faintly color the water on the map in Box 6. Notice how the sea makes inland harbors in the land that makes up Greece.

Then, use a light brown pencil to faintly color the mountains shown on the map in Box 6 throughout Greece's various kingdoms.

Key Idea: Greece is surrounded by many islands with good harbors for trading. The land of Greece has jagged cliffs and mountains, making travel between cities more difficult.

Bible Quiet Time　[I]

Reading: Choose one option below.

★ *The Illustrated Family Bible* p. 198-199 Optional extension: p. 196-197

★ Your own Bible: Psalms 8 and 121

Scripture Focus: Highlight Psalm 121:1-2.

Prayer Focus: Pray a prayer of confession to admit or acknowledge your sins to God. Begin by reading the highlighted verses out loud as a prayer. End by praying, *I confess I need to ask you for help more often, rather than failing on my own. Help me to...*

Scripture Review: Recite Philippians 2:1-16.
Music: *Philippians 2* CD: Tracks 1-4 (all)

Key Idea: The Lord is the maker of heaven and earth. He created all things.

Independent History Study　[I]

Open your *Student Notebook* to Unit 18. Look at the map in Box 7. Find the Phoenician port city of Tyre. Trace the green arrows on the map with your finger to follow the routes of the Phoenician traders. Notice which products were traded along the route. Find Greece on the route.

Key Idea: The Phoenicians sailed their triremes west on the Mediterranean Sea to trade with the Greeks.

Learning the Basics
Focus: Language Arts, Math, Geography, Bible, and Science

Geography [T]

Read aloud to the students the following pages:

 A Child's Geography Vol. II middle of p. 105-110

Discuss with the students "Field Notes" p. 110

<u>Key Idea</u>: Many tourists travel to Egypt each year to see the Pyramids of Giza. The Great Pyramid of Pharaoh Khufu (or Cheops) is the only one of the Seven Wonders of the Ancient World that is still standing. The city of Cairo, Egypt's capital city, sprawls close to the pyramids. It is the largest city on the continent of Africa.

Poetry [I]

Today, you will copy the last half of the Robert Frost poem from *Paint Like a Poet* that you chose to memorize this week.

Beneath the first part of the poem that you copied in the last unit, copy the rest of the poem in cursive in your *Common Place Book*.

Practice the portion of the poem that you copied today by reading it aloud.

<u>Key Idea</u>: Copy and memorize classic poetry.

Language Arts [S]

Help students complete one lesson from the following reading program:

 Drawn into the Heart of Reading

Work with the students to complete **one** of the writing options listed below:

 Writing & Rhetoric Book 1: Fable p. 121-124 (Note: Read aloud the text and guide students through the lesson. Wait to write the fable until Day 3.)

 Your own writing program

<u>Key Idea</u>: Practice language arts skills.

Math Exploration [S]

Choose **one** of the math options listed below.

 Singapore Primary Mathematics 4A/4B or 5A/5B (see Appendix for schedules), or *Math with Confidence,* or *Apologia Math*

 Your own math program

<u>Key Idea</u>: Use a step-by-step math program.

Science Exploration [I]

 Read *Birds of the Air* p. 66-70. Orally retell or narrate to an adult the portion of text that you read today. Use the *Narration Tips* in the Appendix for help as needed.

<u>Key Idea</u>: Gulls, Cormorants, Grebes, and Ducks are swimming birds that live mostly on the water. They are web-footed, meaning their feet have skin between their toes to join them together. This skin can fold up like a fan or spread out like a paddle. Ducks smear their outer feathers with oil to keep them waterproof.

Learning through History
Focus: The Geography and Beginning of Greece

Reading about History [I]

Read about history in the following resource:

★ *Streams of History: Ancient Greece* bottom of p. 4-9

You will be adding to your timeline in your *Student Notebook* today. In Unit 18 – Box 1, draw and color the Parthenon (from the cover of the book). Label it, *Founding of Athens, Greece (approx. 1556 B.C.)*. In Box 2, draw and color a shield. Label it, *Founding of Sparta (approx. 1490 B.C.)*. In Box 3, draw and color a harp or lyre. Label it, *Homer composes the Illiad and Odyssey (approx. 800 B.C.)*.

Key Idea: Greece did not have a large river, which made travel by boat within Greece impossible. This further divided the city-states. Each city-state had its own government.

History Project [S]

Open your *Student Notebook* to Unit 18. On the map in Box 6, find the place where Mt. Parnassus would be, near Delphi. Label it. Shade over Mt. Parnassus with a light red colored pencil. Then, shade over Mt. Olympus in light red. Shade the city-states light red that were mentioned in our reading today: Delphi, Athens, Sparta. Olympia was the site of the first Olympic games. You will read about it soon. Shade it in a different color. Thebes was an ancient Phoenician city. Shade it a different color. Last, use colored pencils to lightly shade the rest of your map. Try saying the names of the places on the map out loud.

Key Idea: Each city-state was independent.

Storytime [T]

Choose one of the following read aloud options:

★ *Archimedes and the Door...* p. 9-15

★ Read aloud the next portion of the mystery that you selected.

After the reading, students will give a summary oral narration. The oral narration must be no longer than 5 sentences and should summarize the reading. As students narrate, have them hold up one finger for each sentence shared. Remind students that the focus should be on the big ideas, rather than on the details.

Key Idea: Summarize the story by narrating.

Bible Quiet Time [I]

Reading: Choose one option below.

★ *The Illustrated Family Bible* p. 200-201

★ Your own Bible: Proverbs chapter 3

Scripture Focus: Highlight Proverbs 3:3-4.

Prayer Focus: Pray a prayer of thanksgiving to express gratitude for God's divine goodness. Begin by reading the highlighted verses out loud as a prayer. End by praying, *Thank you for showing me how to live my life according to your word. Help me to be loving and faithful with my words and actions and to find favor in your sight.*

Scripture Review: Recite Philippians 2:1-16.
Music: *Philippians 2* CD: Tracks 1-4 (all)

Key Idea: Proverbs guides us in living for God.

Independent History Study [I]

Look at the timeline entries in today's "Reading About History" box. Then, open your *Student Notebook* and look at your past timeline entries to see what was happening in history at the same time as the founding of Athens and Sparta and at the time of Homer.

Key Idea: Sparta was founded around the time the Israelites were entering Canaan and Jericho fell.

Learning the Basics

Focus: Language Arts, Math, Geography, Bible, and Science

Bible Study [T]

Read aloud and discuss with the students the following pages:

 The Radical Book for Kids p. 135-137

Key Idea: One-third of the Old Testament is filled with songs and poetry. There are Psalms of praise, Psalms of thanksgiving, and Psalms of lament. The Psalms express emotion and help draw us closer to God. They remind us of who God is and that He is always with us.

Poetry [I]

Using the actions that you added on Day 1, practice reading aloud the poem from *Paint Like a Poet* that you chose to memorize. Do this 2 times.

Then, recite the poem without looking at the words.

You should have your chosen poem memorized by Day 4 of this unit.

Key Idea: Memorize classic poetry.

Language Arts [S]

Have students complete one studied dictation exercise (see Appendix for directions and passages).

Work with the students to complete **one** of the writing options listed below:

 Writing & Rhetoric Book 1: Fable p. 125 (Note: Guide students to use the plan on the bottom of p. 124, so they are successful writing their fable on p 125. Omit p. 126.)

 Your own writing program

Key Idea: Practice language arts skills.

Math Exploration [S]

Choose **one** of the math options listed below.

 Singapore Primary Mathematics 4A/4B or *5A/5B* (see Appendix for schedules), or *Math with Confidence*, or *Apologia Math*

 Your own math program

Key Idea: Use a step-by-step math program.

Science Exploration [I]

 Read *Birds of the Air* p. 71-74. Write the answer to each numbered question on lined paper. You do not need to copy the question. Use the listed page to help you answer each question.
1. List some of the bird's natural enemies. (p. 71-72)
2. Why have laws been made about birds? (p. 73)
3. Write the words *grouse* and *stoat* and give their definitions. (p. 71-72)
4. What good work do birds do? (p. 74)
5. When should birds be driven away? (p. 74)

Key Idea: Birds have many enemies, such as cats, owls, stoats, weasels, and foxes. Even other birds, such as Hawks, can be enemies.

Reading about History | I

Read about history in the following resource:

★ *Streams of History: Ancient Greece*
p. 10 – middle of p. 16

You will be writing a narration about the first part of the chapter *Greece in Her Infancy or the Time of Homer,* which is today's history reading.

To prepare for writing your narration, think about the questions below. If you do not know the answers, find them on p. 10-16 of *Streams of History: Ancient Greece.* Ask yourself, *What country did Harold learn about in today's reading? In the doma, or the gathering room, what did Harold see? After breakfast, where did Phoenix and Harold go? Describe what the mother and sisters were doing in the thalium, or women's room. Why was the dark-haired little girl wiping away tears? Describe dinner time. Why did the man come with a drove of white oxen?*

After you have thought about the answers to the questions, turn to Unit 18 in your *Student Notebook.* In Box 5, write a 5-8 sentence narration. When you have finished writing, read your sentences out loud to catch any mistakes. Check for the following things: *Did you include **who** the reading was mainly about? Did you include **what** important thing(s) happened? Did you include **how** it ended? If not, add those things.*

Then, underline or highlight the main idea sentence in the narration. Use the *Written Narration Skills* in the Appendix as a guide for editing the narration.

Key Idea: Greece changed much as it grew and struggled for its freedom. This part of Greece's history took place during the time of the Israelites in Canaan.

Storytime | T

Choose one of the following read aloud options:

★ *Archimedes and the Door...* p. 16-23

★ Read aloud the next part of the mystery.

After the reading, have each person get a Bible and open it anywhere in Proverbs. Explain, *We will have 5 minutes to skim through the verses in Proverbs to find any connections to today's story. When a connection is found, read the verse out loud and quickly share the connection. At the end of 5 minutes, anyone who has not shared yet must read aloud one verse and make the best connection possible.*

Key Idea: Seek God's word for His guidance.

Bible Quiet Time | I

Reading: Choose one option below.

★ *The Illustrated Family Bible* p. 202-203

★ Your own Bible: Malachi chapter 3

Scripture Focus: Highlight Malachi 3:6-7.

Prayer Focus: Pray a prayer of supplication to make a humble and earnest request of God. Begin by reading the highlighted verses out loud as a prayer. End by praying, *Help me stay close to you Lord, so I do not get far away from you or your words. Thank you for continuing to forgive me when I go astray. Draw me nearer to you each day.*

Scripture Review: Recite Philippians 2:1-16.
Music: *Philippians 2* CD: Tracks 1-4 (all)

Key Idea: Malachi prophecied about John the Baptist and the coming Messiah. Malachi is the last book in the Old Testament.

Independent History Study | I

Open your *Student Notebook* to Unit 18. On the map in Box 6 color Chios (a possible home of Homer).

Key Idea: Homer was a Greek bard or a poet who is credited with writing *The Illiad* and *The Odyssey.*

Learning the Basics

Focus: Language Arts, Math, Geography, Bible, and Science

Geography [T]

Have students get both the blank map and the labeled map of **Egypt, Iraq & Saudi Arabia** that they began in Unit 16.

Then, assign students the following page:

 ⭐ *A Child's Geography Vol. II* p. 111

Note: Do only the "Map Notes" section.

Key Idea: Practice finding and recording the locations of various places on a map of Egypt.

Language Arts [S]

Have students complete one dictation exercise.

Guide students to complete one reading lesson.
⭐ *Drawn into the Heart of Reading*

Help students complete **one** English lesson.
⭐ *Building with Diligence:* Lesson 34
⭐ *Following the Plan:* Lesson 30 (Last half)
⭐ Your own grammar program

Key Idea: Practice language arts skills.

Poetry [I]

Today, you will be performing a poetry recitation of the Robert Frost poem that you chose to memorize from *Paint Like a Poet.* You will recite your poem for an audience of your choosing, without looking at the words.

Before reciting, practice saying the poem aloud using an expression that matches the mood of the poem. Then, stand and recite the poem aloud in front of your chosen audience.

At the end of the recitation, share the following, *I decided to choose this poem of Robert Frost's to memorize because...* Then, call on your audience to comment on what they liked about the poem that you shared.

Key Idea: Share the poetry of Robert Frost.

Math Exploration [S]

Choose **one** of the math options listed below.

⭐ *Singapore Primary Mathematics 4A/4B* or *5A/5B* (see Appendix for schedules), or *Math with Confidence,* or *Apologia Math*

⭐ Your own math program

Key Idea: Use a step-by-step math program.

Science Exploration [I]

Turn to the science experiment section in your science binder or sketchbook. At the top of a blank page, write: *How do Ducks stay dry when they are swimming?* Under the question, write: *'Guess'.* Write down your guess. Fill a bowl partway full of water. Then, cut 2 feathers out of brown paper. Use a paper towel to lightly coat both sides of one feather with vegetable shortening or lard. Then, place both feathers on the surface of the water. What do you notice? Why did water soak into the uncoated feather? What did the water do to the oil-coated feather? Remove both feathers. Discard the uncoated feather. Now, add laundry detergent to the water and stir. Rub the coated feather between your fingers to feel it. Then, place it back on the surface of the water. What happened to the feather? Rub it between your fingers again. What difference do you notice in how it feels? Next, on the paper write: *'Procedure'.* Draw a labeled picture of the experiment. At the bottom of the paper, write: *'Conclusion'.* Explain what you learned from the experiment.

Key Idea: Ducks oil their feathers to keep them waterproof, which helps them stay afloat. Soap breaks down the oil, allowing water to penetrate the feather. Without the oil, the feathers are not waterproof.

Learning through History
Focus: The Greeks Resist the Persians

Reading about History   I

Read about history in the following resource:

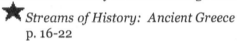 *Streams of History: Ancient Greece*
p. 16-22

The Battle of Marathon was a historic battle fought between Persia and Greece. Where could you look to research more about the **Battle of Marathon**? Use a reference book or an online resource like www.wikipedia.org.

Answer one or more of the following questions from your research: *What events led up to the Battle of Marathon? Who aided Ionia in a revolt against Persia? When did the Battle of Marathon take place? Where was it fought? Who was the battle between? What was a hoplite? Name the athletic event inspired by the Battle of Marathon and the story of a runner carrying the victory message to Athens. Who was king of Persia at the time of the Battle of Marathon?*

Key Idea: Homer was a blind poet who sang and told Greek stories of bravery and heroism.

History Project   S

In this unit you will act out Phidippides' historic run and the message delivered from the Athenians to the Spartans. During this time period the Greeks used a method called scytale to send their messages. To make a scytale message, cut strips of white paper that are each ½ inch wide. Tape the ends of the strips together to make one long strip that is at least 72 inches long. Save the long strip of paper for Day 2.

Key Idea: Phidippides was a famous runner.

Storytime   T

Choose one of the following read aloud options:

 Archimedes and the Door... p. 24-32

Read at least one mystery for the next 8 days of plans.

After the reading, students will give a detailed oral narration. Select one paragraph from the story to read out loud to the students. This will be the starting point for the narration. Set a timer for 3-5 minutes. When the timer rings the narration is over, even if it isn't complete. A detailed, descriptive narration is the goal. See *Narration Tips* in the Appendix as needed.

Key Idea: Use oral narration to retell the story.

Bible Quiet Time   I

Bible Reading: Choose one option below.

The Illustrated Family Bible p. 212-215
Optional extension: p. 207

Your own Bible: Luke 1:1-38

Scripture Focus: Highlight Luke 1:30-33.

Prayer Focus: Pray a prayer of adoration to worship and honor God. Begin by reading the highlighted verses out loud as a prayer. End by praying, *I give you praise and adoration for your Son Jesus, who left the splendors of heaven to dwell on earth. Thank you that His kingdom will never end.*

Scripture Memory: Recite Philippians 2:17.
Music: *Philippians 2* CD: Track 5 (verse 17)

Key Idea: Jesus is the promised Savior.

Independent History Study   I

Open your *Student Notebook* to Unit 19 – Box 7. Follow the directions from *Draw and Write Through History* p. 14-17 to draw a Greek soldier. You will color your drawing on Day 2.

Key Idea: The Greeks city-states often fought amongst themselves and eventually fought the Persians too.

Learning the Basics
Focus: Language Arts, Math, Geography, Bible, and Science

Bible Study $\boxed{T}$

Read aloud and discuss with the students the following pages:

 The Radical Book for Kids p. 138-141

Key Idea: In Bible times, the stars were used for navigation and for keeping track of the days and seasons. The constellations Pleiades, Ursa Major, Orion, and the Mazzaroth are mentioned in the book of Job. It is possible that the "star" that led the wise men to Bethlehem was actually a comet.

Language Arts $\boxed{S}$

Have students complete one studied dictation exercise (see Appendix for directions and passages).

Help students complete one lesson from the following reading program:

 Drawn into the Heart of Reading

Work with the students to complete **one** of the English options listed below:

⭐ *Building with Diligence:* Lesson 35

⭐ *Following the Plan:* Lesson 31

⭐ Your own grammar program

Key Idea: Practice language arts skills.

Poetry $\boxed{I}$

Open *Paint Like a Poet* to Lesson 15. Read aloud the poem *"The Birthplace"*. On a 3 x 5 index card, neatly copy in black ink or in pencil the following highlighted lines from the poem:

Here further up the mountain slope
Than there was ever any hope,
My father built, enclosed a spring,
Strung chains of wall round everything,
Subdued the growth of earth to grass,
And brought our various lives to pass.
                              -Robert Frost

Check your work to make sure it is correctly copied. Then, cut around your copywork. You may choose to outline the edge of the cut-out with a light gray marker. Save it for Day 3.

Key Idea: Read and appreciate classic poetry.

Math Exploration $\boxed{S}$

Choose **one** of the math options listed below.

⭐ *Singapore Primary Mathematics 4A/4B* or *5A/5B* (see Appendix for schedules), or *Math with Confidence,* or *Apologia Math*

⭐ Your own math program

Key Idea: Use a step-by-step math program.

Science Exploration $\boxed{I}$

⭐ Read *Plant Life in Field and Garden* p. 1 -4. Today, you will begin a book about plants in your area. You will add to this book for the next 4 units. You may make your book either by adding a "Plants" section to your hardcover "Tracks" and "Birds" book, or you may make a paper book for "Plants" similar to the one described in Unit 2 – Day 1. At the top of a clean page in your book, copy Genesis 1:11 in cursive. Beneath the verse, sketch the Shepherd's Purse shown on p. 3. Color your sketch and label it. You may also like to refer to www.wikipedia.org to see a photograph of the Shepherd's Purse. To see a photograph, type "Shepherd's Purse" in the "Search" feature at www.wikipedia.org. Click on the picture to make it larger. You may choose to write a few facts under your sketch. Does the Shepherd's Purse grow where you live?

Key Idea: Plants have roots, a stem, leaves, flowers, and seed-boxes. The *stock* is the place where the leaves join the stem. The Shepherd's Purse is a weed that has seed-pods.

Reading about History   I

Read about history in the following resource:

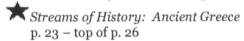 *Streams of History: Ancient Greece* p. 23 – top of p. 26

You will be choosing a portion from today's reading that you found memorable or worthy of being reread to copy. Open your *Student Notebook* to Unit 19. In Box 4, carefully copy in cursive the portion from today's reading that you selected. Then, compare your written work to the original. Last, draw a small colorful picture in Box 4 to illustrate your sentences.

Key Idea: In the hundreds of years after Homer, Greece changed in many ways.

Storytime   T

Choose one of the following read aloud options:

⭐ *Archimedes and the Door...* p. 33-38

⭐ Read aloud the next portion of the mystery that you selected.

After reading, work with the students to plan a 3 minute skit with simple props to act out part of today's reading. Set a timer for 3 minutes to quickly prepare for the skit. Make sure that you participate in the skit along with the students. When the timer rings, set it again for 3 minutes and perform the skit. You do not need an audience, as the goal is the retelling.

Key Idea: Use a skit to retell part of the story.

History Project   S

Get the long slip of paper that you made on Day 1. Wrap the long strip of paper in a spiral around a rolling pin. As you wind, make sure the edges of the paper touch, but do not overlap. Tape the top and bottom ends of the paper strip to the rolling pin. Lay the rolling pin horizontally on a table. Write the message by going across placing one letter on each strip. Leave a strip blank between words. Each time you reach the end of the rolling pin, start over on the left side of the row beneath. Write the following message Phidippides carried: *Men of Sparta, the Athenians ask you to help them and not to stand by while the most ancient city of Greece is crushed and subdued by a foreign invader; for even now Eretria has been enslaved, and Greece is the weaker for the loss of one fine city.* When your message is complete, unwind the paper. Save it for Day 3.

Key Idea: Greece is richer and stronger now.

Bible Quiet Time   I

Reading: Choose one option below.

⭐ *The Illustrated Family Bible* p. 216-217

⭐ Your own Bible: Luke 1:39-80

Scripture Focus: Highlight Luke 1:66.

Prayer Focus: Pray a prayer of confession to admit or acknowledge your sins to God. Begin by reading the highlighted verse out loud as a prayer. End by praying, *I confess that I wonder sometimes what I will grow up to be. I pray for your hand to be with me as I...*

Scripture Memory: Recite Philippians 2:17.
Music: *Philippians 2* CD: Track 5 (verse 17)

Key Idea: It was evident that God's hand was with John the Baptist. Zechariah prophecied that John would prepare the way for the Savior.

Independent History Study   I

Open your *Student Notebook* to Unit 19 – Box 7. Use *Draw and Write Through History* p. 18 as a guide to color your sketch of the Greek soldier. You may finish coloring on Day 3, if needed.

Key Idea: The Greeks wanted to rule themselves and were willing to fight for their freedom from Persia.

Geography [T]

Go to the website link listed on p. 6 of *A Child's Geography Vol. II*. At the link, select "History & Geography". Then, under "Knowledge Quest" select ACG2-Extra Activities". Print the "Travel Log Template" of your choice from p. 39-42. Also at the link, for older students, print and assign the "Chapter Eight Review" on p. 75.

Assign all students the following page:

 A Child's Geography Vol. II p. 111
Note: Do only the "Travel Notes" section. The "Books" and "Poetry" on p. 112 are optional.

Key Idea: Share three sights from Egypt.

Poetry [I]

Open *Paint Like a Poet* to Lesson 15. Read aloud the poem *"The Birthplace"* by Robert Frost.

Today, you will be painting a mountain backdrop. You will need painting paper, a palette, water, a small flat paintbrush, a pencil, and blue, grey, green, and white paint.

After gathering your supplies, turn to the "Step-by-Step Watercolor Tutorial" for Lesson 15 in *Paint Like a Poet*. Follow steps 1-3 to complete "Part One: Mountain Backdrop". Then, let your background dry. You will complete "Part Two" of the tutorial on Day 3.

Key Idea: Use painting to illustrate poetry.

Language Arts [S]

Help students complete one lesson from the following reading program:

 *Drawn into the Heart of Reading*

Work with the students to complete **one** of the writing options listed below:

 Writing & Rhetoric Book 1: Fable p. 127-129 (Note: Read aloud the text while the students follow along. Then, discuss. You will finish the rest of "Writing Time" on Day 3.)

 Your own writing program

Key Idea: Practice language arts skills.

Math Exploration [S]

Choose **one** of the math options listed below.

 Singapore Primary Mathematics 4A/4B or *5A/5B* (see Appendix for schedules), or *Math with Confidence*, or *Apologia Math*

Your own math program

Key Idea: Use a step-by-step math program.

Science Exploration [I]

Read *Plant Life in Field and Garden* p. 5-8. Orally retell or narrate to an adult the portion of text that you read today. Use the *Narration Tips* in the Appendix for help as needed.

Key Idea: Plants make their own food. The leaves need sunshine and air to do the work of making food, which is called photosynthesis. Plants take in carbon dioxide and give off oxygen. A plant's leaves are carefully arranged on its stem to be able to get needed light and air. It is interesting to study different plants to see how their leaves grow upon the stem.

Learning through History
Focus: The Greeks Resist the Persians

Reading about History | I |

Read about history in the following resource:

★ *Streams of History: Ancient Greece*
p. 26 – middle p. 29

You will be adding to your timeline in your *Student Notebook* today. In Unit 19 – Box 1, draw and color a burning torch. Label it, *First Olympic Games in Olympia, Greece (776 B.C.)*. In Box 2, draw and color a stone tablet. Label it, *Solon's laws reform Athens (593 B.C.)*. In Box 3, draw and color a sword. Label it, *Battle of Marathon (Greeks win) and Battle of Thermopylae (Persians win – 490 B.C.)*.

Key Idea: Some of the Grecian cities revolted.

Storytime | T |

Choose one of the following read aloud options:

★ *Archimedes and the Door...* p. 39-46

★ Read aloud the next portion of the mystery that you selected.

After the reading, students will give a summary oral narration. The oral narration must be no longer than 5 sentences and should summarize the reading. As students narrate, have them hold up one finger for each sentence shared. Remind students that the focus should be on the big ideas, rather than on the details.

Key Idea: Summarize the story by narrating.

History Project | S |

Phidippides ran 150 miles from Athens to Sparta in 2 days! Each mile equals 5,280 feet. Use a measuring tape to measure 52' 8" in an open area of your home or yard. Place a piece of masking tape at the start and finish points of your measurement. Place the scytale message you wrote yesterday in a pocket, pouch, or purse to carry with you. To get a feel for how far Phidippides ran, run back and forth between your start and finish points 100 times. You have now run 1 mile. To equal the distance Phidippides ran, you would need to run the same distance 149 more times! Choose someone to be a Spartan reading your message. Give both the message and the rolling pin used when writing the message to the Spartan. After reading the message, have the Spartan say, *It is against our law to battle before the moon is full.*

Key Idea: Athens and Eretria burned Sardis.

Bible Quiet Time | I |

Reading: Choose one option below.

★ *The Illustrated Family Bible* p. 218-221

★ Your own Bible: Luke 2:1-20

Scripture Focus: Highlight Luke 2:10-11.

Prayer Focus: Pray a prayer of thanksgiving to express gratitude for God's divine goodness. Begin by reading the highlighted verse out loud as a prayer. End by praying, *Through Scripture, I feel the joy that your birth meant for all people. I'm so thankful that you arrived just as God promised, and I thank you for being my Savior!*

Scripture Memory: Recite Philippians 2:17.
Music: *Philippians 2* CD: Track 5 (verse 17)

Key Idea: The angels brought the good news of the Savior's birth to shepherds on the hillside.

Independent History Study | I |

★ Listen to *What in the World?* Disc 3, Track 4: "The Persian Empire". Then, open your *Student Notebook* to Unit 19- Box 7. Finish coloring your drawing from Day 2, if needed.

Key Idea: When the Greeks burned the Persian city of Sardis, Darius decided to punish them at Marathon.

Learning the Basics
Focus: Language Arts, Math, Geography, Bible, and Science

Bible Study   T

Read aloud and discuss with the students the following pages:

 The Radical Book for Kids p. 142-146 (Note: The recipe on p. 144 is optional.)

<u>Key Idea</u>: In Old Testament times, God made rules for His people about what they could and could not eat. These rules set His people apart from the pagan nations that surrounded them. After Jesus' sacrifice on the cross, anyone who turns to Christ in faith is made clean from the inside out. His sacrifice changed all the Old Testament laws about food. As a result, all food is considered clean.

Language Arts   S

Have students complete one dictation exercise. (see Appendix for directions and passages).

Work with the students to complete **one** of the writing options listed below:

★ *Writing & Rhetoric Book 1: Fable* p. 130-132 (Note: Guide students through the lesson, so they are successful writing a fable. Read aloud the example from the Teacher's Guide p. 131 for help.)

★ Your own writing program

<u>Key Idea</u>: Practice language arts skills.

Poetry   I

Open *Paint Like a Poet* to Lesson 15. Read aloud the poem *"The Birthplace"* by Robert Frost.

Get the mountain backdrop that you painted on Day 2. Today, you will be adding mountain ridges and trees. You will need a palette, water, a small round paintbrush, and white, green, and blue paint.

After gathering your supplies, turn to the "Step-by-Step Watercolor Tutorial" for Lesson 15 in *Paint Like a Poet*. Follow steps 4-6 to complete "Part Two: Mountain Ridges and Trees". When your painting is dry, glue your poetry copywork from Day 1 to your painting. Store your completed artwork in the place you have chosen for it.

<u>Key Idea</u>: Explore poetry moods with painting.

Math Exploration   S

Choose **one** of the math options listed below.

★ *Singapore Primary Mathematics 4A/4B or 5A/5B* (see Appendix for schedules), or *Math with Confidence*, or *Apologia Math*

★ Your own math program

<u>Key Idea</u>: Use a step-by-step math program.

Science Exploration   I

★ Read *Plant Life in Field and Garden* p. 9-13. Write the answer to each numbered question on lined paper. You do not need to copy the question. Use the listed page to help you answer each question.

1. Draw a flower according to the description on p. 9, and label the *sepals, calyx, petals, corolla, stamens, anthers,* and *ovary.* (p. 9)
2. List a vegetable of which we eat the roots, one of which we eat the leaves, and one of which we eat the flowers. (p. 10)
3. Tell about the Turnip Flea-beetle. (p. 10-12)
4. Write the words *weevil* and *gall* and give their definitions. (p. 12)
5. In Deuteronomy 28:38-39, what curses does God give as a consequence for Israel's sin?

<u>Key Idea</u>: The Orange Saw-fly, Flea-beetle, rabbit, mouse, and Flower-beetle love to eat the turnip.

Reading about History | I |

Read about history in the following resource:

★ *Streams of History: Ancient Greece*
p. 29 – middle of p. 32

You will be writing a narration about part of the chapter *The Youth of Greece and Her Struggles for Liberty,* which is today's history reading.

To prepare for writing your narration, think about the questions below. If you do not know the answers, find them on p. 29-32 of *Streams of History: Ancient Greece.* Ask yourself a few guided questions such as, *How did it happen that the Greeks ended up with a large fleet of ships? What was the difference between the Greek soldiers and the Persian soldiers? Describe Xerxes' army.*

After you have thought about the answers to the questions, turn to Unit 19 in your *Student Notebook.* In Box 5, write a 5-8 sentence narration. When you have finished writing, read your sentences out loud to catch any mistakes.

Check for the following things: *Did you include **who** the reading was mainly about? Did you include **what** important thing(s) happened? Did you include **how** it ended? If not, add those things.*

Then, underline or highlight the main idea sentence in the narration. Use the *Written Narration Skills* in the Appendix as a guide for editing the narration.

<u>Key Idea:</u> After the Persians were defeated at Marathon, Darius began preparing for another battle with Greece. After his death, his son Xerxes carried out his plans and led the army.

Storytime | T |

Choose one of the following read aloud options:

★ *Archimedes and the Door...* p. 47-53

★ Read aloud the next part of the mystery.

After the reading, have each person get a Bible and open it anywhere in Proverbs. Explain, *We will have 5 minutes to skim through the verses in Proverbs to find any connections to today's story. When a connection is found, read the verse out loud and quickly share the connection. At the end of 5 minutes, anyone who has not shared yet must read aloud one verse and make the best connection possible.*

<u>Key Idea:</u> Seek God's word for His guidance.

Bible Quiet Time | I |

Reading: Choose one option below.

★ *The Illustrated Family Bible* p. 222-225

★ Your own Bible: Luke 2:21-40

Scripture Focus: Highlight Luke 2:30-32.

Prayer Focus: Pray a prayer of supplication to make a humble and earnest request of God. Begin by reading the highlighted verses out loud as a prayer. End by praying, *Help me recognize how blessed I am to be included in your saving grace along with your chosen people the Israelites. Guide me to understand the blessing of salvation through Christ Jesus.*

Scripture Memory: Copy Philippians 2:17 in your Common Place Book.
Music: *Philippians 2* CD: Track 5 (verse 17)

<u>Key Idea:</u> Jesus is the promised Savior.

Independent History Study | I |

★ Listen to *What in the World?* Disc 3, Track 5: "Xerxes". Open your *Student Notebook* to Unit 19. In Box 6, copy in cursive Daniel 11:2.

<u>Key Idea:</u> Xerxes was the son of Darius. Upon Darius' death, Xerxes became king of Persia.

Learning the Basics
Focus: Language Arts, Math, Geography, Bible, and Science

Geography [T]

Read aloud to the students the following pages:

 A Child's Geography Vol. II p. 113-117

Discuss with the students "Field Notes" p. 118.

<u>Key Idea</u>: The mouth of the Nile River empties into the Mediterranean Sea. As the river deposits sand and soil that it has carried from upriver, a delta is formed. This is one of the world's largest deltas. The Israelites made their Exodus out of the Nile Delta area.

Language Arts [S]

Have students complete one dictation exercise.

Guide students to complete one reading lesson.

★ *Drawn into the Heart of Reading*

Help students complete **one** English lesson.

★ *Building with Diligence:* Lesson 36 (Half)

★ *Following the Plan:* Lesson 32

★ Your own grammar program

<u>Key Idea</u>: Practice language arts skills.

Poetry [I]

Open *Paint Like a Poet* to Lesson 15. Today, you will be performing a poetry reading of *"The Birthplace"*. Practice reading the poem aloud with expression that matches the mood of the poem. Then, read the poem aloud in front of your chosen audience.

At the end of the reading, share the following, *When I read this poem by Robert Frost, it made me think of...* Call on your audience to share what thoughts the poem brought to their minds. Last, say, *Did you know that before his son, Eliott, died, Robert was attending college at Harvard? Robert became ill and didn't finish. He left Harvard to move to a farm in Derry, New Hampshire that Grandfather Frost purchased for Robert and his family.*

<u>Key Idea</u>: Share the poetry of Robert Frost.

Math Exploration [S]

Choose **one** of the math options listed below.

★ *Singapore Primary Mathematics 4A/4B* or *5A/5B* (see Appendix for schedules), or *Math with Confidence*, or *Apologia Math*

★ Your own math program

<u>Key Idea</u>: Use a step-by-step math program.

Science Exploration [I]

★ Read *Plant Life in Field and Garden* p. 14-17. Turn to the science experiment section in your science binder or sketchbook. At the top of a blank page, write: *How do plants absorb and transport the nutrients they need?* Under the question, write: *'Guess'*. Write down your guess. Do one of the following experiments. **Experiment 1:** Fill two glasses partway full with water. Label one glass "sweet" and one glass "plain". Add 4 tsp. of sugar to the "sweet" glass and stir. Place one pale, inner stalk of celery with leaves in each glass. Wait 2 days. Then, taste the leaves from each celery stalk. What do you notice? **Experiment 2:** Fill one glass partway full with water. Add several drops of green food coloring. Tightly roll a paper towel into a cylinder and tape it. Use your scissors to slit the bottom of the cylinder in 4 spots, and fan out the cut pieces to be the roots. Then, slit the top edges of the cylinder and fold back the top layers of towel to be flower petals. Leave a center stem to be the pistil. Place the paper towel flower in the green water, fanning out the bottom roots. What do you see? Next, on the paper write: *'Procedure'*. Draw a picture of the experiment. At the bottom of the paper, write: *'Conclusion'*. Explain what you learned.

<u>Key Idea</u>: Through tiny xylem tubes, water and nutrients move up the plant stem and out to the leaf cells.

Learning through History
Focus: The Golden Age of Greece

Reading about History | I

Read about history in the following resource:

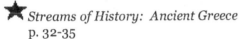★ *Streams of History: Ancient Greece* p. 32-35

The Greeks and the Persians fought a famous battle at Thermopylae. Where could you look to research more about the **Battle of Thermopylae**? Use an online resource like www.wikipedia.org or a reference book.

Answer one or more of the following questions from your research: *What event led up to the Battle of Thermopylae? Who led the Persian army at this time? Who led the Greek army during this battle? How long did the battle last? Why was this such a famous battle? How were the Greeks betrayed? How did the battle end? After the Battle of Thermopylae which famous battle came next? What happened at the Battle of Salamis?*

Key Idea: The Spartan king Leonidas and a small army of Greeks held off the Persian army.

History Project | S

In this unit you will make a Greek style column. Look at p. 45 of *Draw and Write Through History* to see the 3 orders or types of Greek columns. Then, open your *Student Notebook* to Unit 20. Look at Boxes 7-9 for a more detailed view of the capitals, or tops, of the 3 types of columns. Choose one column to sketch on a 9" x 12" piece of white paper. Then, cut the column out, trace around it, and make a second column that looks just like the first one.

Key Idea: Athens was burned by the Persians.

Storytime | T

Choose one of the following read aloud options:

★ *Archimedes and the Door...* p. 54-61

★ Read at least one mystery for the next 4 days of plans.

After the reading, students will give a detailed oral narration. Select one paragraph from the story to read out loud to the students. This will be the starting point for the narration. Set a timer for 3-5 minutes. When the timer rings the narration is over, even if it isn't complete. A detailed, descriptive narration is the goal. See *Narration Tips* in the Appendix as needed.

Key Idea: Use oral narration to retell the story.

Bible Quiet Time | I

Bible Reading: Choose one option below.

★ *The Illustrated Family Bible* p. 226-227

★ Your own Bible: Luke 2:41-52

Scripture Focus: Highlight Luke 2:46-47.

Prayer Focus: Pray a prayer of adoration to worship and honor God. Begin by reading the highlighted verses out loud as a prayer. End by praying, *I am in awe of you Jesus, all throughout Scripture. Even as a boy, people were surprised by your understanding and your answers. You are truly amazing, Lord!*

Scripture Memory: Recite Philippians 2:18.
Music: *Philippians 2* CD: Track 5 (vs. 17-18)

Key Idea: Even when Jesus was a young boy, people were amazed at His wisdom.

Independent History Study | I

★ Listen to *What in the World?* Disc 3, Track 6: "Daniel's Vision". Then, open your *Student Notebook* to Unit 20. In Box 6, copy in cursive the **first** paragraph of p. 28 from *Draw and Write Through History*.

Key Idea: Daniel had prophecied the fall of the Persian Empire and the rise of Greece 200 years earlier.

Learning the Basics
Focus: Language Arts, Math, Geography, Bible, and Science

Bible Study [T]

Read aloud and discuss with the students the following pages:

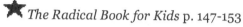 *The Radical Book for Kids* p. 147-153

Key Idea: John Huss, Martin Luther, and John Bunyan were all men who served Christ with their lives. Huss was martyred for his faith. Luther discovered he was saved through Christ's grace alone. Bunyan's heart was changed through Luther's commentary on Galatians. Later, Bunyan was jailed for preaching and wrote *Pilgirm's Progress* in jail.

Language Arts [S]

Have students complete one studied dictation exercise (see Appendix for directions and passages).

Help students complete one lesson from the following reading program:

★ *Drawn into the Heart of Reading*

Work with the students to complete **one** of the English options listed below:

★ *Building with Diligence:* Lesson 36 (Half)

★ *Following the Plan:* Lesson 33

★ Your own grammar program

Key Idea: Practice language arts skills.

Poetry [I]

Open *Paint Like a Poet* to Lesson 16. Read aloud the poem *"Lodged"*. On a 3 x 5 index card, neatly copy in black ink or in pencil the following highlighted lines from the poem:

The rain to the wind said,
'You push and I'll pelt.'
They so smote the garden bed
That the flowers actually knelt,
And lay lodged, though not dead.
I know how the flowers felt.
-Robert Frost

Check your work to make sure it is correctly copied. Then, cut around your copywork. You may choose to outline the edge of the cut-out with a red marker. Save it for Day 3.

Key Idea: Read and appreciate a variety of classic poetry.

Math Exploration [S]

Choose **one** of the math options listed below.

★ *Singapore Primary Mathematics 4A/4B or 5A/5B* (see Appendix for schedules), or *Math with Confidence,* or *Apologia Math*

★ Your own math program

Key Idea: Use a step-by-step math program.

Science Exploration [I]

★ Read *Plant Life in Field and Garden* p. 18-23. Get your book about plants that you began in unit 19. At the top of the next page in your book, copy in cursive 1 Corinthians 15:37-38. Beneath the verse, you will be making sketches of 3 flowers. First, sketch and label the Buttercup shown on p. 18. Second, sketch and label one of the diagrams of the Primrose shown on p. 19. Third, sketch and label one of the diagrams of the Dandelion shown on p. 22. If you wish to see the many different species of Buttercups, Primroses, and Dandelions, you can see full-color photographs of these flowers at www.gardenia.net. To find photographs of these flowers, type the name of the wildflower in the "Search" feature at www.gardenia.net. You may click on the picture to see a larger image of the flower.

Key Idea: Seeds are formed within the flowers of the plant. Each flower's seed box, or ovary, is protected.

Learning through History
Focus: The Golden Age of Greece

Reading about History | I |

Read about history in the following resource:

 Streams of History: Ancient Greece
p. 36 – top of p. 40

You will be choosing a portion from today's reading that you found memorable or worthy of being reread to copy. Open your *Student Notebook* to Unit 20. In Box 4, carefully copy in cursive the portion from today's reading that you selected. Then, compare your written work to the original. Last, draw a small colorful picture in Box 4 to illustrate your sentences.

<u>Key Idea</u>: After the Battle of Salamis, the Athenians rebuilt their city with the help of the cities that surrounded them. Pericles helped make Athens great. This was known as the Golden Age of Athens.

Storytime | T |

Choose one of the following read aloud options:

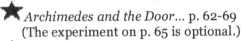 *Archimedes and the Door...* p. 62-69
(The experiment on p. 65 is optional.)

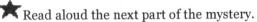 Read aloud the next part of the mystery.

After reading, give students a few minutes to prepare a short advertisement speech for the book. During the speech, students should hold up the book and say the book title and the name of the author. The wording of the advertisement should provide a peek into the book without giving away the ending. The goal should be for listeners to feel like they've "Got to Have This Book"!

<u>Key Idea</u>: Use an ad speech to share the story.

History Project | S |

Get the two Greek columns that you made on Day 1. Use a thin, brown watercolor marker to carefully outline the columns along the pencil lines. Then, dip a fine-tipped paintbrush in water and lightly paint over your column, blurring the edges of the marker's outline to make the column look old. Lay your columns flat to dry for Day 3.

<u>Key Idea</u>: The Golden Age of Greece lasted around 50 years. During that time, many beautiful buildings were built in Athens. You can still visit the ruins of these buildings today. These include the Acropolis, the columnade with gateways called the Propylaea, and the Parthenon to name a few.

Bible Quiet Time | I |

Reading: Choose one option below.

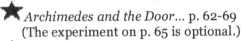 *The Illustrated Family Bible* p. 228-229

Your own Bible: Luke 3:1-23

Scripture Focus: Highlight Luke 3:15-16.

Prayer Focus: Pray a prayer of confession to admit or acknowledge your sins to God. Begin by reading the highlighted verses out loud as a prayer. End by praying, *I confess that without faith in your word, it is easy to wonder about Christ and about my salvation. I ask for the calm, faithful assurance that comes from the Holy Spirit.*

Scripture Memory: Recite Philippians 2:18.
Music: *Philippians 2* CD: Track 5 (vs. 17-18)

<u>Key Idea</u>: John prepared the way for Christ.

Independent History Study | I |

Open your *Student Notebook* to Unit 20 – Box 10. Follow the directions from *Draw and Write Through History* p. 11-13 (through step 6) to draw the Parthenon. You will color your drawing on Day 3.

<u>Key Idea</u>: The Parthenon was built to honor the goddess Athena and included many carvings by Phidias.

Learning the Basics
Focus: Language Arts, Math, Geography, Bible, and Science

Geography   [T]

Read aloud to the students the following pages:

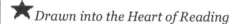 *A Child's Geography Vol. II* p. 118 (second column) – p. 123

Discuss with the students "Field Notes" p. 123.

<u>Key Idea</u>: The Western Desert covers two-thirds of Egypt. It is part of the Sahara Desert. In the desert, travelers go from oasis to oasis. The desert's colors change as you travel from the Black Desert to the White Desert. The colors change again as you cross the Great Sand Sea with its field of silica glass.

Language Arts   [S]

Help students complete one lesson from the following reading program:

★ *Drawn into the Heart of Reading*

Work with the students to complete **one** of the writing options listed below:

★ *Writing & Rhetoric Book 1: Fable* p. 133 – middle of p. 137 (Note: Read aloud the text while the students follow along. Then, discuss.)

★ Your own writing program

<u>Key Idea</u>: Practice language arts skills.

Poetry   [I]

Open *Paint Like a Poet* to Lesson 16. Read aloud the poem *"Lodged"* by Robert Frost.

Today, you will be painting a rainy backdrop. You will need painting paper, a palette, water, a large flat paintbrush, and blue and grey paint.

After gathering your supplies, turn to the "Step-by-Step Watercolor Tutorial" for Lesson 16 in *Paint Like a Poet*. Follow steps 1-3 to complete "Part One: Rainy Backdrop". Then, let your background dry. You will complete "Part Two" of the tutorial on Day 3.

<u>Key Idea</u>: Use painting to illustrate poetry.

Math Exploration   [S]

Choose **one** of the math options listed below.

★ *Singapore Primary Mathematics 4A/4B* or *5A/5B* (see Appendix for schedules), or *Math with Confidence,* or *Apologia Math*

★ Your own math program

<u>Key Idea</u>: Use a step-by-step math program.

Science Exploration   [I]

★ Read *Plant Life in Field and Garden* p. 24-29. Orally retell or narrate to an adult the portion of text that you read today. Use the *Narration Tips* in the Appendix for help as needed.

<u>Key Idea</u>: Unless pollen grows down into the ovary, or seed-box, plants cannot make seeds. In return for honey from the plants, bees and insects carry the pollen from one flower to another. Some flowers, like the "Parson-in-the-pulpit", shut the flies in until their dust-flags burst open, and the stamens and hairs wither away. Then, the flies can get out again.

Reading about History [I]

Read about history in the following resource:

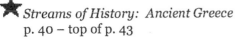 ⭐ *Streams of History: Ancient Greece* p. 40 – top of p. 43

You will be adding to your timeline in your *Student Notebook* today. In Unit 20 – Box 1, draw and color a sword. Label it, *Battle of Salamis (Greeks win - 480 B.C.)*. In Box 2, draw and color a golden pillar. Label it, *Pericles rules during the Golden Age of Athens (461-429 B.C.)*. In Box 3, draw and color the Parthenon. Label it, *Parthenon is built and dedicated to Athena (438 B.C.)*.

Key Idea: Socrates was a famous Greek philosopher who lived during the Golden Age.

Storytime [T]

Choose one of the following read aloud options:

⭐ *Archimedes and the Door...* p. 70-80

⭐ Read aloud the next portion of the mystery that you selected.

After the reading, students will give a summary oral narration. The oral narration must be no longer than 5 sentences and should summarize the reading. As students narrate, have them hold up one finger for each sentence shared. Remind students that the focus should be on the big ideas, rather than on the details.

Key Idea: Summarize the story by narrating.

History Project [S]

Get the two Greek columns that you painted on Day 2. You will be taping these two columns together to make one 3-dimensional column. Place the two columns back-to-back with the painted side of each column facing out. Then, use clear tape to tape the columns together down the sides, leaving the tops and bottoms of the columns untaped.

Gently squeeze the sides of the columns to cause an empty space in the center of the column. In this empty space in center of the column, stuff tightly wadded up tissues or paper towels to make the column puff out 3-dimensionally. Bend the top, or the capital of your column, slightly out.

Key Idea: The boys in Athens were sent to a gymnasium outside Athens each day. These gymnasiums were designed to be beautiful.

Bible Quiet Time [I]

Reading: Choose one option below.

⭐ *The Illustrated Family Bible* p. 230-231

⭐ Your own Bible: Luke 4:1-13, 37

Scripture Focus: Highlight Luke 3:21-22.

Prayer Focus: Pray a prayer of thanksgiving to express gratitude for God's divine goodness. Begin by reading the highlighted verses out loud as a prayer. End by praying, *God, thank you for showing us that Jesus is your Son. I see all three parts of you in these verses, as the Father speaks, the Son is baptized, and the Holy Spirit descends like a dove.*

Scripture Memory: Recite Philippians 2:18.
Music: *Philippians 2* CD: Track 5 (vs. 17-18)

Key Idea: Jesus is God's only Son.

Independent History Study [I]

Open your *Student Notebook* to Unit 20 – Box 10. Use *Draw and Write Through History* p. 13 (step 7) as a guide to color your sketch of the Parthenon. You may finish coloring on Day 4, if needed.

Key Idea: The Parthenon overlooked the Acropolis and was built with Doric style columns.

Learning the Basics
Focus: Language Arts, Math, Geography, Bible, and Science

Bible Study [T]

Read aloud and discuss with the students the following pages:

 The Radical Book for Kids p. 154-155

Key Idea: God has a good plan for your family. Parents make mistakes, because they are sinners just like you. Often parents try to do their best, but no parent is perfect. If you need help or are in danger, you can talk to a doctor, a pastor, a teacher, or a school counselor. Flawed parents remind us that we need a perfect Father like our Father in heaven.

Language Arts [S]

Have students complete one studied dictation exercise (see Appendix for directions and passages).

Work with the students to complete **one** of the writing options listed below:

 Writing & Rhetoric Book 1: Fable p. 139-142 (Note: Omit bottom p. 137 – 138. Guide students through the lesson, so they are successful writing a fable from a different point of view. They may choose to be **either** the Grasshopper **or** the Ant.)

 Your own writing program

Key Idea: Practice language arts skills.

Poetry [I]

Open *Paint Like a Poet* to Lesson 16. Read aloud the poem *"Lodged"* by Robert Frost.

Get the rainy backdrop that you painted on Day 2. Today, you will be adding flowers and raindrops. You will need a palette, water, a small round paintbrush, and green, grey, and rose paint.

After gathering your supplies, turn to the "Step-by-Step Watercolor Tutorial" for Lesson 16 in *Paint Like a Poet*. Follow steps 4-6 to complete "Part Two: Flowers and Raindrops". When your painting is dry, glue your poetry copywork from Day 1 to your painting. Store your completed artwork in the place you have chosen for it.

Key Idea: Explore poetry moods with painting.

Math Exploration [S]

Choose **one** of the math options listed below.

 Singapore Primary Mathematics 4A/4B or *5A/5B* (see Appendix for schedules), or *Math with Confidence*, or *Apologia Math*

Your own math program

Key Idea: Use a step-by-step math program.

Science Exploration [I]

Read *Plant Life in Field and Garden* p. 30-34. Write the answer to each numbered question on lined paper. You do not need to copy the question. Use the listed page to help you answer each question.

1. Name two vegetables of which we eat the seeds and two of which we eat the fruit. (p. 30)
2. Draw and label the parts that the two different Vegetable Marrow flowers need for their seeds to grow. (p. 31)
3. Why does the Vegetable Marrow need bees and insects? (p. 32)
4. Which other vegetables have two kinds of flowers like the Marrow? (p. 32-33)
5. What promise does God make in Genesis 8:22 that shows He is in control of the plant life cycle?

Key Idea: Ripe seed-boxes are called fruit. We eat the seeds of some fruits and the whole fruit of others.

Reading about History | I |

Read about history in the following resource:

 Streams of History: Ancient Greece p. 43 – middle of p. 46

You will be writing a narration about part of the chapter *A Visit to Athens When Greece Was in Her Greatest Beauty,* which is part of today's history reading.

To prepare for writing your narration, choose to describe either an assembly meeting or the Greek theater. You may wish to look back over p. 43-46 of *Streams of History: Ancient Greece* to guide you as you write your narration.

After you have thought about which topic you will choose and how you will begin your narration, turn to Unit 20 in your *Student Notebook*. In Box 5, write a 5-8 sentence narration.

When you have finished writing, read your sentences out loud to catch any mistakes. Check for the following things: *Did you include **who** or **what topic** the reading was mainly about? Did you include **descriptors** of the important thing(s) that happened? Did you include a **closing sentence**? If not, add those things.*

Then, underline or highlight the main idea sentence in the narration.

Use the *Written Narration Skills* in the Appendix as a guide for editing the narration.

Key Idea: At the time of Pericles, Athens was a democracy. Citizens who were 18 or older met to vote and pass laws for their city. Another important Athenian pasttime was attending the theater. This was done in honor of their gods.

Storytime | T |

Choose one of the following read aloud options:

 Archimedes and the Door... p. 81-85

 Read aloud the next portion of the mystery that you selected.

After the reading, have each person get a Bible and open it anywhere in Proverbs. Explain, *We will have 5 minutes to skim through the verses in Proverbs to find any connections to today's story. When a connection is found, read the verse out loud and quickly share the connection. At the end of 5 minutes, anyone who has not shared yet must read aloud one verse and make the best connection possible.*

Key Idea: Seek God's word for His guidance.

Bible Quiet Time | I |

Reading: Choose one option below.

 The Illustrated Family Bible p. 234-235 Optional extension: p. 206

 Your own Bible: Luke 4:14-44

Scripture Focus: Highlight Luke 4:18-22.

Prayer Focus: Pray a prayer of supplication to make a humble and earnest request of God. Begin by reading the highlighted verses out loud as a prayer. End by praying, *Help me to recognize you as the fulfillment of Scripture and as my Savior. Help me not to miss seeing you as Lord, like those in your own hometown.*

Scripture Memory: Copy Philippians 2:18 in your Common Place Book.
Music: *Philippians 2* CD: Track 5 (vs. 17-18)

Key Idea: Jesus fulfilled the Scriptures.

Independent History Study | I |

 Listen to *What in the World?* Disc 3, Track 7: "Athens & Sparta".

Key Idea: Greece's Golden Age advanced architecture, medicine, philosophy, government, and science.

Learning the Basics

Focus: Language Arts, Math, Geography, Bible, and Science

Geography [T]

Have students get both the blank map and the labeled map of **Egypt, Iraq & Saudi Arabia** that they began in Unit 16.

Then, assign students the following page:

 A Child's Geography Vol. II p. 125

Note: Do only the "Map Notes" section. Then, save both the blank map and the labeled map of **Egypt, Iraq & Saudi Arabia** to use with the units on Iraq and Saudi Arabia.

<u>Key Idea</u>: Practice finding and recording the locations of various places on a map of Egypt.

Language Arts [S]

Have students complete one dictation exercise.

Guide students to complete one reading lesson.

 Drawn into the Heart of Reading

Help students complete **one** English lesson.

⭐ *Building with Diligence:* Lesson 37

⭐ *Following the Plan:* Lesson 34 (Half)

⭐ Your own grammar program

<u>Key Idea</u>: Practice language arts skills.

Poetry [I]

Open *Paint Like a Poet* to Lesson 16. Today, you will be performing a poetry reading of *"Lodged"*. Practice reading the poem aloud with expression that matches the mood of the poem. Then, read the poem aloud in front of your chosen audience.

At the end of the reading, share the following, *When I read this poem by Robert Frost, it made me think of...* Call on your audience to share what thoughts the poem brought to their minds. Last, say, *Did you know that Robert Frost's farm was a poultry farm? Along with raising chickens, he also had orchard trees. He continued to write poetry during his ten years on the farm. During this time, his mother died of cancer, and his daughter, Elinor Bettina, died shortly after birth.*

<u>Key Idea</u>: Share the poetry of Robert Frost.

Math Exploration [S]

Choose **one** of the math options listed below.

 Singapore Primary Mathematics 4A/4B or 5A/5B (see Appendix for schedules), or *Math with Confidence,* or *Apologia Math*

⭐ Your own math program

<u>Key Idea</u>: Use a step-by-step math program.

Science Exploration [I]

⭐ Read *Plant Life in Field and Garden* p. 35-38. Turn to the science experiment section in your science binder or sketchbook. At the top of a blank page, write: *Which parts of plants do you often eat?* Under the question, write: *'Guess'.* Write down your guess. Plan a "Plant Part Meal" or make a "Plant Part Salad". Try to use a vegetable from as many different plant parts as possible. **Seeds:** corn, peas, peanuts, sunflower seeds, lima beans, or pinto beans; **Roots:** carrots, radishes, turnips, or beets; **Stems:** celery, onions, asparagus, potatoes, or rhubarb; **Leaves:** cabbage, lettuce, spinach, collards, or brussel sprouts; **Fruits:** apple, orange, tomato, watermelon, strawberries, or blueberries; **Flowers:** broccoli, cauliflower, squash blossoms, or artichokes. Write your menu under the "Procedure" section of your lab sheet. Make sure to label each plant part. Serve your meal for lunch and have your guests try to guess which plant part each item represents. At the bottom of the paper, write: *'Conclusion'.* Explain what you learned.

<u>Key Idea</u>: We eat many different parts of plants each day. As plants grow, it's important to keep them free from enemies like creatures and insects who feed on the plants.

Learning through History
Focus: Alexander the Great Conquers Persia

Reading about History | I |

Read about history in the following resource:

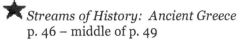 *Streams of History: Ancient Greece*
p. 46 – middle of p. 49

Olympia, Greece was the site of the first Olympic Games around 776 B.C. Where could you look to research more about **Olympia, Greece**? Use an online resource like www.wikipedia.org or a reference book.

Answer one or more of the following questions from your research: *Where was Olympia located? How often were the Olympic games held in Olympia? Who were the games honoring? Which of the Seven Wonders of the Ancient World was in Olympia? What was the hippodrome? Which buildings were part of the ancient Olympic site? How is the modern-day Olympic torch lit at Olympia?*

<u>Key Idea</u>: Olympia held the Olympic Games.

History Project | S |

In this unit you will have Olympic Game Trials with 2 events each day. Begin with prayer to honor the one true God. Place a piece of masking tape on the floor as a starting line. On paper, write the event "Shot Put". Number from 1-3 under the title. Stand behind the line and throw a cotton ball shot put as far as you can. Measure each throw from the starting line and record it on your paper. You have 3 trials. Next, write "Broad Jump" and number 1-3 beneath it. Stand behind the line and jump as far as you can with both feet together. Place a piece of tape where your back heel landed. Measure and record each trial. Save the paper.

<u>Key Idea</u>: The main contest was on the 3rd day.

Storytime | T |

Choose one of the following read aloud options:

 Archimedes and the Door... p. 86-91

Read at least one nonfiction book for the next 16 days of plans (see Appendix).

After the reading, students will give a detailed oral narration. Select one paragraph from the story to read out loud to the students. This will be the starting point for the narration. Set a timer for 3-5 minutes. When the timer rings the narration is over, even if it isn't complete. A detailed, descriptive narration is the goal. See *Narration Tips* in the Appendix as needed.

<u>Key Idea</u>: Use oral narration to retell the story.

Bible Quiet Time | I |

Bible Reading: Choose one option below.

The Illustrated Family Bible p. 240-241

Your own Bible: Luke 5:1-39

Scripture Focus: Highlight Luke 5:15-16.

Prayer Focus: Pray a prayer of adoration to worship and honor God. Begin by reading the highlighted verses out loud as a prayer. End by praying, *I praise you as the Lord who can heal and forgive sins. You know my needs and care for me so much. Help me to follow your example and spend time each day in prayer.*

Scripture Review: Philippians 2:1-18.
Music: *Philippians 2* CD: Tracks 1-5 (all)

<u>Key Idea</u>: Jesus is truly the Son of God.

Independent History Study | I |

Open your *Student Notebook* to Unit 21 – Box 7. Follow the directions from *Draw and Write Through History* p. 19-21 (through step 7) to draw Bucephalus. You will color your drawing on Day 2.

<u>Key Idea</u>: Alexander the Great's father, Philip II of Macedon, grew up in Greece and learned Greek ways.

Learning the Basics
Focus: Language Arts, Math, Geography, Bible, and Science

Bible Study $\boxed{\text{T}}$

Read aloud and discuss with the students the following pages:

 The Radical Book for Kids p. 156-157

<u>Key Idea</u>: In Bible times, the daytime hours were divided into twelve equal parts. The first hour began at sunrise and the last hour ended at sunset. The hours varied in length depending on the length of the daytime. Night was also divided into twelve equal parts. Midnight was at the end of the sixth hour. Sunrise signalled the end of the twelfth hour.

Language Arts $\boxed{\text{S}}$

Have students complete one studied dictation exercise (see Appendix for directions and passages).

Help students complete one lesson from the following reading program:

 Drawn into the Heart of Reading

Work with the students to complete **one** of the English options listed below:

 Building with Diligence: Lesson 38

 Following the Plan: Lesson 34 (Last half)

 Your own grammar program

<u>Key Idea</u>: Practice language arts skills.

Poetry $\boxed{\text{I}}$

Open *Paint Like a Poet* to Lesson 17. Read aloud the poem *"Acceptance"*. On a 3 x 5 index card, neatly copy in black ink or in pencil the following highlighted lines in the poem:

When the spent sun throws up its rays on cloud
And goes down burning into the gulf below,
No voice in nature is heard to cry aloud
At what has happened. Birds, at least must know...

      -Robert Frost

Check your work to make sure it is correctly copied. Then, cut around your copywork. You may choose to outline the edge of the cut-out with a yellow marker. Save it for Day 3.

<u>Key Idea</u>: Read and appreciate classic poetry.

Math Exploration $\boxed{\text{S}}$

Choose **one** of the math options listed below.

 Singapore Primary Mathematics 4A/4B or *5A/5B* (see Appendix for schedules), or *Math with Confidence,* or *Apologia Math*

 Your own math program

<u>Key Idea</u>: Use a step-by-step math program.

Science Exploration $\boxed{\text{I}}$

 Read *Plant Life in Field and Garden* p. 39-43. Get your book about plants that you began in unit 19. At the top of the next page in your book, copy in cursive Isaiah 40:8. Beneath the verse, choose one or more of the flowers shown on p. 42 to sketch. If you prefer, you may photocopy these flowers instead, and then glue them in your "Plants" book and color them. If you choose to color, refer to another source to make sure to color the flowers accurately. For each flower, draw an arrow pointing to the flower and describe the way it protects itself. You can see full-color photographs of the Ragged Robin and the Teasel at www.wikipedia.org. To find photographs of these flowers, type the name of the wildflower in the "Search" feature at www.wikipedia.org. You may click on the picture to see a larger image of each flower.

<u>Key Idea</u>: Flowers such as the Anemone, Buttercup, and Geranium have bitter leaves. Gorse has thorns on its stem. The Teasel collects rain in its "basin", which stop ants. Campions have sticky stems.

Learning through History
Focus: Alexander the Great Conquers Persia

Unit 21 - Day 2

Reading about History | I

Read about history in the following resource:

 Streams of History: Ancient Greece p. 50 – middle of p. 53

You will be choosing a portion from today's reading that you found memorable or worthy of being reread to copy. Open your *Student Notebook* to Unit 21. In Box 4, carefully copy in cursive the portion from today's reading that you selected. Then, compare your written work to the original. Last, draw a small colorful picture in Box 4 to illustrate your sentences.

Key Idea: Philip II grew up in Thebes. He returned to Macedonia to be king when his father died. Philip taught his soldiers to fight in a phalanx. He conquered Greece.

History Project | S

You will continue the Olympic Game Trials with 2 more events today. Begin with prayer to honor the one true God. Place a piece of masking tape on the floor as a starting line. On paper, write the event "Discus Throw". Number from 1-3 under the title. Stand behind the line and throw a paper plate discus as far as you can. Measure each throw from the starting line and record it on your paper. You have 3 trials. Next, write "High Jump" and number 1-3 beneath it. Stand next to a blank section of the wall. Holding a small piece of masking tape in your fingers, jump as high as you can, placing the tape on the wall when you jump. Measure from the floor to the tape mark and record each trial. Save the paper for Day 3.

Key Idea: The Greeks took pride in winning.

Storytime | T

Choose one of the following read aloud options:

 Archimedes and the Door... p. 92-98

Read aloud the next portion of the nonfiction book that you selected.

After reading, give each person a white piece of paper or a markerboard and a marker. Set a timer for 3-5 minutes and instruct each person to do a quick outline sketch about the story. Ideas for sketches include settings, characters, actions, important objects, or symbols. When the timer rings, briefly share the sketches.

Key Idea: Use sketching to share the story.

Bible Quiet Time | I

Reading: Choose one option below.

The Illustrated Family Bible p. 242

Your own Bible: Luke 6:1-26

Scripture Focus: Highlight Luke 6:5.

Prayer Focus: Pray a prayer of confession to admit or acknowledge your sins to God. Begin by reading the highlighted verse out loud as a prayer. End by praying, *I confess that I need to be more focused on you and less worried about what other people think. Help me to focus on you Lord when I...*

Scripture Review: Philippians 2:1-18.
Music: *Philippians 2* CD: Tracks 1-5 (all)

Key Idea: As Lord, Jesus is the Creator of the Sabbath. He rules over all things.

Independent History Study | I

Open your *Student Notebook* to Unit 21 – Box 7. Use *Draw and Write Through History* p. 21-22 (steps 8-9) as a guide to color your sketch of Bucephalus. You may finish coloring on Day 3, if needed.

Key Idea: When Philip's son Alexander was 13, he was able to tame a wild horse when he realized it was afraid of its own shadow. He named the horse Bucephalus and later rode him through many battles.

Learning the Basics
Focus: Language Arts, Math, Geography, Bible, and Science

Geography [T]

Go to the website link listed on p. 6 of *A Child's Geography Vol. II*. At the link, select "History & Geography". Then, under "Knowledge Quest" select ACG2-Extra Activities". Print the "Travel Log Template" of your choice from p. 39-42. Also at the link, for older students, print and assign the "Chapter Nine Review" on p. 76. Assign all students the following pages:

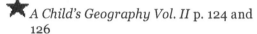 *A Child's Geography Vol. II* p. 124 and 126

Note: Do the "Travel Notes" section on p. 124 and the "Walk of Prayer" on p. 126. The "Food" section on p. 125 is an optional extra.

Key Idea: Share three sights from Egypt.

Language Arts [S]

Help students complete one lesson from the following reading program:

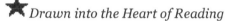 *Drawn into the Heart of Reading*

Work with the students to complete **one** of the writing options listed below:

⭐ *Writing & Rhetoric Book 2: Narrative I* p. 1 – bottom of p. 6 (Note: Today's text includes references to magic, Greek gods, and witches as examples from literature. Read aloud the text while the students follow along. Then, discuss.)

⭐ Your own writing program

Key Idea: Practice language arts skills.

Poetry [I]

Open *Paint Like a Poet* to Lesson 17. Read aloud the poem *"Acceptance"* by Robert Frost.

Today, you will be painting a sunset backdrop. You will need painting paper, a palette, water, a large flat paintbrush, a pencil, masking tape, and blue, orange, red, and white paint.

After gathering your supplies, turn to the "Step-by-Step Watercolor Tutorial" for Lesson 17 in *Paint Like a Poet*. Follow steps 1-3 to complete "Part One: Sunset Backdrop". Then, let your background dry. You will complete "Part Two" of the tutorial on Day 3.

Key Idea: Use painting to illustrate poetry.

Math Exploration [S]

Choose **one** of the math options listed below.

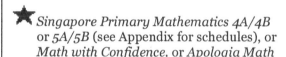 *Singapore Primary Mathematics 4A/4B or 5A/5B* (see Appendix for schedules), or *Math with Confidence,* or *Apologia Math*

⭐ Your own math program

Key Idea: Use a step-by-step math program.

Science Exploration [I]

⭐ Read *Plant Life in Field and Garden* p. 44-48. Orally retell or narrate to an adult the portion of text that you read today. Use the *Narration Tips* in the Appendix for help as needed.

Key Idea: Garden plants were once wild plants. They have been carefully tended so that their flowers are larger and more beautiful. Only the best seeds are sown the next year. The flowers have good soil and plenty of water, making it easier for the plants to produce more seeds. Pinks and carnations are part of the Pink Family of flowers. Ragged Robins and Campions are the wild flower version of the Pink Family.

Reading about History | I |

Read about history in the following resource:

★ *Streams of History: Ancient Greece*
p. 53 – middle of p. 57

You will be adding to your timeline in your *Student Notebook* today. In Unit 21 – Box 1, draw and color two crossed swords. Label it, *Athens vs. Sparta (Peloponnesian War 431-404 B.C.)*. In Box 2, draw and color a a long spear. Label it, *Philip II of Macedon gains control of Greece (338 B.C.)*. In Box 3, draw and color a knot. Label it, *Reign of Alexander the Great (336-323 B.C.)*

Key Idea: Alexander fought Darius and Persia.

Storytime | T |

Choose one of the following read aloud options:

★ *Archimedes and the Door...* p. 99-104

★ Read aloud the next portion of the nonfiction book that you selected.

After the reading, students will give a summary oral narration. The oral narration must be no longer than 5 sentences and should summarize the reading. As students narrate, have them hold up one finger for each sentence shared. Remind students that the focus should be on the big ideas, rather than on the details.

Key Idea: Summarize the story by narrating.

History Project | S |

You will complete the Olympic Game Trials with 2 more events today. Have an adult help you. Begin with prayer to honor the one true God. Place a piece of masking tape on the floor as a starting line. On paper, write the event "Javelin Toss". Number from 1-3 under the title. Stand behind the line and throw a drinking straw javelin as far as you can. Measure each throw from the starting line to the spot where the javelin first touched down and record it on your paper. You have 3 trials. Next, write "Long Jump" and number 1-3 beneath it. Take a running start from behind the line and jump as far as you can. Do not cross the line with your run. Place a piece of tape where your back heel landed. Measure and record each trial. Circle your best trial in each event. Which trial number was the best most often? Which event was your favorite?

Key Idea: The Greek games were every 4 years.

Bible Quiet Time | I |

Reading: Choose one option below.

★ *The Illustrated Family Bible* p. 244-247

★ Your own Bible: Luke 6:27-49

Scripture Focus: Highlight Matt. 6:31-34.

Prayer Focus: Pray a prayer of thanksgiving to express gratitude for God's divine goodness. Begin by reading the highlighted verses out loud as a prayer. End by praying, *Thank you for my food, drink, clothing, and my home. I know each one is a gift from you. Help me to seek your kingdom first and not to worry about gaining the riches of the earth instead.*

Scripture Review: Philippians 2:1-18.
Music: *Philippians 2* CD: Tracks 1-5 (all)

Key Idea: It is important to seek God first.

Independent History Study | I |

Open your *Student Notebook* to Unit 21. In Box 6, copy in cursive the **second** paragraph of p. 28 from *Draw and Write Through History*. Then, finish coloring your drawing in Box 7 if needed.

Key Idea: Alexander became king when he was 20 years old. He studied under the Greek Aristotle.

Learning the Basics
Focus: Language Arts, Math, Geography, Bible, and Science

Bible Study [T]

Read aloud and discuss with the students the following pages:

 The Radical for Kids p. 158-159

Key Idea: We can glimpse God's creativity through the things He has made. His invisible qualities, divine nature, and eternal power are reflected in His Creation. The Bible gives us an even clearer picture of God through Jesus Christ. Jesus shows us more clearly what God is like.

Language Arts [S]

Have students complete one studied dictation exercise (see Appendix for directions and passages).

Work with the students to complete **one** of the writing options listed below:

 Writing & Rhetoric Book 2: Narrative I bottom of p. 6-9 (Note: Omit "Myth of the Minotaur" bottom of p. 8 – top of p. 9. Guide students through the lesson as needed.)

 Your own writing program

Key Idea: Practice language arts skills.

Poetry [I]

Open *Paint Like a Poet* to Lesson 17. Read aloud the poem *"Acceptance"* by Robert Frost.

Get the sunset backdrop that you painted on Day 2. Today, you will be adding a sun, clouds, and water. You will need a palette, water, a small flat paintbrush, a toothpick, and yellow, red, purple, blue, and white paint.

Next, turn to the "Step-by-Step Watercolor Tutorial" for Lesson 17 in *Paint Like a Poet*. Follow steps 4-6 to complete "Part Two: Sun, Clouds, and Water". When your painting is dry, glue your poetry copywork from Day 1 to your painting. Store your completed artwork in the place you have chosen for it.

Key Idea: Explore poetry moods with painting.

Math Exploration [S]

Choose **one** of the math options listed below.

 Singapore Primary Mathematics 4A/4B or 5A/5B (see Appendix for schedules), or *Math with Confidence,* or *Apologia Math*

 Your own math program

Key Idea: Use a step-by-step math program.

Science Exploration [I]

 Read *Plant Life in Field and Garden* p. 49-53. Write the answer to each numbered question on lined paper. You do not need to copy the question. Use the listed pages to help you answer each question.
1. What is the difference between wild roses and garden roses? (p. 49)
2. List 10 or more fruits that belong to the Rose Family. (p. 50)
3. Describe the seed-boxes in a strawberry and a blackberry. (p. 52)
4. Draw the seed-boxes and the seeds inside an apple. (p. 52)
5. In Joshua 5:12, after the Passover when the manna ceased, what did the Israelites eat?

Key Idea: Many wonderful fruits come from the Rose Family. The seeds can be found within each fruit.

Reading about History | I |

Read about history in the following resource:

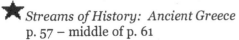 *Streams of History: Ancient Greece*
p. 57 – middle of p. 61

You will be writing a narration about part of the chapter *The Story of Alexander the Great,* which is part of today's history reading.

To prepare for writing your narration, think about the questions below. If you do not know the answers, find them on p. 57-61 of *Streams of History: Ancient Greece.* Ask yourself a few guided questions such as, *How did Alexander conquer Tyre in Phoenicia? What happened when Alexander faced King Darius? When Alexander entered Babylon, Susa and Persepolis, what did he do?*

After you have thought about the answers to the questions, turn to Unit 21 in your *Student Notebook.* In Box 5, write a 5-8 sentence narration. When you have finished writing, read your sentences out loud to catch any mistakes. Check for the following things: *Did you include **who** the reading was mainly about? Did you include **what** important thing(s) happened? Did you include **how** it ended? If not, add those things.* Then, underline or highlight the main idea sentence in the narration. Use the *Written Narration Skills* in the Appendix as a guide for editing the narration.

Key Idea: Alexander was victorious over Darius and the Persians. Next, he beseiged the Phoenician city of Tyre by building a road to the island. Then, the soldiers battered the walls until they broke through and conquered the city. He moved on to Egypt next and built the city of Alexandria. Then, he headed for the Persian capitals of Babylon, Susa, and Persepolis.

Storytime | T |

Choose one of the following read aloud options:

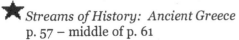 *Archimedes and the Door...* p. 105-109

★ Read aloud the next portion of the nonfiction book that you selected.

After the reading, have each person get a Bible and open it anywhere in Proverbs. Explain, *We will have 5 minutes to skim through the verses in Proverbs to find any connections to today's story. When a connection is found, read the verse out loud and quickly share the connection. At the end of 5 minutes, anyone who has not shared yet must read aloud one verse and make the best connection possible.*

Key Idea: Seek God's word for His guidance.

Bible Quiet Time | I |

Reading: Choose one option below.

★ *The Illustrated Family Bible* p. 248-249

★ Your own Bible: Luke 7:1-50

Scripture Focus: Highlight Luke 7:48-50.

Prayer Focus: Pray a prayer of supplication to make a humble and earnest request of God. Begin by reading the highlighted verse out loud as a prayer. End by praying, *I know I have many sins and pray that you would forgive them. Help me have a strong faith in you and guide me to overcome my sins with your help.*

Scripture Review: Philippians 2:1-18.
Music: *Philippians 2* CD: Tracks 1-5 (all)

Key Idea: Jesus has the power to forgive sins.

Independent History Study | I |

★ Listen to *What in the World?* Disc 3, Track 8: "Alexander the Great". Then, turn to your *Student Notebook* Unit 21. On a modern world map or globe, locate Alexander's Empire as shown in Box 8.

Key Idea: Alexander pursued Darius until he came upon him dying. Alexander was now king of Persia.

Learning the Basics
Focus: Language Arts, Math, Geography, Bible, and Science

Geography [T]

Read aloud to the students the following pages:

 A Child's Geography Vol. II p. 127 – first paragraph on p. 131

Discuss with the students "Field Notes" p. 130.

Key Idea: Iraq is in Mesopotamia. The ancient Biblical places Shinar, Babylon, Chaldea, and Assyria are all found in the land we now call Iraq. Iraq is almost completely surrounded by land. It is located at the northern end of the Persian Gulf. The Tigris and Euphrates Rivers cross Iraq.

Language Arts [S]

Have students complete one dictation exercise.

Guide students to complete one reading lesson.

⭐ *Drawn into the Heart of Reading*

Help students complete **one** English lesson.

⭐ *Building with Diligence:* Lesson 39

⭐ *Following the Plan:* Lesson 35

⭐ Your own grammar program

Key Idea: Practice language arts skills.

Poetry [I]

Open *Paint Like a Poet* to Lesson 17. Today, you will be performing a poetry reading of "Acceptance". Practice reading the poem aloud with expression that matches the poem's mood. Then, read the poem aloud in front of your chosen audience. At the end of the reading, share the following, *When I read this poem by Robert Frost, it made me think of...* Call on your audience to share what thoughts the poem brought to their minds. Last, say, *Did you know that Robert Frost's poems were rejected for 20 years by editors in America? The Atlantic Monthly returned his poems with a note that read: "We regret that the Atlantic has no place for your vigorous verse." They would later request to print his then popular poems, and Frost would submit the exact same poems that they had previously rejected!*

Key Idea: Share the poetry of Robert Frost.

Math Exploration [S]

Choose **one** of the math options listed below.

 *Singapore Primary Mathematics 4A/4B or 5A/5B* (see Appendix for schedules), or *Math with Confidence,* or *Apologia Math*

⭐ Your own math program

Key Idea: Use a step-by-step math program.

Science Exploration [I]

Turn to the science experiment section in your science binder or sketchbook. At the top of a blank page, write: *In the fruits within the Rose Family, where are the seed-boxes and seeds located?* Under the question, write: *'Guess'*. Write down your guess.

Gather any of the following fruits from the Rose Family that you happen to have in your house: strawberry, raspberry, blackberry, plum, cherry, pear, apple, peach, quince, nectarine, or apricot. Now, look to find the seed-boxes. You may have to cut the fruit open to see them. Refer to p. 52-53 in *Plant Life in Field and Garden* for help in finding the seed-boxes and seeds in each fruit. Next, on the paper write: *'Procedure'*. Draw and label the fruits that you examined and label the seed-boxes. At the bottom of the paper, write: *'Conclusion'*. Explain what you learned from the experiment.

Key Idea: Each fruit has seed-boxes in which its seeds are stored. By examining the various fruits, you can locate the seed-boxes. Without seeds, the plant cannot reproduce.

Learning through History
Focus: The Empire of Alexander the Great

Reading about History [I]

Read about history in the following resource:

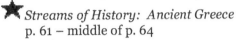 *Streams of History: Ancient Greece* p. 61 – middle of p. 64

Alexander the Great made Alexandria his capital city. Where could you look to research **Alexandria**? Use an online resource like www.wikipedia.org or a reference book. Answer one or more of the following questions: *Where is Alexandria located? When was Alexandria founded? How many years was it the capital of Egypt? For what things was the ancient city of Alexandria known? Describe the Library of Alexandria. Where was the island of Pharos? Describe the Pharos of Alexandria (or the Lighthouse of Alexandria).*

Key Idea: Alexander's tomb was in Alexandria.

History Project [S]

In this unit you will be making paper to remind you of the papyrus used in the library in Alexandria. Place a piece of waxed paper on your work surface. Mix ¼ cup glue and ¼ cup water in a bowl. Cut a paper bag into strips that are ½" wide and 12" long. Dip one strip in the glue mixture. Then, lay it on the waxed paper vertically. Dip a second strip and lay it next to the first strip, overlapping it slightly so the two strips are joined. Continue dipping and adding more strips until you have 12 strips joined on the waxed paper. Press the strips so that they feel smooth. Next, start at the top, making a second layer by adding strips horizontally across the first layer. Press this layer so it's smooth. Then, lay it flat to dry.

Key Idea: Alexandria was the capital of Egypt.

Storytime [T]

Choose one of the following read aloud options:

 Archimedes and the Door... p. 110-123

⭐ Read at least one nonfiction book for the next 12 days of plans.

After the reading, students will give a detailed oral narration. Select one paragraph from the story to read out loud to the students. This will be the starting point for the narration. Set a timer for 3-5 minutes. When the timer rings the narration is over, even if it isn't complete. A detailed, descriptive narration is the goal. See *Narration Tips* in the Appendix as needed.

Key Idea: Use oral narration to retell the story.

Bible Quiet Time [I]

Bible Reading: Choose one option below.

⭐ *The Illustrated Family Bible* p. 250-251

⭐ Your own Bible: Luke 8:1-21

Scripture Focus: Highlight Luke 8:11-15.

Prayer Focus: Pray a prayer of adoration to worship and honor God. Begin by reading the highlighted verses out loud as a prayer. End by praying, *I glory in your words and teachings. You are Almighty, yet you explained your words to me. Help me to be like the seed sown on good soil and produce a crop for you.*

Scripture Memory: Recite Philippians 2:19.
Music: *Philippians 2* CD: Track 6 (verse 19)

Key Idea: Jesus taught with parables.

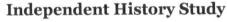

Independent History Study [I]

⭐ Open your *Student Notebook* to Unit 22 – Box 7. Follow the directions from *Draw and Write Through History* p. 23-25 (through step 7) to draw the Lighthouse of Alexandria. Finish on Day 3.

Key Idea: The Lighthouse of Alexandria was one of the Seven Wonders of the Ancient World.

Learning the Basics
Focus: Language Arts, Math, Geography, Bible, and Science

Bible Study [T]

Read aloud and discuss with the students the following pages:

 The Radical Book for Kids p. 160-163

Key Idea: Approximately 1/3 of the Bible is "prophecy." Old Testament prophets were messengers sent by God to remind Israel to listen and follow God's law. The prophets also carried warnings and promises of blessing. Israel often rejected God's prophets.

Language Arts [S]

Have students complete one studied dictation exercise (see Appendix for directions and passages).

Help students complete one lesson from the following reading program:

 Drawn into the Heart of Reading

Work with the students to complete **one** of the English options listed below:

 Building with Diligence: Lesson 40

 Following the Plan: Lesson 36

 Your own grammar program

Key Idea: Practice language arts skills.

Poetry [I]

Open *Paint Like a Poet* to Lesson 18. Read aloud the poem *"In Hardwood Groves"*. On a 3 x 5 index card, neatly copy in black ink or in pencil the following highlighted lines from the poem:

The same leaves over and over again!
They fall from giving shade above
To make one texture of faded brown
And fit the earth like a leather glove.
                                    -Robert Frost

Check your work to make sure it is correctly copied. Then, cut around your copywork. You may choose to outline the edge of the cut-out with a brown marker. Save it for Day 3.

Key Idea: Read and appreciate a variety of classic poetry.

Math Exploration [S]

Choose **one** of the math options listed below.

 Singapore Primary Mathematics 4A/4B or 5A/5B (see Appendix for schedules), or *Math with Confidence,* or *Apologia Math*

 Your own math program

Key Idea: Use a step-by-step math program.

Science Exploration [I]

 Read *Plant Life in Field and Garden* p. 54-58. Get your book about plants that you began in unit 19. At the top of the next page in your book, copy in cursive Psalm 103:15-16. Beneath the verse, choose one or more of the following flowers to sketch: Dead-nettle p. 54, Meadow-sage p. 56, and/or Pea-flower p. 57. Make sure to label each part of the flower, as shown on the listed page(s). For each flower, draw labeled arrows as shown in the diagram(s). If you choose, you may color the flowers. However, before coloring, refer to another source to make sure to color the flowers accurately. You can see full-color photographs of the Dead-nettle, Meadow-sage, and Pea-flower at www.wikipedia.org. To find photographs of these flowers, type the name of the wildflower in the "Search" feature at www.wikipedia.org. You may click on the picture to see a larger image of the flower.

Key Idea: Dead-nettle flowers have lips. Sage have swinging anthers. Pea-flowers have keels.

Reading about History I

Read about history in the following resource:

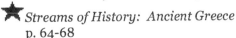 *Streams of History: Ancient Greece* p. 64-68

You will be choosing a portion from today's reading that you found memorable or worthy of being reread to copy. Open your *Student Notebook* to Unit 22. In Box 4, carefully copy in cursive the portion from today's reading that you selected. Then, compare your written work to the original. Last, draw a small colorful picture in Box 4 to illustrate your sentences.

Key Idea: After Alexander's death, one of his Macedonian generals, Ptolemy I, ruled in Egypt and lived in Alexandria. He later chose to be called Pharaoh.

History Project S

Take out the "papyrus" that you made on Day 1. Open your *Student Notebook* to Unit 22-Box 8. Using a permanent marker and the map numbered 8 as your guide, draw a map of the Seven Wonders of the Ancient World on your papyrus. Your map should include an outline of the countries, colored dots for the cities, and a written label for each of the Seven Wonders of the Ancient World. You will not need to draw the Seven Wonders themselves on your map, unless you choose to do so.

Key Idea: At the time of Alexander the Great's death, five of the Seven Wonders of the world were still standing. Two had not yet been built. The Lighthouse of Alexandria and the Colossus of Rhodes were both built after his death.

Storytime T

Choose one of the following read aloud options:

⭐ *Archimedes and the Door...* p. 124-131

⭐ Read aloud the next portion of the nonfiction book that you selected.

After reading, give each person 2 slips of paper. Each person must think of 2 questions to ask about the book and write one question on each slip of paper. Next, fold up the slips of paper and place them in a container. Each person must select at least one question from the container to answer.

Key Idea: Use questioning to share the story.

Bible Quiet Time I

Reading: Choose one option below.

⭐ *The Illustrated Family Bible* p. 252-253

⭐ Your own Bible: Luke 8:22-38

Scripture Focus: Highlight Luke 8:24-25.

Prayer Focus: Pray a prayer of confession to admit or acknowledge your sins to God. Begin by reading the highlighted verses out loud as a prayer. End by praying, *Lord, I confess that sometimes I am afraid of storms too. Help me to remember that you control the wind, the rain, and the waves, and you can protect me!*

Scripture Memory: Recite Philippians 2:19.
Music: *Philippians 2* CD: Track 6 (verse 19)

Key Idea: Jesus calmed the wind and waves.

Independent History Study I

⭐ Listen to *What in the World?* Disc 4, Track 1: "The Hellenistic Empire". Open your *Student Notebook* to Unit 22-Box 6. Notice the division on the map of Alexander the Great's Empire (after his death) among his generals as they fought one another for control over it. Read Daniel 11:4 to see this was prophecied.

Key Idea: Two hundred years earlier, Daniel had prophecied the rise of Alexander the Great and the eventual division of his kingdom. God allowed Daniel to glimpse His plan for the future.

Learning the Basics
Focus: Language Arts, Math, Geography, Bible, and Science

Geography [T]

Read aloud to the students the following pages:

 A Child's Geography Vol. II first paragraph on p. 131-137

Discuss with the students "Field Notes" p. 137.

Key Idea: In Iraq, archeologists have discovered the remains of Babylon. The *Ishtar Gate* has been reconstructed, so people can see what it looked like. Walking through the ruins brings to mind Daniel, Nebuchadnezzar, and Belshazzar. Archeologists have also unearthed ancient Ur, once home to Abraham; and ancient Nineveh, the site of Jonah's burial.

Language Arts [S]

Help students complete one lesson from the following reading program:

 Drawn into the Heart of Reading

Work with the students to complete **one** of the writing options listed below:

 Writing & Rhetoric Book 2: Narrative I p. 10-16 (Note: Read aloud the text while the students follow along. Then, discuss.)

★ Your own writing program

Key Idea: Practice language arts skills.

Poetry [I]

Open *Paint Like a Poet* to Lesson 18. Read aloud the poem *"In Hardwood Groves"* by Robert Frost.

Today, you will be painting a green backdrop. You will need painting paper, a palette, water, a large flat paintbrush, a paper towel, and green and yellow paint.

After gathering your supplies, turn to the "Step-by-Step Watercolor Tutorial" for Lesson 18 in *Paint Like a Poet*. Follow steps 1-3 to complete "Part One: Green Backdrop". Then, let your background dry. You will complete "Part Two" of the tutorial on Day 3.

Key Idea: Use painting to illustrate poetry.

Math Exploration [S]

Choose **one** of the math options listed below.

 Singapore Primary Mathematics 4A/4B or 5A/5B (see Appendix for schedules), or *Math with Confidence,* or *Apologia Math*

 Your own math program

Key Idea: Use a step-by-step math program.

Science Exploration [I]

★ Read *Plant Life in Field and Garden* p. 59-64. Orally retell or narrate to an adult the portion of text that you read today. Use the *Narration Tips* in the Appendix for help as needed.

Key Idea: Climbing plants, like peas and scarlet-runners, have weak stems. They must cling to other plants, sticks, bushes, hedges, walls, or porches. Often, climbing tendrils hold the plants up toward the light, air, and bees. Climbing plants may use their hooks, roots, or threads to climb. Or, the whole plant may twine as it climbs.

Learning through History
Focus: The Empire of Alexander the Great

Unit 22 - Day 3

Reading about History | I

Read about history in the following resource:

★ *Streams of History: Ancient Rome*
p. 1-7

You will be adding to your timeline in your *Student Notebook* today. In Unit 22 – Box 1, draw a red star and next to it write *Alexandria*. Label it, *Ptolemy rules Egypt (and later Syria) (323 B.C.)*. In Box 2, draw and color a crown. Label it, *Seleucus rules Persia/Syria*. In Box 3, draw and color a laurel wreath. Label it, *Antigonus rules Macedonia/Greece*.

Key Idea: Italy is shaped like a boot. It is located near Greece, has the mountainous Alps, and opens to the Mediterranean and Adriatic Seas. Near the mouth of the Tiber River, Rome grew and became the capital city of Italy.

History Project | S

Take out your papyrus that you made on Day 1. On your papyrus map, label the following modern-day countries near the locations of the Seven Wonders of the Ancient World. Write, "Greece" by the Temple of Zeus. Write, "Turkey" by the Temple of Artemis, the Mausoleum of Halicarnassus, and the Colossus of Rhodes. Write, "Iraq" by the Hanging Gardens of Babylon. Write, "Egypt" by the Great Pyramid at Giza.

Key Idea: The Seven Wonders of the Ancient World were all located near the Mediterranean Sea. Five of the seven wonders were Greek creations. The Great Pyramid at Giza is the only one of the seven wonders still standing.

Storytime | T

Choose one of the following read aloud options:

★ *Cleopatra: Preface – Map*

★ Read aloud the next portion of the nonfiction book that you selected.

After the reading, students will give a summary oral narration. The oral narration must be no longer than 5 sentences and should summarize the reading. As students narrate, have them hold up one finger for each sentence shared. Remind students that the focus should be on the big ideas, rather than on the details.

Key Idea: Summarize the story by narrating.

Bible Quiet Time | I

Reading: Choose one option below.

★ *The Illustrated Family Bible* p. 254-255

★ Your own Bible: Luke 8:40-56

Scripture Focus: Highlight Luke 8:45-48.

Prayer Focus: Pray a prayer of thanksgiving to express gratitude for God's divine goodness. Begin by reading the highlighted verses out loud as a prayer. End by praying, *Thank you for your healing power and your love for others. I pray for a strong faith like the woman in today's story.*

Scripture Memory: Recite Philippians 2:19.
Music: *Philippians 2* CD: Track 6 (verse 19)

Key Idea: Jesus knew healing power had gone out of Him, when the woman touched Him.

Independent History Study | I

★ Open your *Student Notebook* to Unit 22 – Box 7. Follow the directions from *Draw and Write Through History* p. 25-26 (steps 8-11) to finish drawing the Lighthouse of Alexandria. You will color your drawing on Day 4.

Key Idea: The Lighthouse of Alexandria, in the Pharos' harbor, was a project begun by Ptolemy I of Egypt.

Learning the Basics

Focus: Language Arts, Math, Geography, Bible, and Science

Bible Study [T]

Read aloud and discuss with the students the following pages:

 The Radical Book for Kids p. 164-167

Key Idea: Human DNA and the complexity of a single cell give evidence that we are "fearfully and wonderfully made" by an amazing Creator. The predictable patterns of the universe show a careful Designer. The precise laws of gravity which hold the universe together reveal an all-knowing, all-powerful Creator.

Language Arts [S]

Have students complete one studied dictation exercise (see Appendix for directions and passages).

Work with the students to complete **one** of the writing options listed below:

 Writing & Rhetoric Book 2: Narrative I p. 17 – top of p. 20 (Note: Refer to the parable on p. 12-15 as needed to complete today's lesson.)

 Your own writing program

Key Idea: Practice language arts skills.

Poetry [I]

Open *Paint Like a Poet* to Lesson 18. Read aloud the poem *"In Hardwood Groves"* by Robert Frost.

Get the green backdrop that you painted on Day 2. Today, you will be adding leafy branches. You will need a palette, water, a small flat paintbrush, a paper towel, and green, dark blue, and brown paint.

Next, turn to the "Step-by-Step Watercolor Tutorial" for Lesson 18 in *Paint Like a Poet*. Follow steps 4-6 to complete "Part Two: Leafy Branches". When your painting is dry, glue your poetry copywork from Day 1 to your painting. Store your completed artwork in the place you have chosen for it.

Key Idea: Explore poetry moods with painting.

Math Exploration [S]

Choose **one** of the math options listed below.

 Singapore Primary Mathematics 4A/4B or 5A/5B (see Appendix for schedules), or *Math with Confidence,* or *Apologia Math*

 Your own math program

Key Idea: Use a step-by-step math program.

Science Exploration [I]

 Read *Plant Life in Field and Garden* p. 65-69. Write the answer to each numbered question on lined paper. You do not need to copy the question. Use the listed page to help you answer each question.
1. List several plants that store their food in their roots. (p. 66)
2. Where do the Yellow Flag and Solomon's Seal store their food? What will you see if you look at their stems? (p. 67-68)
3. Write the words *bulb* and *stalk* and give their definitions. (p. 68)
4. Describe how some plants store their food inside a bulb. (p. 68-69)
5. In Isaiah 11:1, which parts of a flower do you read about? Which part is referring to Jesus?

Key Idea: Plants store their food in their roots, their stems, or within their bulbs.

Reading about History | I |

Read about history in the following resource:

 Streams of History: Ancient Rome
p. 8– bottom of p. 12

You will be writing a narration about the chapter *Rome in Her Infancy,* which is part of today's history reading.

To prepare for writing your narration, think about the questions below. If you do not know the answers, find them on p. 8-12 of *Streams of History: Ancient Rome.* Ask yourself a few guided questions such as, *Why was the location of the city of Rome so important? Tell what you read about a small Roman farm.*

After you have thought about the answers to the questions, turn to Unit 22 in your *Student Notebook.* In Box 5, write a 5-8 sentence narration. When you have finished writing, read your sentences out loud to catch any mistakes.

Check for the following things: *Did you include* **who** *the reading was mainly about? Did you include* **what** *important thing(s) happened? Did you include* **how** *it ended? If not, add those things.*

Then, underline or highlight the main idea sentence in the narration. Use the *Written Narration Skills* in the Appendix as a guide for editing the narration.

<u>Key Idea</u>: The stories about the founding of Rome are legends, meaning that they are not all true. The city of Rome grew as Greece was fighting for her freedom and Alexander the Great was conquering cities in the Far East. On its west side, Italy had good harbors and flat plains for growing crops. On the hills above the Tiber River, the city of Rome grew.

Storytime | T |

Choose one of the following read aloud options:

Cleopatra: Read 10 pages from the start of the story (count pictures as pages too)

Read aloud part of the nonfiction book.

After the reading, have each person get a Bible and open it anywhere in Proverbs. Explain, *We will have 5 minutes to skim through the verses in Proverbs to find any connections to today's story. When a connection is found, read the verse out loud and quickly share the connection. At the end of 5 minutes, anyone who has not shared yet must read aloud one verse and make the best connection possible.*

<u>Key Idea</u>: Seek God's word for His guidance.

Bible Quiet Time | I |

Reading: Choose one option below.

The Illustrated Family Bible p. 256-257

Your own Bible: Luke 9:1-27

Scripture Focus: Highlight Luke 9:1-5.

Prayer Focus: Pray a prayer of supplication to make a humble and earnest request of God. Begin by reading the highlighted verses out loud as a prayer. End by praying, *Help me to learn and understand your teachings. Train me to be a disciple you can use for your purpose. Help me to glorify you with my life.*

Scripture Memory: Copy Philippians 2:19 in your Common Place Book.
Music: *Philippians 2* CD: Track 6 (verse 19)

<u>Key Idea</u>: Jesus taught and led His disciples.

Independent History Study | I |

Open your *Student Notebook* to Unit 22 – Box 7. Use *Draw and Write Through History* p. 27 as a guide to color your sketch of the Lighthouse of Alexandria.

<u>Key Idea</u>: The Lighthouse of Alexandria stood for almost 1500 years before being toppled by earthquakes.

Learning the Basics
Focus: Language Arts, Math, Geography, Bible, and Science

Geography [T]

Get both the blank map and the labeled map of **Egypt, Iraq & Saudi Arabia** that you saved from the study of Egypt. Or, you may print a new map at the link shown on p. 6 of *A Child's Geography Vol. II*. At the link, select "History & Geography". Then, under "Knowledge Quest" select ACG2-Extra Activities". Print p. 48. Then, assign the following page:

★ *A Child's Geography Vol. II* p. 138
Note: Do only the "Map Notes" section. If desired, play "Music" from the links on p. 139.

Key Idea: Practice finding locations in Iraq.

Language Arts [S]

Have students complete one dictation exercise.

Guide students to complete one reading lesson.

★ *Drawn into the Heart of Reading*

Help students complete **one** English lesson.

★ *Building with Diligence:* Lesson 41

★ *Following the Plan:* Lesson 37

★ Your own grammar program

Key Idea: Practice language arts skills.

Poetry [I]

Open *Paint Like a Poet* to Lesson 18. Today, you will be performing a poetry reading of *"In Hardwood Groves"*. Practice reading the poem aloud with expression that matches the poem's mood. Then, read the poem aloud in front of your chosen audience. At the end of the reading, share the following, *When I read this poem by Robert Frost, it made me think of...* Call on your audience to share what thoughts the poem brought to their minds.
Last, say, *Did you know that after ten years Robert sold his poultry farm and moved his family to England? The farming had never gone well, and Robert's grandfather had died, leaving him an annuity that along with the sale of the farm helped pay for the move and life in England. Within a year in England, Frost had published his first book of poetry.*

Key Idea: Share the poetry of Robert Frost.

Math Exploration [S]

Choose **one** of the math options listed below.

★ *Singapore Primary Mathematics 4A/4B* or *5A/5B* (see Appendix for schedules), or *Math with Confidence*, or *Apologia Math*

★ Your own math program

Key Idea: Use a step-by-step math program.

Science Exploration [I]

★ Read *Plant Life in Field and Garden* p. 70-74. Turn to the science experiment section in your science binder or sketchbook. At the top of a blank page, write: *Why is the part of the potato plant that we eat a tuber and not a root?* Under the question, write: *'Guess'.* Write down your guess. **Experiment 1:** Wash a potato and look at the dark spots on it, which are called eyes. Each eye is a growing tip, or bud that is the beginning of leaves. So, the potato cannot be a root. A potato is the swollen part at the end of a stem called a tuber. If desired, place one potato inside a dark cabinet. Eventually, you should see small white growths on the potato. **Experiment 2:** Place a potato on a plate on the counter in the sun. Watch for the potato to turn green. This means that the exposure to the sun has caused photosynthesis to occur. Leaves use photosynthesis to manufacture food for the plant, so for photosynthesis to occur the potato cannot be a root. Green potatoes will taste bitter and can be poisonous, so do not eat green potatoes. To prevent them from turning green, keep them stored away from light. Next, on the paper write: *'Procedure'.* Draw a picture of the experiment. At the bottom of the paper, write: *'Conclusion'.* Explain what you learned.

Key Idea: The part of the potato plant that we eat is called a tuber. This plant's seed-box is poisonous.

Learning through History
Focus: Rome in Her Infancy

Reading about History $\boxed{I}$

Read about history in the following resource:

★ *Streams of History: Ancient Rome*
p. 12 – top of p. 17 (On p. 13-15, the stories about the gods and goddesses are not true. They are Roman myths and legends.)

Rome was (and still is) the capital city of Italy. Where could you look to research more about **Rome**? Use an online resource like www.wikipedia.org or a reference book.

Answer one or more of the following questions from your research: *Describe where Rome is located. What are the names of the seven hills on which Rome is situated? Describe the climate of Rome. Which famous ancient structures can be seen in Rome? When was the Roman Empire at the height of its power?*

Key Idea: Rome became known as the city of seven hills. The early kings of Rome were Romulus, Numa, and Tarquin.

History Project $\boxed{S}$

In this unit you will study the geography of Rome. Open your *Student Notebook* to Unit 23. Use the map in Box 7 to help you find Rome on a globe or a world map. In which country is Rome located? On which continent is it found? Find the seas that surround Italy and give their names. Rome was founded near the Tiber River. Find the Tiber River, which flows to the Tyrrhenian Sea. Which mountain ranges are in Italy? Which countries border Italy on the north?

Key Idea: Rome is still the capital of Italy today. It is filled with a very rich history.

Storytime $\boxed{T}$

Choose one of the following read aloud options:

★ *Cleopatra*: Read from the stabbing of Caesar through Antony with the fish.

★ Read at least one nonfiction book for the next 8 days of plans.

After the reading, students will give a detailed oral narration. Select one paragraph from the story to read out loud to the students. This will be the starting point for the narration. Set a timer for 3-5 minutes. When the timer rings the narration is over, even if it isn't complete. A detailed, descriptive narration is the goal. See *Narration Tips* in the Appendix as needed.

Key Idea: Use oral narration to retell the story.

Bible Quiet Time $\boxed{I}$

Bible Reading: Choose one option below.

★ *The Illustrated Family Bible* p. 260-261 and p. 274-275

★ Your own Bible: Luke 9:28-62

Scripture Focus: Highlight Luke 9:18-20.

Prayer Focus: Pray a prayer of adoration to worship and honor God. Begin by reading the highlighted verses out loud as a prayer. End by praying, *I worship you Lord as the Christ, the Son of the living God! I thank you for revealing yourself to me, and I bow down before you.*

Scripture Memory: Recite Philippians 2:20.
Music: *Philippians 2* CD: Track 6 (vs. 19-20)

Key Idea: Jesus is the Son of the living God.

Independent History Study $\boxed{I}$

★ Listen to *What in the World?* Disc 4, Track 2: "Early Rome".

Key Idea: During its early years, Rome was at war most of the time. The early history of Rome is made up of fictional myths, legends, and stories of gods and goddesses woven together with real facts.

Learning the Basics
Focus: Language Arts, Math, Geography, Bible, and Science

Bible Study   [T]

Read aloud and discuss with the students the following pages:

 The Radical Book for Kids p. 168-171

Key Idea: "The Lord's Prayer" is a model for how we are to pray. The Bible is filled with other examples of prayer as well. We can learn much about how we should pray by reading and thinking about the prayers provided in Scripture.

Language Arts   [S]

Have students complete one studied dictation exercise (see Appendix for directions and passages).

Help students complete one lesson from the following reading program:

 Drawn into the Heart of Reading

Work with the students to complete **one** of the English options listed below:

⭐ *Building with Diligence:* Lesson 42

⭐ *Following the Plan:* Lesson 38

⭐ Your own grammar program

Key Idea: Practice language arts skills.

Poetry   [I]

Open *Paint Like a Poet* to Lesson 19. Read aloud the poem *"After Apple-Picking"*. On a 3 x 5 index card, neatly copy in black ink or in pencil the following highlighted lines from the poem:

My long two-pointed ladder's
sticking through a tree
Toward heaven still,
And there's a barrel that I didn't fill
Beside it, and there may be two or three
Apples I didn't pick upon some bough.
But I am done with apple-picking now.
                              -Robert Frost

Check your work to make sure it is correctly copied. Then, cut around your copywork. You may choose to outline the edge of the cut-out with a red marker. Save it for Day 3.

Key Idea: Read and appreciate classic poetry.

Math Exploration   [S]

Choose **one** of the math options listed below.

⭐ *Singapore Primary Mathematics 4A/4B* or *5A/5B* (see Appendix for schedules), or *Math with Confidence*, or *Apologia Math*

⭐ Your own math program

Key Idea: Use a step-by-step math program.

Science Exploration   [I]

⭐ Read *Plant Life in Field and Garden* p. 75-79. Get your book about plants that you began in unit 19. At the top of the next page in your book, copy in cursive Genesis 3:18-19. Beneath the verse, choose one or both of the following flowers to sketch: Burdock p. 78 and/or Wild Geranium p. 78. Make sure to label the flower as shown on p. 78. If you choose, you may color the flowers. However, before coloring, refer to another source to make sure to color the flowers accurately. You can see full-color photographs of the Burdock and the Wild Geranium at www.wikipedia.org. To find photographs of these flowers, type the name of the wildflower in the "Search" feature at www.wikipedia.org. You may click on each picture to see a larger image of each flower. You may also wish to view the Sow-thistle, Groundsel, Teasel, Goose-grass, and Wild Rose.

Key Idea: Seeds travel by wind, water, and animals. Fruit and bright colors help attract birds and animals.

Learning through History
Focus: Rome in Her Infancy

Reading about History | I

Read about history in the following resource:

 Streams of History: Ancient Rome p. 17 – top of p. 20 (Note: p. 17-18 discuss worship of pagan gods and goddesses in which the Romans believed.)

You will be choosing a portion from today's reading that you found memorable or worthy of being reread to copy. Open your *Student Notebook* to Unit 23. In Box 4, carefully copy in cursive the portion from today's reading that you selected. Then, compare your written work to the original. Last, draw a small colorful picture in Box 4 to illustrate your sentences.

<u>Key Idea</u>: The plebians were poor common farmers, while the patricians were wealthy landowners. The plebians fought for over 400 years to be equal citizens with the patricians.

History Project | S

Open your *Student Notebook* to Unit 23. Refer to the map in Box 7 to guide you and use a light blue pencil to faintly color the water on the map in Box 8. Then, use a darker pencil to label the Mediterranean Sea, the Black Sea, the Adriatic Sea, the Red Sea, the Baltic Sea, and the Atlantic Ocean.

Also, draw and label in blue the following major rivers: The Rhine River, the Danube River, and the Nile River.

Last, use a red colored pencil to label the continents of Africa, Europe, and Asia.

<u>Key Idea</u>: Rome would one day unite Italy.

Storytime | T

Choose one of the following read aloud options:

 Cleopatra: Read from the three children on thrones through the ships sailing away.

 Read the next part of the nonfiction book.

After reading, work with the students to plan a 3 minute skit with simple props to act out part of today's reading. Set a timer for 3 minutes to quickly prepare for the skit. Make sure that you participate in the skit along with the students. When the timer rings, set it again for 3 minutes and perform the skit. You do not need an audience, as the goal is the retelling.

<u>Key Idea</u>: Use a skit to retell part of the story.

Bible Quiet Time | I

Reading: Choose one option below.

 The Illustrated Family Bible p. 266-267 Optional extension: p. 262

 Your own Bible: Luke 10:1-41

Scripture Focus: Highlight Luke 10:27.

Prayer Focus: Pray a prayer of confession to admit or acknowledge your sins to God. Begin by reading the highlighted verse out loud as a prayer. End by praying, *Help me to love you with all of my heart, soul, and strength. I confess I need to work on being more loving to others too. Help me to be loving to...*

Scripture Memory: Recite Philippians 2:20.
Music: *Philippians 2* CD: Track 6 (vs. 19-20)

<u>Key Idea</u>: We should love the Lord above all.

Independent History Study | I

Open your *Student Notebook* to Unit 23. Use the map in Box 7 to help you draw and label the following places in Box 8: Draw 7 brown hills and label them Rome. Draw and label the Alps Mountain Range. Draw a blue line to be the Tiber River near Rome and label the river.

<u>Key Idea</u>: Italy had mountain ranges, plains, rivers, and sea harbors. The people were either poor or rich.

Learning the Basics
Focus: Language Arts, Math, Geography, Bible, and Science

Geography [T]

Go to the website link listed on p. 6 of *A Child's Geography Vol. II*. At the link, select "History & Geography". Then, under "Knowledge Quest" select ACG2-Extra Activities". Print the "Travel Log Template" of your choice from p. 39-42. Also at the link, for older students, print and assign the "Chapter Ten Review" on p. 77.

Assign all students the following page:

 A Child's Geography Vol. II p. 138
Note: Do only the "Travel Notes" section. The "Art" section of p. 139 is an optional extra.

Key Idea: Share three sights from Iraq.

Language Arts [S]

Help students complete one lesson from the following reading program:

 Drawn into the Heart of Reading

Work with the students to complete **one** of the writing options listed below:

⭐ *Writing & Rhetoric Book 2: Narrative I* middle of p. 22-27 (Note: Omit p. 20 – top of p. 22. Guide students through the lesson, so they are successful writing from a different point of view.)

⭐ Your own writing program

Key Idea: Practice language arts skills.

Poetry [I]

Open *Paint Like a Poet* to Lesson 19. Read aloud the poem *"After Apple-Picking"* by Robert Frost.

Today, you will be painting a table and wallpaper. You will need painting paper, a palette, water, a large flat paintbrush, a pencil, masking tape, and brown, white, and blue paint.

After gathering your supplies, turn to the "Step-by-Step Watercolor Tutorial" for Lesson 19 in *Paint Like a Poet*. Follow steps 1-3 to complete "Part One: Table and Wallpaper". Then, let your background dry. You will complete "Part Two" of the tutorial on Day 3.

Key Idea: Use painting to illustrate poetry.

Math Exploration [S]

Choose **one** of the math options listed below.

 Singapore Primary Mathematics 4A/4B or 5A/5B (see Appendix for schedules), or *Math with Confidence,* or *Apologia Math*

 Your own math program

Key Idea: Use a step-by-step math program.

Science Exploration [I]

⭐ Read *Galen and the Gateway to Medicine* p. 1-8. Orally retell or narrate to an adult the portion of text that you read today. Use the *Narration Tips* in the Appendix for help as needed.

Key Idea: Galen was a doctor who lived almost 2,000 years ago in the Roman Empire. He eventually became the doctor for four different Roman emperors. Since dissecting a human body was forbidden, Galen based much of his learning about the human body on his dissections of pigs and monkeys! Galen thought of new ways to treat patients and invented new medicines. For almost 1500 years after his death, doctors all over the world read Galen's books and accepted his medical theories as facts.

Reading about History I

Read about history in the following resource:

★ *Streams of History: Ancient Rome*
p. 20 – bottom of p. 22

You will be adding to your timeline in your *Student Notebook* today. In Unit 23 – Box 1, draw and color a river. Label it, *Romulus founds Rome by the Tiber River (753 B.C.).* In Box 2, draw and color 7 hills. Label it, *Numa reigns in Rome (715 B.C.).* In Box 3, draw and color a sword. Label it, *Horatius at the bridge (509 B.C.).*

Key Idea: The Roman laws were finally written on tablets and placed in the Forum so that the plebians could read them just like the patricians.

Storytime T

Choose one of the following read aloud options:

★ *Cleopatra*: Read from Cleopatra dictating a letter through the Epilogue.

★ Read aloud the next portion of the nonfiction book that you selected.

After the reading, students will give a summary oral narration. The oral narration must be no longer than 5 sentences and should summarize the reading. As students narrate, have them hold up one finger for each sentence shared. Remind students that the focus should be on the big ideas, rather than on the details.

Key Idea: Summarize the story by narrating.

History Project S

Open your *Student Notebook* to Unit 23. Refer to the map in Box 7 to guide you. Use a light orange pencil to faintly color the Roman Empire on the map in Box 8. This is what the Roman Empire looked like when it reached its greatest glory.

Last, in Box 8, use a darker pencil to label the remaining cities and nations shown on the map in Box 7.

Key Idea: Rome would first conquer Sicily and then eventually Carthage. After that, Rome would continue to conquer those cities and nations that surrounded her, until she ruled the world around the Mediterranean Sea.

Bible Quiet Time I

Reading: Choose one option below.

★ *The Illustrated Family Bible* p. 268-269
Optional extension: p. 263

★ Your own Bible: Luke 11:1-54

Scripture Focus: Highlight John 3:16.

Prayer Focus: Pray a prayer of thanksgiving to express gratitude for God's divine goodness. Begin by reading the highlighted verse out loud as a prayer. End by praying, *Thank you for loving me enough to send your only Son to save me, so that I may have eternal life.*

Scripture Memory: Recite Philippians 2:20.
Music: *Philippians 2* CD: Track 6 (vs. 19-20)

Key Idea: Belief in Jesus is the way to heaven.

Independent History Study I

Look at the timeline entries in today's "Reading About History" box. Then, open your *Student Notebook* and look at your past timeline entries to see what was happening in history at the same time that Horatius was defending the bridge over the Tiber River.

Key Idea: When Rome rebelled against her kings, Greece also became a republic at about the same time. Meanwhile, the Jews were rebuilding the Temple in Jerusalem after an exile in Babylon.

Learning the Basics

Focus: Language Arts, Math, Geography, Bible, and Science

Bible Study   [T]

Read aloud and discuss with the students the following pages:

 The Radical Book for Kids p. 172-174

<u>Key Idea</u>: God has much to teach us about work. God is a worker. Since we are made in God's image, we should be workers too. Work was part of God's design for man. Sin makes work difficult, but work is still part of God's design for us. When you are working for someone, be sure to work as if you were working for the Lord. Ultimately, you are doing what God has planned for you to do!

Language Arts   [S]

Have students complete one studied dictation exercise (see Appendix for directions and passages).

Work with the students to complete **one** of the writing options listed below:

 Writing & Rhetoric Book 2: Narrative I p. 28 – middle of p. 32 (Note: Read aloud the text while the students follow along. Then, discuss.)

 Your own writing program

<u>Key Idea</u>: Practice language arts skills.

Poetry   [I]

Open *Paint Like a Poet* to Lesson 19. Read aloud the poem *"After Apple-Picking"* by Robert Frost.

Get the table and wallpaper backdrop that you painted on Day 2. Today, you will be adding an apple and its shadow. You will need a palette, water, a small flat paintbrush, a toothpick, and yellow, red, brown, and white paint.

After gathering your supplies, turn to the "Step-by-Step Watercolor Tutorial" for Lesson 19 in *Paint Like a Poet*. Follow steps 4-6 to complete "Part Two: Apple and Shadow". When your painting is dry, glue your poetry copywork from Day 1 to your painting. Store your completed artwork in the place you have chosen for it.

<u>Key Idea</u>: Explore poetry moods with painting.

Math Exploration   [S]

Choose **one** of the math options listed below.

 Singapore Primary Mathematics 4A/4B or 5A/5B (see Appendix for schedules), or *Math with Confidence*, or *Apologia Math*

 Your own math program

<u>Key Idea</u>: Use a step-by-step math program.

Science Exploration   [I]

 Read *Galen and the Gateway to Medicine* p. 9-18. Write the answer to each numbered question on lined paper. You do not need to copy the question. Use the listed page to help you answer each question.

1. What did Galen's father, Nicon, do? (p. 10)
2. Why were hours different lengths of time during the year? (p. 12)
3. Write the words *chiton* and *agora* and give their definitions. (p. 12)
4. Describe the city of Pergamum at the time of Galen. (p. 14-16)
5. Galen lived about 75 years after Paul spoke to the Greeks in Athens. Pergamum was a Greek city fashioned to be like Athens. What can you learn from Paul's words to the Greeks in Acts 17:23-25?

<u>Key Idea</u>: Galen grew up in a wealthy family in the city of Pergamum. Although Pergamum was a part of the Roman Empire, it remained a mainly Greek city. Galen was surrounded by beauty and learning.

Reading about History | I

Read about history in the following resource:

⭐ *Streams of History: Ancient Rome* p. 22-25

You will be writing a narration about the last part of the chapter *Rome in Her Infancy,* which is part of today's history reading.

To prepare for writing your narration, describe how the forming of "Little Romes" and the building of roads united people under the Roman government. You may wish to look back over p. 22-25 of *Streams of History: Ancient Rome* to guide you as you write your narration.

After you have thought about the topic and how you will begin your narration, turn to Unit 23 in your *Student Notebook.* In Box 5, write a 5-8 sentence narration.

When you have finished writing, read your sentences out loud to catch any mistakes. Check for the following things: *Did you include **who** or **what topic** the reading was mainly about? Did you include **descriptors** of the important thing(s) that happened? Did you include a **closing sentence**? If not, add those things.*

Then, underline or highlight the main idea sentence in the narration.

Use the *Written Narration Skills* in the Appendix as a guide for editing the narration.

<u>Key Idea:</u> Whenever a place was conquered by Rome, citizens from Rome were sent to live on part of the conquered land. These citizens formed a state and gradually those people around the state became more like Romans.

Storytime | T

Choose one of the following read aloud options:

⭐ *City* p. 5-19

⭐ Read aloud the next part of the nonfiction book that you selected.

After the reading, have each person get a Bible and open it anywhere in Proverbs. Explain, *We will have 5 minutes to skim through the verses in Proverbs to find any connections to today's story. When a connection is found, read the verse out loud and quickly share the connection. At the end of 5 minutes, anyone who has not shared yet must read aloud one verse and make the best connection possible.*

<u>Key Idea:</u> Seek God's word for His guidance.

Bible Quiet Time | I

Reading: Choose one option below.

⭐ *The Illustrated Family Bible* p. 292-293

⭐ Your own Bible: Luke 12:1-59

Scripture Focus: Highlight Matt. 24:42-44.

Prayer Focus: Pray a prayer of supplication to make a humble and earnest request of God. Begin by reading the highlighted verses out loud as a prayer. End by praying, *I know that you could return at any time. Help me continually seek to please you more each day so that I am ready for your return.*

Scripture Memory: Copy Philippians 2:20 in your Common Place Book.
Music: *Philippians 2* CD: Track 6 (vs. 19-20)

<u>Key Idea:</u> Are you ready for Jesus to return?

Independent History Study | I

Open your *Student Notebook* to Unit 23. Look at the map in Box 6 to see all of the Roman roads that were built during the time of the Roman Empire. After the death and resurrection of Christ, how would these roads help Christianity to spread very quickly throughout the Roman Empire?

<u>Key Idea:</u> As Rome conquered other nations, roads were built leading back to Rome.

Geography | T |

Read aloud to the students the following pages:

⭐ *A Child's Geography Vol. II* p. 140 – middle of p. 144

Discuss with the students "Field Notes" p. 144.

Key Idea: Iraq's two main mountain chains are the Taurus Mountains and the Zagros Mountains. The Kurdish people make up one-fifth of Iraq's population. They are thought to be descendents of the Medes. Across from the ruins of ancient Nineveh lies the city of Mosul.

Language Arts | S |

Have students complete one dictation exercise.

Guide students to complete one reading lesson.

⭐ *Drawn into the Heart of Reading*

Help students complete **one** English lesson.

⭐ *Building with Diligence:* Lesson 43

⭐ *Following the Plan:* Lesson 39

⭐ Your own grammar program

Key Idea: Practice language arts skills.

Poetry | I |

Open *Paint Like a Poet* to Lesson 19. Today, you will be performing a poetry reading of *"After Apple-Picking"*. Practice reading the poem aloud with expression that matches the mood of the poem. Then, read the poem aloud in front of your chosen audience. At the end of the reading, share the following, *When I read this poem by Robert Frost, it made me think of...* Call on your audience to share what thoughts the poem brought to their minds. Last, say, *After Frost's first book of poetry was published in England, he published a second book of poetry. Until World War I began, the Frosts continued to live in England in a cottage outside London. Robert was amused by local concern that he might be a spy.*

Key Idea: Share the poetry of Robert Frost.

Math Exploration | S |

Choose **one** of the math options listed below.

⭐ *Singapore Primary Mathematics 4A/4B or 5A/5B* (see Appendix for schedules), or *Math with Confidence,* or *Apologia Math*

⭐ Your own math program

Key Idea: Use a step-by-step math program.

Science Exploration | I |

⭐ Read *Galen and the Gateway to Medicine* p. 19-24. Turn to the science experiment section in your science binder or sketchbook. At the top of a blank page, write: *How can geometry be used to test what the eye is really seeing?* Under the question, write: *'Guess'*. Write down your guess. **Experiment 1:** On paper, use a ruler to draw two parallel lines that are each 3 inches long. Draw the lines about 1 inch apart. At both ends of one line draw a 'v' pointing out. At both ends of the other line, draw a 'v' pointing in. Does one line appear to be longer than the other? How do you know that both lines are actually the same length? **Experiment 2:** Fold a clean sheet of paper in half like a greeting card. In the center of each half, trace around a quarter. Trace around a dime 6 or more times to form a ring around one quarter. Trace around a milk jug lid or juice jug lid 5 or more times to form a ring around the other quarter. Do the inside circles appear to be the same size? How do you know they are the same size? Under *'Procedure'*, draw a picture of the experiment. At the bottom of the paper, write: *'Conclusion'*. Explain what you learned.
Note: To see other optical illusions online, visit https://faculty.washington.edu/chudler/chvision.html
To make an optical illusion spinner, see this link: https://faculty.washington.edu/chudler/benham.html

Key Idea: Galen loved geometry because he loved studying problems and trying to solve them.

Learning through History
Focus: The Struggle Between Rome and Carthage

Reading about History · I

Read about history in the following resource:

★ *Streams of History: Ancient Rome* p. 26 – top of p. 30

The Phoenicians founded Carthage almost 100 years before Rome was founded. Where could you look to research more about **Carthage**? Use an online resource like www.wikipedia.org or a reference book.

Answer one or more of the following questions from your research: *Where was Carthage located? What modern-day city is located where Carthage once stood? Carthage was on an isthmus. What is an isthmus? For what was Carthage known? What kinds of riches were traded in Carthage's harbor? How did Carthage treat her citizens differently from the way Rome treated her citizens? How did the Punic Wars affect Carthage? When was the city of Carthage destroyed? After being rebuilt, when was it destroyed again?*

Key Idea: Carthage was a busy trading port.

History Project · S

In this unit you will make a trading card game. You will need 21 index cards cut in half and 14 different colored pencils to make your cards. Use the same colored pencil to make 3 cards that each say *Linen from Egypt*. Next, use a different color to make 3 cards that each say *Gold and pearls from the East*. Make 3 cards for each of the following, using a new color each time: *Frankincense from Arabia, Oil and wine from India, Copper from Cyprus, Pottery and wine from Greece,* and *Silver from Spain*.

Key Idea: Many ships traded in Carthage.

Storytime · T

Choose one of the following read aloud options:

★ *City* p. 20-31

★ Read at least one nonfiction book for the next 4 days of plans.

After the reading, students will give a detailed oral narration. Select one paragraph from the story to read out loud to the students. This will be the starting point for the narration. Set a timer for 3-5 minutes. When the timer rings the narration is over, even if it isn't complete. A detailed, descriptive narration is the goal. See *Narration Tips* in the Appendix as needed.

Key Idea: Use oral narration to retell the story.

Bible Quiet Time · I

Bible Reading: Use the option below.

★ Your own Bible: Luke 13:22-35

Scripture Focus: Highlight Luke 13:29-30.

Prayer Focus: Pray a prayer of adoration to worship and honor God. Begin by reading the highlighted verses out loud as a prayer. End by praying, *I give you praise and adoration for your kingdom and the way to heaven you've given us through Jesus Christ. Help me desire to be more like Jesus, so I can join Him in your kingdom one day.*

Scripture Memory: Recite Philippians 2:21.
Music: *Philippians 2* CD: Track 6 (vs. 19-21)

Key Idea: Knowing about Jesus is not enough to gain entrance into heaven. You must believe He is the Son of God and repent of your sin.

Independent History Study · I

★ Open your *Student Notebook* to Unit 24 – Box 6. Follow the directions from *Draw and Write Through History* p. 36-37 (through step 5) to draw Hannibal's war elephant. Finish drawing on Day 2.

Key Idea: The city of Carthage's thick walls housed soldiers, armor, war elephants, and horses.

Learning the Basics
Focus: Language Arts, Math, Geography, Bible, and Science

Bible Study T

Read aloud and discuss the following pages:

 The Radical Book for Kids p. 175-181

Key Idea: History is the story of God's love for His Son and for His creation. God's perfect creation displayed His love. When Adam and Eve rejected God's love, sin entered the world. Then, God's world was no longer perfect, but God still loved Adam and Eve. God judged sin but rescued sinners through His Son's perfect sacrifice. Ultimately, God's love spreads and triumphs.

Language Arts S

Have students complete one studied dictation exercise (see Appendix for directions and passages).

Help students complete one lesson from the following reading program:

⭐ *Drawn into the Heart of Reading*

Work with the students to complete **one** of the English options listed below:

⭐ *Building with Diligence:* Lesson 44

⭐ *Following the Plan:* Lesson 40

⭐ Your own grammar program

Key Idea: Practice language arts skills.

Poetry I

Open *Paint Like a Poet* to Lesson 20. Read aloud the poem *"Stopping by Woods on a Snowy Evening"*. On a 3 x 5 index card, neatly copy in black ink or in pencil the following highlighted lines from the poem:

Whose woods these are I think I know.
His house is in the village, though;
He will not see me stopping here
To watch his woods fill up with snow.
                    -Robert Frost

Check your work to make sure it is correctly copied. Then, cut around your copywork. You may choose to outline the edge of the cut-out with a gray marker. Save it for Day 3.

Key Idea: Read and appreciate a variety of classic poetry.

Math Exploration S

Choose **one** of the math options listed below.

⭐ *Singapore Primary Mathematics 4A/4B* or *5A/5B* (see Appendix for schedules), or *Math with Confidence*, or *Apologia Math*

⭐ Your own math program

Key Idea: Use a step-by-step math program.

Science Exploration I

⭐ Read *Galen and the Gateway to Medicine* p. 25-36. Today, you will add to your science notebook. At the top of an unlined paper, copy in cursive Genesis 2:7. Beneath the verse, write the following two headings: "Greek ideas about the body that are true" and "Greek ideas about the body that are not true". Under each heading list ideas from p. 25-36 of *Galen and the Gateway of Medicine* that fit each category.

Key Idea: Galen studied under doctors at the temple to Aesculapius in Pergamum. At that time, doctors believed that a patient's dreams could help diagnose the problem and cure a patient. Various types of tea were a common treatment. The doctors observed and took notes about patients' symptoms and well-being.

Reading about History | I |

Read about history in the following resource:

★ *Streams of History: Ancient Rome* p. 30 – top of p. 33

You will be choosing a portion from today's reading that you found memorable or worthy of being reread to copy. Open your *Student Notebook* to Unit 24. In Box 4, carefully copy in cursive the portion from today's reading that you selected. Then, compare your written work to the original. Last, draw a small colorful picture in Box 4 to illustrate your sentences.

<u>Key Idea</u>: Over time, Carthage developed trading ports around the Mediterranean Sea. As Carthage extended her rule beyond her shores, Rome was watching.

Storytime | T |

Choose one of the following read aloud options:

★ *City* p. 32-43

★ Read aloud the next portion of the nonfiction book that you selected.

After reading, give students a few minutes to prepare a short advertisement speech for the book. During the speech, students should hold up the book and say the book title and the name of the author. The wording of the advertisement should provide a peek into the book without giving away the ending. The goal should be for listeners to feel like they've "Got to Have This Book"!

<u>Key Idea</u>: Use an ad speech to share the story.

History Project | S |

Get out the index cards and colored pencils that you were using to make your trading cards on Day 1. Use a new color to make 3 cards that each say *Ivory and salt from Africa.* Make 3 cards for each of the following, using a new color each time: *Iron from Elba, Amber from the Baltic Sea, Tin from England,* and *Honey and wax from Corsica.* Then, use a different color to make one of each of the following cards: *Storm – Move one card of cargo to the bottom of deck; Attacked – Move one card of stolen cargo to bottom of deck; Hole in the Ship – One card of cargo "floats away" to bottom of deck.* Then, use one final color to make one of each of the following cards: *Smooth sailing, arrive early – Make one more trade; Profitable journey – Make one more trade; Extra money – Make one more trade.*

<u>Key Idea</u>: Carthage's main focus was on trade.

Bible Quiet Time | I |

Reading: Choose one option below.

★ *The Illustrated Family Bible* p. 272-273

★ Your own Bible: Luke 14:1-34

Scripture Focus: Highlight Luke 14:11.

Prayer Focus: Pray a prayer of confession to admit or acknowledge your sins to God. Begin by reading the highlighted verse out loud as a prayer. End by praying, *I confess that sometimes I am prideful and talk or think highly of myself, exalting myself. Help me remember to be humble and to exalt you instead.*

Scripture Memory: Recite Philippians 2:21.
Music: *Philippians 2* CD: Track 6 (vs. 19-21)

<u>Key Idea</u>: Jesus is to be exalted above us.

Independent History Study | I |

★ Open your *Student Notebook* to Unit 24 – Box 6. Follow the directions from *Draw and Write Through History* p. 38-40 (through step 10) to draw Hannibal's war elephant. You will color it on Day 3.

<u>Key Idea</u>: Since Carthage was based in North Africa, Carthaginians used war elephants for fighting battles.

Learning the Basics

Focus: Language Arts, Math, Geography, Bible, and Science

Geography | T |

Read aloud to the students the following pages:

 A Child's Geography Vol. II bottom of p. 144-149

Discuss with the students "Field Notes" p. 149.

Key Idea: Iraq is one of the largest producers of oil in the world. Yet, many Iraqis live in poverty, and their children are hungry. In Iraq, Muslims are either *Sunni* Muslims or *Shiite* Muslims. These two groups formed after the death of Mohammed. The tomb of Ali, Mohammed's cousin, is a Muslim shrine today.

Language Arts | S |

Help students complete one lesson from the following reading program:

 Drawn into the Heart of Reading

Work with the students to complete **one** of the writing options listed below:

⭐ *Writing & Rhetoric Book 2: Narrative I* bottom of p. 33-38 (Note: Omit bottom of p. 32 – top of p. 33. Guide students through the lesson, so they are successful writing an amplification.)

⭐ Your own writing program

Key Idea: Practice language arts skills.

Poetry | I |

Open *Paint Like a Poet* to Lesson 20. Read aloud the poem *"Stopping by Woods on a Snowy Evening"* by Robert Frost.

Today, you will be painting a winter backdrop. You will need painting paper, a palette, water, a large flat paintbrush, a pencil, a paper towel, and light blue, grey, and white paint.

After gathering your supplies, turn to the "Step-by-Step Watercolor Tutorial" for Lesson 20 in *Paint Like a Poet*. Follow steps 1-3 to complete "Part One: Winter Backdrop". Then, let your background dry. You will complete "Part Two" of the tutorial on Day 3.

Key Idea: Use painting to illustrate poetry.

Math Exploration | S |

Choose **one** of the math options listed below.

⭐ *Singapore Primary Mathematics 4A/4B* or *5A/5B* (see Appendix for schedules), or *Math with Confidence,* or *Apologia Math*

⭐ Your own math program

Key Idea: Use a step-by-step math program.

Science Exploration | I |

⭐ Read *Galen and the Gateway to Medicine* p. 37-42. Orally retell or narrate to an adult the portion of text that you read today. Use the *Narration Tips* in the Appendix for help as needed.

Key Idea: Hippocrates is known as the "Father of Medicine". He came from a long line of doctors and started a medical school in Cos that was famous throughout the ancient world. Hippocrates lived long before Galen, but Galen modeled much of his writing and study after Hippocrates. The Hippocratic Oath was used for thousands of years after Hippocrates' death. Some medical schools still use it today.

Learning through History
Focus: The Struggle Between Rome and Carthage

Reading about History   I

Read about history in the following resource:

★ *Streams of History: Ancient Rome*
   p. 33 – top of p. 38

You will be adding to your timeline in your *Student Notebook* today. In Unit 24 – Box 1, draw and color an outline of Italy. Label it, *Rome gains all of Italy (266 B.C.).* In Box 2, draw and color the island of Sicily. Label it, *1st Punic War (Rome vs. Carthage 264-241 B.C.).* In Box 3, draw an elephant. Label it, *2nd Punic War – Hannibal crosses Alps (218-202 B.C).*

<u>Key Idea</u>: Rome fought Carthage for Sicily.

Storytime   T

Choose one of the following read aloud options:

★ *City* p. 44-53

★ Read aloud the next portion of the nonfiction book that you selected.

After the reading, students will give a summary oral narration. The oral narration must be no longer than 5 sentences and should summarize the reading. As students narrate, have them hold up one finger for each sentence shared. Remind students that the focus should be on the big ideas, rather than on the details.

<u>Key Idea</u>: Summarize the story by narrating.

History Project   S

Get the 42 trading cards that you made. You will need two people to play the game "Go Trade". Shuffle the deck. Deal 4 cards to each player. Place the rest of the cards face down in a pile. The goal is to get 3 cards of one kind of cargo. Each time you have 3 of a kind, lay them down in front of you. The player with the most sets of 3 at the end of the game wins. The player to the right of the dealer goes first. This player asks another player for something in his/her hand (i.e. Cole, do you have any *Silver from Spain*?). If the other player does have the requested card(s), he/she must give **all** of that kind of cargo to the other player. Then, the player asks again. If the other player does not have the requested cards, he/she says, *Go Trade*. Then, the asking player draws one card and the turn ends, unless a specialty card is drawn. If a specialty card is drawn, the player must follow the instructions and then discard the card. It is now the next player's turn.

<u>Key Idea</u>: Syracuse, Sicily was a trading center.

Bible Quiet Time   I

Reading: Choose one option below.

★ *The Illustrated Family Bible* p. 276-277

★ Your own Bible: Luke 15:1-32

Scripture Focus: Highlight Luke 15:31-32.

Prayer Focus: Pray a prayer of thanksgiving to express gratitude for God's divine goodness. Begin by reading the highlighted verses out loud as a prayer. End by praying, *Thank you for forgiving a sinner like me. Help me to rejoice when others are saved and not to be jealous of others.*

Scripture Memory: Recite Philippians 2:21.
Music: *Philippians 2* CD: Track 6 (vs. 19-21)

<u>Key Idea</u>: Sinners who are lost and come to Jesus are given the same grace that we receive.

Independent History Study   I

★ Open your *Student Notebook* to Unit 24 – Box 6. Use *Draw and Write Through History* p. 41 as a guide to color your sketch of Hannibal's war elephant. You will finish coloring your sketch on Day 4.

<u>Key Idea</u>: Hannibal was the son of the Carthaginian general Hamilcar. Hamilcar lost Sicily to Rome.

Learning the Basics

Focus: Language Arts, Math, Geography, Bible, and Science

Bible Study [T]

Read aloud and discuss with the students the following pages:

 The Radical Book for Kids p. 182-184

Key Idea: Friendship was designed by God. It is important to choose friends who love the Lord. There are warnings in the Bible about the types of friends to avoid. You should avoid friends who are easily angered, who steal, who reject God's ways, who are arrogant, who gossip, and who stir up trouble. As a friend, you have responsibilities too.

Language Arts [S]

Have students complete one studied dictation exercise (see Appendix for directions and passages).

Work with the students to complete **one** of the writing options listed below:

 Writing & Rhetoric Book 2: Narrative I p. 39-40 (Note: Reread the parable on p. 29 first. Then, guide students as needed to successfully write the parable from the wise man's point of view. Omit "Speak It" on p. 40.)

 Your own writing program

Key Idea: Practice language arts skills.

Poetry [I]

Open *Paint Like a Poet* to Lesson 20. Read aloud the poem *"Stopping by Woods on a Snowy Evening"* by Robert Frost.

Get the winter backdrop that you painted on Day 2. Today, you will be adding a path and trees. You will need a palette, water, a small round paintbrush, a paper towel, and light blue, green, and brown paint.

After gathering your supplies, turn to the "Step-by-Step Watercolor Tutorial" for Lesson 20 in *Paint Like a Poet*. Follow steps 4-6 to complete "Part Two: Path and Trees". When your painting is dry, glue your poetry copywork from Day 1 to your painting. Store your completed artwork in the place you have chosen for it.

Key Idea: Explore poetry moods with painting.

Math Exploration [S]

Choose **one** of the math options listed below.

 Singapore Primary Mathematics 4A/4B or *5A/5B* (see Appendix for schedules), or *Math with Confidence*, or *Apologia Math*

 Your own math program

Key Idea: Use a step-by-step math program.

Science Exploration [I]

 Read *Galen and the Gateway to Medicine* p. 43-51. Write the answer to each numbered question on lined paper. You do not need to copy the question. Use the listed page to help you answer each question.

1. Why did Galen leave Pergamum? (p. 43)
2. Who was Dioscorides? For what did he become famous? (p. 46-47)
3. What did Galen study in Smyrna? (p. 46)
4. Write the words *botany* and *pharmacology* and give their definitions. (p. 46)
5. What things did Solomon use his wisdom to study and describe in 1 Kings 4:29-33?

Key Idea: After his father died, Galen left Pergamum and traveled to Smyrna. He studied botany and collected plants for medicine. Next, he traveled to Corinth. Later, he traveled to Alexandria in Egypt.

Reading about History | I |

Read about history in the following resource:

⭐ *Streams of History: Ancient Rome* p. 38-43

You will be writing a narration about part of the chapter *The Struggle Between Rome and Carthage,* which is today's history reading.

To prepare for writing your narration, choose to describe either Hannibal's army or some of Hannibal's adventures as he advanced toward Rome. You may wish to look back over p. 38-43 of *Streams of History: Ancient Rome* to guide you as you write your narration.

After you have thought about which topic you will choose and how you will begin your narration, turn to Unit 24 in your *Student Notebook.* In Box 5, write a 5-8 sentence narration.

When you have finished writing, read your sentences out loud to catch any mistakes. Check for the following things: *Did you include* **who** *or* **what topic** *the reading was mainly about? Did you include* **descriptors** *of the important thing(s) that happened? Did you include a* **closing sentence**? *If not, add those things.*

Then, underline or highlight the main idea sentence in the narration. Use the *Written Narration Skills* in the Appendix as a guide for editing the narration.

Key Idea: After the death of Hamilcar, Hannibal became the general of Carthage's army. First, he attacked and conquered much of Spain, and then Carthage declared war on Rome. Hannibal meant to gain the help of the Gauls in fighting against Rome, so he crossed the Pyrenees Mountains and later the Alps.

Storytime | T |

Choose one of the following read aloud options:

⭐ *City* p. 54-65

⭐ Read the last part of the nonfiction book.

After the reading, have each person get a Bible and open it anywhere in Proverbs. Explain, *We will have 5 minutes to skim through the verses in Proverbs to find any connections to today's story. When a connection is found, read the verse out loud and quickly share the connection. At the end of 5 minutes, anyone who has not shared yet must read aloud one verse and make the best connection possible.*

Key Idea: Seek God's word for His guidance.

Bible Quiet Time | I |

Reading: Choose the option below.

⭐ *The Illustrated Family Bible* p. 278-279

⭐ Your own Bible: Luke 16:1-31

Scripture Focus: Highlight Luke 16:10.

Prayer Focus: Pray a prayer of supplication to make a humble and earnest request of God. Begin by reading the highlighted verse out loud as a prayer. End by praying, *Forgive me for the times when I haven't been honest. Help me to be honest and to be known as a person who can be trusted. Help others to see you in me.*

Scripture Memory: Copy Philippians 2:21 in your Common Place Book.
Music: *Philippians 2* CD: Track 6 (vs. 19-21)

Key Idea: Jesus expects us to be trustworthy.

Independent History Study | I |

⭐ Open your *Student Notebook* to Unit 24 – Box 6. Use *Draw and Write Through History* p. 42 as a guide to finish coloring your sketch of Hannibal's war elephant.

Key Idea: Hannibal's war elephants were used to carry archers and slingers while charging their enemies.

Learning the Basics
Focus: Language Arts, Math, Geography, Bible, and Science

Geography　[T]

Have students get both the blank map and the labeled map of **Egypt, Iraq & Saudi Arabia** that they used in Unit 22.

Then, assign students the following page:

 A Child's Geography Vol. II p. 150

Note: Do only the "Map Notes" section to map **Iraq.**

Key Idea: Practice finding and recording the locations of various places on a map of Iraq.

Language Arts　[S]

Have students complete one dictation exercise.

Guide students to complete one reading lesson.

 Drawn into the Heart of Reading

Help students complete **one** English lesson.

★ *Building with Diligence:* Lesson 45

★ *Following the Plan:* Lesson 41

★ Your own grammar program

Key Idea: Practice language arts skills.

Poetry　[I]

Open *Paint Like a Poet* to Lesson 20. Today, you will be performing a poetry reading of *"Stopping by Woods on a Snowy Evening"*. Practice reading the poem aloud with expression that matches the mood of the poem. Then, read the poem aloud in front of your chosen audience. At the end of the reading, share the following, *When I read this poem by Robert Frost, it made me think of...* Call on your audience to share what thoughts the poem brought to their minds. Last, say, *Did you know that upon hearing that his poetry would be published in the United States, Robert Frost decided to return home? His second book of poetry was a best seller and the sudden fame embarrassed Frost, who had always avoided crowds.*

Key Idea: Share the poetry of Robert Frost.

Math Exploration　[S]

Choose **one** of the math options listed below.

★ *Singapore Primary Mathematics 4A/4B or 5A/5B* (see Appendix for schedules), or *Math with Confidence*, or *Apologia Math*

★ Your own math program

Key Idea: Use a step-by-step math program.

Science Exploration　[I]

★ Read *Galen and the Gateway to Medicine* p. 52-61. Turn to the science experiment section in your science binder or sketchbook. At the top of a blank page, write: *How does blood flow throughout the body?* Under the question, write: *'Guess'*. Write down your guess. Stand in front of a mirror, and raise your tongue to look at the underside. You may use a flashlight to help you see better. Do you see thin red vessels? These are called capillaries, and the red capillaries connect to the arteries, which contain oxygen rich blood coming from the heart. Do you see large blue blood vessels? These are called veins, and they carry blood that is low in oxygen and high in carbon dioxide back to the heart to be "cleaned".

Compare Galen's diagram of circulation on p. 59 with the one shown on p. 20 of *An Illustrated Adventure in Human Anatomy*. What do you notice?

Next, write: *'Procedure'*. Draw and label the veins and the red capillaries on the tongue, leading to arteries. Write: *'Conclusion'*. Explain what you learned.

Key Idea: Galen's ideas about how blood circulated throughout the body were accepted for 1500 years.

Learning through History
Focus: Rome Conquers Carthage

Reading about History [I]

Read about history in the following resource:

★ *Streams of History: Ancient Rome*
p. 44 – top of p. 48

As Hannibal fought his way toward Rome, the Romans appointed Fabius Maximus as their dictator. Where could you look to research more about **Fabius Maximus**? Use an online resource like www.wikipedia.org or a reference book. Answer one or more of the following questions from your research: *Who were the Fabii? What was Fabius Maximus like as a child? For what victory did Fabius Maximus receive a triumph? What strategy did Fabius Maximus use to fight Hannibal? What problems did Fabius have with Minucius, another Roman commander? How was this resolved? For what is Fabius best known?*

Key Idea: Hannibal was a threat to Rome.

History Project [S]

Catapults were used by the Romans in their siege of Carthage. In this unit you will make and test several catapults. For today's activities, gather a plastic spoon or a ruler, a small rectangular or square block, and several tightly wadded paper balls or miniature marshmallows. Use the items that you gathered to make a catapult that can launch the paper balls or marshmallows across the room. Experiment with several different styles of catapults. Then, set out a bowl and try to catapult your ball or marshmallow into the bowl. Next, make a paper bulls-eye and lay it flat on the floor. Try to hit the bulls-eye.

Key Idea: The Roman army used catapults.

Storytime [T]

Choose one of the following read aloud options:

★ *City* p. 66-77

★ Read at least one humorous book for the next 16 days of plans (see Appendix).

After the reading, students will give a detailed oral narration. Select one paragraph from the story to read out loud to the students. This will be the starting point for the narration. Set a timer for 3-5 minutes. When the timer rings the narration is over, even if it isn't complete. A detailed, descriptive narration is the goal. See *Narration Tips* in the Appendix as needed.

Key Idea: Use oral narration to retell the story.

Bible Quiet Time [I]

Bible Reading: Choose one option below.

★ *The Illustrated Family Bible* p. 294-295

★ Your own Bible: Luke 17:1-37

Scripture Focus: Highlight Matt. 25:31-32.

Prayer Focus: Pray a prayer of adoration to worship and honor God. Begin by reading the highlighted verses out loud as a prayer. End by praying, *I know one day you will return in all your glory with the angels to take those to heaven who believe in you. I worship you as the Son of God, and I look forward to heaven.*

Scripture Memory: Recite Philippians 2:22.
Music: *Philippians 2* CD: Track 6 (vs. 19-22)

Key Idea: Jesus will return in all of His glory.

Independent History Study [I]

Open your *Student Notebook* to Unit 25. In Box 6, copy in cursive the **second** paragraph of p. 43 from *Draw and Write Through History*. Then, use colored pencils to lightly color Hannibal's route shown in steps 1-5 on the map in Box 7.

Key Idea: As Hannibal won battles and drew close to Rome, frightened Romans chose Fabius as dictator.

Learning the Basics
Focus: Language Arts, Math, Geography, Bible, and Science

Bible Study | T |

Read aloud and discuss with the students the following pages:

 The Radical Book for Kids p. 185-189

<u>Key Idea</u>: There are summary passages in the Bible that summarize what the Bible teaches. Passages like 1 Corinthians 15:1-5, 1 Timothy 3:16, and 2 Timothy 2:8 are summary passages about the Gospels. "The Apostles' Creed" is a brief summary of the apostles' teachings.

Language Arts | S |

Have students complete one studied dictation exercise (see Appendix for directions and passages).

Help students complete one lesson from the following reading program:

 Drawn into the Heart of Reading

Work with the students to complete **one** of the English options listed below:

★ *Building with Diligence:* Lesson 46

★ *Following the Plan:* Lesson 42 (Half)

★ Your own grammar program

<u>Key Idea</u>: Practice language arts skills.

Poetry | I |

Open *Paint Like a Poet* to Lesson 21. Read aloud the poem *"The Door in the Dark"*. On a 3 x 5 index card, neatly copy in black ink or in pencil the following highlighted lines from the poem:

In going from room to room in the dark,
I reached out blindly to save my face,
But neglected, however lightly, to lace
My fingers and close my arms in an arc.
A slim door got in past my guard,
And hit me a blow in the head so hard
I had my native smile jarred.
So people and things don't pair any more
With what they used to pair with before.
                    -Robert Frost

Check your work to make sure it is correctly copied. Then, cut around your copywork. You may outline the edge with a dark blue marker.

<u>Key Idea</u>: Read and appreciate classic poetry.

Math Exploration | S |

Choose **one** of the math options listed below.

★ *Singapore Primary Mathematics 4A/4B or 5A/5B* (see Appendix for schedules), or *Math with Confidence,* or *Apologia Math*

★ Your own math program

<u>Key Idea</u>: Use a step-by-step math program.

Science Exploration | I |

★ Read *Galen and the Gateway to Medicine* p. 62-70.

Today, you will add to your science notebook. At the top of an unlined paper, copy in cursive 3 John 1:2. Beneath the verse, write the following heading: "Galen's Surgical Tools". Under the heading either draw, trace, or photocopy the tools shown on p. 68-69 of *Galen and the Gateway to Medicine*. Make sure to label each tool with its name. Then, number each tool and make a key below the tools to list each tool's use. Descriptions of each tool's use are given on p. 69-70.

<u>Key Idea</u>: After nine years of being away from home, Galen returned to Pergamum to be a doctor. He worked as a doctor at the ludi, or school for gladiators. Galen learned much about the body by doctoring gladiators.

Learning through History
Focus: Rome Conquers Carthage

Reading about History `I`

Read about history in the following resource:

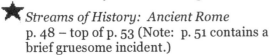 *Streams of History: Ancient Rome*
p. 48 – top of p. 53 (Note: p. 51 contains a brief gruesome incident.)

You will be choosing a portion from today's reading that you found memorable or worthy of being reread to copy. Open your *Student Notebook* to Unit 25. In Box 4, carefully copy in cursive the portion from today's reading that you selected. Then, compare your written work to the original. Last, draw a small colorful picture in Box 4 to illustrate your sentences.

Key Idea: Fabius Maximus wore down Hannibal's army, without openly confronting him. This plan continued for years.

History Project `S`

Today you will experiment with using different materials to make a catapult. Gather 4 index cards, a clothespin, several large paper clips, up to 10 craft sticks or tinker toys, rubber bands of various sizes, 2 straws, a plastic spoon, a ruler, string, a small cardboard box, tightly wadded paper balls or mini-marshmallows, and masking tape. If you don't have some of the listed items that is fine, just make do with what you have. Spend some time thinking or sketching ideas for making a catapult using any combination of the items you gathered. You do not need to use all of the items. Once you have a good plan, begin constructing your catapult. When you have built a catapult, test it by firing a ball or a marshmallow into a bowl. You may also try to hit a flat paper bulls-eye target.

Key Idea: A Roman catapult was a war device.

Storytime `T`

Choose one of the following read aloud options:

 City p. 78-87

Read aloud the next portion of the humorous book that you selected.

After reading, give each person a white piece of paper or a markerboard and a marker. Set a timer for 3-5 minutes and instruct each person to do a quick outline sketch about the story. Ideas for sketches include settings, characters, actions, important objects, or symbols. When the timer rings, briefly share the sketches.

Key Idea: Use sketching to share the story.

Bible Quiet Time `I`

Reading: Choose one option below.

The Illustrated Family Bible p. 270-271

Your own Bible: Luke 18:1-43

Scripture Focus: Highlight Luke 18:26-27.

Prayer Focus: Pray a prayer of confession to admit or acknowledge your sins to God. Begin by reading the highlighted verses out loud as a prayer. End by praying, *I confess that I need to make you more important in my life than anything else that I own or love. Only you can save me from my sins.*

Scripture Memory: Recite Philippians 2:22.
Music: *Philippians 2* CD: Track 6 (vs. 19-22)

Key Idea: Jesus needs to be the most important part of our lives. He is the only way to heaven, and He makes salvation possible.

Independent History Study `I`

Open your *Student Notebook* to Unit 25. Then, use colored pencils to lightly color the map of Hannibal's route from steps 6-9 on the map in Box 7.

Key Idea: When General Scipio Africanus invaded Africa, Hannibal was called home to defend Carthage.

Learning the Basics
Focus: Language Arts, Math, Geography, Bible, and Science

Geography [T]

Go to the website link listed on p. 6 of *A Child's Geography Vol. II*. At the link, select "History & Geography". Then, under "Knowledge Quest" select ACG2-Extra Activities". Print the "Travel Log Template" of your choice from p. 39-42. Also at the link, for older students, print and assign the "Chapter Eleven Review" on p. 78.

Assign all students the following page:

 A Child's Geography Vol. II p. 150
Note: Do only the "Travel Notes" section. The "Books" and "Poetry" on p. 151 are optional.

Key Idea: Share three sights from Iraq.

Language Arts [S]

Help students complete one lesson from the following reading program:

 Drawn into the Heart of Reading

Work with the students to complete **one** of the writing options listed below:

 Writing & Rhetoric Book 2: Narrative I p. 41-43 (Note: Read aloud the text while the students follow along. Then, discuss.)

⭐ Your own writing program

Key Idea: Practice language arts skills.

Poetry [I]

Open *Paint Like a Poet* to Lesson 21. Read aloud the poem *"The Door in the Dark"* by Robert Frost.

Today, you will be painting a cloudy night sky. You will need painting paper, a palette, water, a large flat paintbrush, masking tape, a coin, a paper towel, and dark blue and grey paint.

After gathering your supplies, turn to the "Step-by-Step Watercolor Tutorial" for Lesson 21 in *Paint Like a Poet*. Follow steps 1-3 to complete "Part One: Cloudy Night Sky". Then, let your background dry. You will complete "Part Two" of the tutorial on Day 3.

Key Idea: Use painting to illustrate poetry.

Math Exploration [S]

Choose **one** of the math options listed below.

 Singapore Primary Mathematics 4A/4B or 5A/5B (see Appendix for schedules), or *Math with Confidence,* or *Apologia Math*

 Your own math program

Key Idea: Use a step-by-step math program.

Science Exploration [I]

⭐ Read *Galen and the Gateway to Medicine* p. 71-82. Orally retell or narrate to an adult the portion of text that you read today. Use the *Narration Tips* in the Appendix for help as needed.

Key Idea: When he was 31, Galen left Pergamum to go to Rome. Rome was the chief city of the Roman Empire. It was crowded and busy. Galen visited the Circus Maximus, the Colosseum, and the Forum. He bought a house in the hills. Rome had good aqueducts for carrying clean water and a good sewage system. The Roman baths were beautiful. Galen treated Eudemus, and became sought after as a doctor. Galen gave medical lectures and demonstrations. He wrote books, articles, and "guide-books" for others.

Learning through History
Focus: Rome Conquers Carthage

Unit 25 - Day 3

Reading about History 〔 I 〕

Read about history in the following resource:

★ *Streams of History: Ancient Rome*
p. 53-57

You will be adding to your timeline in your *Student Notebook* today. In Unit 25 – Box 1, draw and color a battering ram. Label it, *Scipio Africanus marches on Carthage (204 B.C.)*. In Box 2, draw and color a laurel leaf crown. Label it, *Scipio defeats Hannibal at Zama (202 B.C.)*. In Box 3, draw and color a burning city. Label it, *Third Punic War (Carthage destroyed by Scipio Aemilianus 149-146 B.C.)*.

<u>Key Idea</u>: During the 3rd Punic War, Carthage was burned to the ground by the Romans.

Storytime 〔 T 〕

Choose one of the following read aloud options:

★ *City* p. 88-100

★ Read aloud the next portion of the humorous book that you selected.

After the reading, students will give a summary oral narration. The oral narration must be no longer than 5 sentences and should summarize the reading. As students narrate, have them hold up one finger for each sentence shared. Remind students that the focus should be on the big ideas, rather than on the details.

<u>Key Idea</u>: Summarize the story by narrating.

History Project 〔 S 〕

If you have access to the internet, go to one of the following websites to experiment with trebuchets (or catapults):

Option 1:
www.pbs.org/wgbh/nova/lostempires/trebuchet

Option 2:
https://gizmos.explorelearning.com (Note: At the site, search for "trebuchet".)

If you do not have access to the internet, or the links above do not work, then continue experimenting with various types of catapults as explained on Day 2 instead.

<u>Key Idea</u>: After the death of Hannibal, Rome attacked Carthage again. This time, Carthage was completely destroyed.

Bible Quiet Time 〔 I 〕

Reading: Choose one option below.

★ *The Illustrated Family Bible* p. 280-281

★ Your own Bible: Luke 19:1-27

Scripture Focus: Highlight Luke 19:10.

Prayer Focus: Pray a prayer of thanksgiving to express gratitude for God's divine goodness. Begin by reading the highlighted verse out loud as a prayer. End by praying, *Thank you for coming to save those who are lost, like me. I know that I can be forgiven and made new through faith in you, just like Zaccheus.*

Scripture Memory: Recite Philippians 2:22.
Music: *Philippians 2* CD: Track 6 (vs. 19-22)

<u>Key Idea</u>: Jesus came to forgive and to save those who are lost.

Independent History Study 〔 I 〕

Open your *Student Notebook* to "Prophecies About Christ". Under "Prophecy" write, *Isaiah 9:6*. Read the Scripture from the Bible to discover the prophecy. Under "Fulfillment" write, *Matthew 28:18*. Read the fulfillment Scripture. Under "Description", write a few phrases to describe the prophecy about Jesus.

<u>Key Idea</u>: All authority in heaven and earth is given to Christ, and the government is upon His shoulders.

Learning the Basics
Focus: Language Arts, Math, Geography, Bible, and Science

Bible Study | T

Read aloud and discuss with the students the following pages:

 The Radical Book for Kids p. 190-191

Key Idea: In the Bible, God is compared to a potter. God created man from the dust of the ground. As the Potter, God made you the way you are. He shaped and molded you. God has a special plan for each of His children.

Language Arts | S

Have students complete one studied dictation exercise (see Appendix for directions and passages).

Work with the students to complete **one** of the writing options listed below:

 Writing & Rhetoric Book 2: Narrative I bottom p. 44-46 (Note: Omit top of p. 44. It includes a nude statue of the parable. Read aloud today's text while the students Follow along. Then, discuss.)

 Your own writing program

Key Idea: Practice language arts skills.

Poetry | I

Open *Paint Like a Poet* to Lesson 21. Read aloud the poem *"The Door in the Dark"* by Robert Frost.

Get the cloudy night sky backdrop that you painted on Day 2. Today, you will be adding a moon and stars. You will need a palette, water, a small flat paintbrush, a toothpick, and white and grey paint.

After gathering your supplies, turn to the "Step-by-Step Watercolor Tutorial" for Lesson 21 in *Paint Like a Poet*. Follow steps 4-6 to complete "Part Two: Moon and Stars". When your painting is dry, glue your poetry copywork from Day 1 to your painting. Store your completed artwork in the place you have chosen for it.

Key Idea: Explore poetry moods with painting.

Math Exploration | S

Choose **one** of the math options listed below.

 Singapore Primary Mathematics 4A/4B or 5A/5B (see Appendix for schedules), or *Math with Confidence,* or *Apologia Math*

 Your own math program

Key Idea: Use a step-by-step math program.

Science Exploration | I

 Read *Galen and the Gateway to Medicine* p. 83-95. Write the answer to each numbered question on lined paper. You do not need to copy the question. Use the listed page to help you answer each question.
1. How did Galen diagnose a patient's illness? (p. 85)
2. Name some diseases that Galen recognized. (p. 86)
3. What problems do you notice with Galen's explanation of how the organs' work on p. 88?
4. List the four humors and explain how Galen used them to diagnose patients. (p. 34)
5. How does Psalm 139:16 show that astrology charts and the movement of the heavenly bodies have nothing to do with how our days or lives on earth go?

Key Idea: Galen became the doctor to the emperor, Marcus Aurelius, and to other important Romans.

Learning through History
Focus: Rome Conquers Carthage

Reading about History I

Read about history in the following resource:

★ *Streams of History: Ancient Rome* p. 58-63

You will be writing a narration about part of the chapter *How Rome Conquered the World, but Destroyed Herself,* which is part of today's history reading.

To prepare for writing your narration, choose either to tell about Aemilius Paulus as commander of the Roman army or to describe a Roman triumph. You may wish to look back over p. 58-63 of *Streams of History: Ancient Rome* to guide you as you write your narration.

After you have thought about which topic you will choose and how you will begin your narration, turn to Unit 25 in your *Student Notebook.* In Box 5, write a 5-8 sentence narration.

When you have finished writing, read your sentences out loud to catch any mistakes. Check for the following things: *Did you include **who** or **what topic** the reading was mainly about? Did you include **descriptors** of the important thing(s) that happened? Did you include a **closing sentence**? If not, add those things.*

Then, underline or highlight the main idea sentence in the narration. Use the *Written Narration Skills* in the Appendix as a guide for editing the narration.

Key Idea: Aemilius Paulus was named after his father, who had the same name. His father had been killed at Cannae in the battle with Hannibal. Aemilius Paulus (the son) was sent to battle King Perseus of Macedonia. For his victory in Macedonia, Aemilius Paulus received a Roman triumph.

Storytime T

Choose one of the following read aloud options:

★ *City* p. 101-111

★ Read aloud part of the humorous book.

After the reading, have each person get a Bible and open it anywhere in Proverbs. Explain, *We will have 5 minutes to skim through the verses in Proverbs to find any connections to today's story. When a connection is found, read the verse out loud and quickly share the connection. At the end of 5 minutes, anyone who has not shared yet must read aloud one verse and make the best connection possible.*

Key Idea: Seek God's word for His guidance.

Bible Quiet Time I

Reading: Choose one option below.

★ *The Illustrated Family Bible* p. 286-287

★ Your own Bible: Luke 19:28-48

Scripture Focus: Highlight Matthew 21:22.

Prayer Focus: Pray a prayer of supplication to make a humble and earnest request of God. Begin by reading the highlighted verse out loud as a prayer. End by praying, *I ask you to help me believe in you more and more. Help me to pray wisely and to only ask for those things that fit your will for my life.*

Scripture Memory: Copy Philippians 2:22 in your Common Place Book.
Music: *Philippians 2* CD: Track 6 (vs. 19-22)

Key Idea: Jesus is truly the Son of God. He is our King.

Independent History Study I

★ Listen to *What in the World?* Disc 4, Track 3: "The Punic Wars".

Key Idea: In the 1st Punic War, Carthage and Rome fought over Sicily. In the 2nd Punic War, Rome eventually defeated Hannibal and Carthage's army. In the 3rd Punic War, Rome destroyed Carthage.

Learning the Basics

Focus: Language Arts, Math, Geography, Bible, and Science

Geography [T]

Read aloud to the students the following pages:

⭐ *A Child's Geography Vol. II* p. 152-157
Discuss with students "Field Notes" p. 157.

Key Idea: The Tigris and Euphrates rivers have often overflowed their banks, creating an alluvial plain. Iraq has little rainfall, so crops on the alluvial plain must be irrigated. Marshlands form where the Tigris and Euphrates rivers' distributaries cross the land. The Ma'dans have lived in the marshes of Iraq for thousands of years.

Language Arts [S]

Have students complete one dictation exercise.

Guide students to complete one reading lesson.

⭐ *Drawn into the Heart of Reading*

Help students complete **one** English lesson.

⭐ *Building with Diligence:* Lesson 47

⭐ *Following the Plan:* Lesson 42 (Last half)

⭐ Your own grammar program

Key Idea: Practice language arts skills.

Poetry [I]

Open *Paint Like a Poet* to Lesson 21. Today, you will be performing a poetry reading of *"the Door in the Dark"*. Practice reading the poem aloud with expression that matches the mood of the poem. Then, read the poem aloud in front of your chosen audience.

At the end of the reading, share the following, *When I read this poem by Robert Frost, it made me think of...* Call on your audience to share what thoughts the poem brought to their minds. Last, say, *Did you know that Robert Frost conquered his shyness and became a popular American performer, whose folksy and simple style of speaking endeared him to listeners everywhere? He also was quite tall and was known for his watchful eyes.*

Key Idea: Share the poetry of Robert Frost.

Math Exploration [S]

Choose **one** of the math options listed below.

⭐ *Singapore Primary Mathematics 4A/4B* or *5A/5B* (see Appendix for schedules), or *Math with Confidence*, or *Apologia Math*

⭐ Your own math program

Key Idea: Use a step-by-step math program.

Science Exploration [I]

⭐ Read *Galen and the Gateway to Medicine* p. 96-101. Turn to the science experiment section in your science binder or sketchbook. At the top of a blank page, write: *In which types of products is aloe vera used today?* Under the question, write: *'Guess'*. Write down your guess. In Galen's time, aloe was used for cuts, burns, and bruises. Check the ingredient labels on your lotions, sunblocks, anti-itch creams, antibacterial gels, or cooling gels for burns to see if you have any products that contain aloe vera. Is aloe vera still used for cuts, burns, and bruises today? Next, write: *'Procedure'*. List the products that you found that contain aloe vera. Write: *'Conclusion'*. Explain what you learned.

Here's a few easy home remedies you can try: For a sore throat, mix one-half teaspoon of salt with one cup of warm water and gargle. To heal a hoarse throat, drink hot tea with honey. For a stuffy nose, take a hot shower and stand in the steam until you can breathe more freely. For a cut or a scrape, clean it, apply antibiotic ointment, and bandage it. If you have dry lips, drink more water and don't lick your lips. For a headache, drink a glass of water, lie down in a dark room, and place a cool compress on the forehead.

Key Idea: We still use many remedies today that doctors in the ancient world used to treat their patients.

Reading about History   I

Read about history in the following resource:

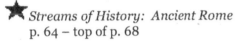 *Streams of History: Ancient Rome* p. 64 – top of p. 68

Roman General Mummius burned the Greek city of Corinth. Where could you look to research more about **Corinth**? Use an online resource like www.wikipedia.org or a reference book. Answer one or more of the following questions: *Where was ancient Corinth located? Which type of ship was originally designed in Corinth? For what exports was Corinth known? What is a Corinthian column? When was Corinth destroyed? Who had Corinth rebuilt? When did the Apostle Paul visit Corinth? Which books of the Bible contain Paul's letters to the church at Corinth? What were some of the problems in Corinth?*

Key Idea: Rome destroyed Corinth.

History Project   S

In this unit you will plan a Roman meal for Day 3. This will include 3 courses, as was customary. Have a parent help you plan your meal. Choose one (or more) of the following suggestions for each course. Then, write down your menu on a sheet of paper. Appetizers: lettuce greens with vinegar and oil; focaccia bread, garlic bread or bread rolls; cut up celery, cucumbers, or broccoli. Main course: tuna (can be canned), sliced hard boiled eggs, cheese (mozzarella, provolone, or ricotta), and/or hot sausage (can be bratwurst or hot dogs). Dessert (choose one from Day 2): cheesecake, custard, and/or fruit.

Key Idea: The Romans learned Greek ways.

Storytime   T

Choose one of the following read aloud options:

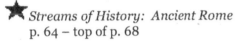 *Traveling the Way* p. 11-17

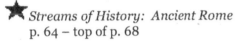 Read at least one humorous book for the next 12 days of plans.

After the reading, students will give a detailed oral narration. Select one paragraph from the story to read out loud to the students. This will be the starting point for the narration. Set a timer for 3-5 minutes. When the timer rings the narration is over, even if it isn't complete. A detailed, descriptive narration is the goal. See *Narration Tips* in the Appendix as needed.

Key Idea: Use oral narration to retell the story.

Bible Quiet Time   I

Bible Reading: Choose one option below.

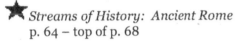 *The Illustrated Family Bible* p. 288-289

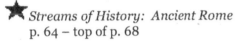 Your own Bible: Luke 20:1-47

Scripture Focus: Highlight Luke 20:13-15.

Prayer Focus: Pray a prayer of adoration to worship and honor God. Begin by reading the highlighted verses out loud as a prayer. End by praying, *Lord, I know you do not have to answer to men, but men do have to answer to you. The Pharisees did not see you as God's Son, but I worship you as the Son of God.*

Scripture Memory: Recite Philippians 2:23.
Music: *Philippians 2* CD: Track 6 (vs. 19-23)

Key Idea: Jesus was (and is) rejected by many.

Independent History Study   I

Open your *Student Notebook* to Unit 26. In Box 6, copy in cursive the following Epicurus' quote that was found on his garden gate: *Stranger, here you will do well to tarry; here our highest good is pleasure.*

Key Idea: Epicurus believed that pleasure was man's goal. He didn't believe in God or life after death.

Learning the Basics
Focus: Language Arts, Math, Geography, Bible, and Science

Bible Study [T]

Read aloud and discuss with the students the following pages:

 The Radical Book for Kids p. 192-193

Key Idea: In Bible times, coins such as a mite and a quadran were used. A mite was equal to about 50 cents. A quadran was equal to about one dollar. A denarius equaled approximately $64.00, and one mina equaled approximately $6,400.00. One talent was equal to about $384,000.00.

Language Arts [S]

Have students complete one studied dictation exercise (see Appendix for directions and passages).

Help students complete one lesson from the following reading program:

 Drawn into the Heart of Reading

Work with the students to complete **one** of the English options listed below:

★ *Building with Diligence:* Lesson 48

★ *Following the Plan:* Lesson 43

★ Your own grammar program

Key Idea: Practice language arts skills.

Poetry [I]

Choose one of Robert Frost's poems from Lessons 19-25 in *Paint Like a Poet* to memorize.

You will have 2 weeks (units) to memorize the entire poem. So, you should have half of your chosen poem memorized by Day 4 of this unit.

After you have chosen your poem to memorize, read it three times, adding actions to help you remember the words.

Key Idea: Read and appreciate classic poetry.

Math Exploration [S]

Choose **one** of the math options listed below.

★ *Singapore Primary Mathematics 4A/4B or 5A/5B* (see Appendix for schedules), or *Math with Confidence*, or *Apologia Math*

★ Your own math program

Key Idea: Use a step-by-step math program.

Science Exploration [I]

★ Read *Galen and the Gateway to Medicine* p. 102-109. Today, you will add to your science notebook. At the top of an unlined paper, copy in cursive Job 33:4. Beneath the verse, write the following heading: "Facts About Galen". Under the heading, either write a narration about Galen or list facts that you have learned about him.

Key Idea: Galen left Rome about the time of the plagues, and then Emperor Marcus Aurelius summoned Galen to Aquileia in northern Italy. Galen didn't like camp life or the battlefield. So, he returned to Rome to take care of Commodus, the emperor's son. Commodus went on to be emperor, and Galen was his doctor. He was also the doctor to the next emperor, Septimius Severus. During that time, part of Galen's writings were burned in a fire in the Temple of Peace. The rest of his works were circulated widely long after his death.

Reading about History [I]

Read about history in the following resource:

⭐ *Streams of History: Ancient Rome* p. 68 – top of p. 72

You will be choosing a portion from today's reading that you found memorable or worthy of being reread to copy. Open your *Student Notebook* to Unit 26. In Box 4, carefully copy in cursive the portion from today's reading that you selected. Then, compare your written work to the original. Last, draw a small colorful picture in Box 4 to illustrate your sentences.

Key Idea: The Romans began seeking luxuries.

Storytime [T]

Choose one of the following read aloud options:

⭐ *Traveling the Way* p. 18-24

⭐ Read aloud the next portion of the humorous book that you selected.

After reading, give each person 2 slips of paper. Each person must think of 2 questions to ask about the book and write one question on each slip of paper. Next, fold up the slips of paper and place them in a container. Each person must select at least one question from the container to answer.

Key Idea: Use questioning to share the story.

History Project [S]

Choose **one** of the following desserts for your Roman meal. You may either make it today and refrigerate it for Day 3 or make it on Day 3. **Option 1 – Roman Custard:** Whisk together 2 cups milk and ¼ cup honey until blended. In a different bowl, whisk 5 eggs until frothy. Combine the two mixtures, add 1 tsp. vanilla, and blend well. Pour into an 11 x 7 pan. Bake for 25-35 min. at 300 degrees (until a knife inserted comes out clean). **Option 2 – Roman Cheesecake:** Beat 8 oz. ricotta cheese until soft. Stir in 1 cup all-purpose flour. Add 1 beaten egg and stir until a soft dough forms. Divide the dough into 4 parts. Mold each part into a bun and place it on a greased baking tray with a bay leaf underneath. Cover the cakes and bake for 35-40 min. at 425 degrees, until golden brown. Warm ½ cup honey and place warm cakes in it for 30 min. so they absorb it. **Option 3 – Cut up fruit.**

Key Idea: Roman feasts became very lavish.

Bible Quiet Time [I]

Reading: Choose one option below.

⭐ *The Illustrated Family Bible* p. 290-291

⭐ Your own Bible: Luke 21:1-38

Scripture Focus: Highlight Matt. 24:36-42.

Prayer Focus: Pray a prayer of confession to admit or acknowledge your sins to God. Begin by reading the highlighted verses out loud as a prayer. End by praying, *I confess that I don't always live each day as if I'm ready for your return. Help me to live my life according to your word so that I am always ready for your return.*

Scripture Memory: Recite Philippians 2:23.
Music: *Philippians 2* CD: Track 6 (vs. 19-23)

Key Idea: Only the Father knows when Christ will return, so we must be ready at any hour.

Independent History Study [I]

⭐ Open your *Student Notebook* to Unit 26 – Box 7. Follow the directions from *Draw and Write Through History* p. 58-60 (through step 7) to draw a Roman chariot. You will finish drawing on Day 2.

Key Idea: The Romans adopted the Greek's pleasure-seeking ways, such as the theater, baths, and races.

Learning the Basics
Focus: Language Arts, Math, Geography, Bible, and Science

Geography [T]

Read aloud to the students the following pages:

 A Child's Geography Vol. II p. 158-160

Discuss the "Field Notes" on p. 160.

<u>Key Idea</u>: Basrah, one of Iraq's largest cities, is located on the flat-panned deserts of Iraq. Oil flows beneath the surface of the earth here and is found primarily in the Middle East. Iraq is second in the world only to Saudi Arabia in the amount of oil pumped daily out of the earth.

Language Arts [S]

Help students complete one lesson from the following reading program:

 Drawn into the Heart of Reading

Work with the students to complete **one** of the writing options listed below:

 Writing & Rhetoric Book 2: Narrative I p. 47 – top of p. 54 (Note: Today's text includes a witch and Greek gods in the examples from literature. Read aloud the text while the students follow along. Then, discuss.)

 Your own writing program

<u>Key Idea</u>: Practice language arts skills.

Poetry [I]

Today, you will copy half of the Robert Frost poem from *Paint Like a Poet* that you chose to memorize this week.

At the top of a clean page in your *Common Place Book,* copy the title and the author of the poem. Then, copy half of the poem in cursive, leaving the rest of the page blank.

You will copy the remaining half of the poem during the next unit.

Practice the portion of the poem that you copied today by reading it aloud.

<u>Key Idea</u>: Copy and memorize classic poetry.

Math Exploration [S]

Choose **one** of the math options listed below.

 Singapore Primary Mathematics 4A/4B or *5A/5B* (see Appendix for schedules), or *Math with Confidence,* or *Apologia Math*

 Your own math program

<u>Key Idea</u>: Use a step-by-step math program.

Science Exploration [I]

 Read *Galen and the Gateway to Medicine* p. 110-123. Orally retell or narrate to an adult the portion of text that you read today. Use the *Narration Tips* in the Appendix for help as needed.

<u>Key Idea</u>: Galen believed in a perfect Creator who had created a perfect human being. His ideas formed the basis for later medical theories. Galen's writings were preserved and circulated through the centuries. During the Renaissance, Paracelsus began questioning some of Galen's thinking. He was an alchemist or a believer in changing base metals into medicines. Vesalius also questioned Galen when he realized Galen had never dissected a human body and had instead used animals as a basis for describing human anatomy. William Harvey corrected Galen's theories about the heart and how blood moves throughout the body.

Reading about History   I

Read about history in the following resource:

★ *Streams of History: Ancient Rome* p. 72 – middle of p. 76

You will be adding to your timeline in your *Student Notebook* today. In Unit 26 – Box 1, draw and color a Roman shield. Label it, *Rome conquers Corinth and Greece (146 B.C.).* In Box 2, draw and color a spear. Label it, *Rome conquers Spain (133 B.C.).* In Box 3, draw and color a red cape. Label it, *Tiberius and Gaius Gracchus are tribunes in Rome (133-121 B.C.).*

<u>Key Idea</u>: Over time, the city of Rome became more focused on amusement.

Storytime   T

Choose one of the following read aloud options:

★ *Traveling the Way* p. 25-30

★ Read aloud the next portion of the humorous book that you selected.

After the reading, students will give a summary oral narration. The oral narration must be no longer than 5 sentences and should summarize the reading. As students narrate, have them hold up one finger for each sentence shared. Remind students that the focus should be on the big ideas, rather than on the details.

<u>Key Idea</u>: Summarize the story by narrating.

History Project   S

Set up your Roman meal. To recline while eating, either use couches in a 'U'-shape around a coffee table, or place 3 large towels to be couches around a coffee table. If you don't have a coffee table, use trays instead. Place your menu in the center of the area. Put an open napkin in front of each guest's spot. No silverware is used until dessert. Pour water over guests' hands while they wash them over a basin and dry them. Serve the food cut into bite-sized pieces one course at a time. Place each course of food in individual bowls served to each guest on his/her napkin. Between courses, rinse guests' hands with water. Eat while reclining barefoot. Wear a robe (as Romans did over their togas). Women may sit in straight-backed chairs as Roman women did. During dessert, read poetry to the guests.

<u>Key Idea</u>: Dining and bathing filled the day.

Bible Quiet Time   I

Reading: Choose one option below.

★ *The Illustrated Family Bible* p. 296-297

★ Your own Bible: Luke 22:1-46

Scripture Focus: Highlight Luke 22:17-19.

Prayer Focus: Pray a prayer of thanksgiving to express gratitude for God's divine goodness. Begin by reading the highlighted verses out loud as a prayer. End by praying, *Thank you for sacrificing your life for sinners like me. Help me to remember your sacrifice through the Lord's Supper.*

Scripture Memory: Recite Philippians 2:23.
Music: *Philippians 2* CD: Track 6 (vs. 19-23)

<u>Key Idea</u>: Jesus calls us to remember His sacrifice through the Lord's Supper.

Independent History Study   I

★ Open your *Student Notebook* to Unit 26 – Box 7. Follow the directions from *Draw and Write Through History* p. 60-61 (steps 8-10) to finish drawing a Roman chariot. You will color it on Day 4.

<u>Key Idea</u>: Chariot races were held at the Circus Maximus in Rome. Up to 250,000 people could fit inside the arena, and they gambled on the races. The Romans also loved to go to the Colosseum to watch fights.

Learning the Basics
Focus: Language Arts, Math, Geography, Bible, and Science

Bible Study ⬚ T

Read aloud and discuss with the students the following pages:

 The Radical Book for Kids p. 194-195

Key Idea: It is important to make choices based upon God's Word. When we make choices, we should ask God for His wisdom and guidance. Our choices should please God. We might not always make the perfect choice, but the Bible can help us make good decisions.

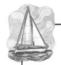

Poetry ⬚ I

Practice reading aloud half of the poem that you chose to memorize from *Paint Like a Poet*, using the actions that you added to help you remember the words. Do this 2 times.

Then, recite half of the poem without looking at the words.

You have 2 weeks (units) to memorize the entire poem. So, you should have half of your chosen poem memorized by Day 4 of this unit.

Key Idea: Memorize classic poetry.

Language Arts ⬚ S

Have students complete one studied dictation exercise (see Appendix for directions and passages).

Work with the students to complete **one** of the writing options listed below:

 Writing & Rhetoric Book 2: Narrative I p. 55 – middle of p. 57 (Note: Omit p. 54. Guide students as needed through the lesson.)

 Your own writing program

Key Idea: Practice language arts skills.

Math Exploration ⬚ S

Choose **one** of the math options listed below.

  Singapore Primary Mathematics 4A/4B or *5A/5B* (see Appendix for schedules), or *Math with Confidence*, or *Apologia Math*

 Your own math program

Key Idea: Use a step-by-step math program.

Science Exploration ⬚ I

⭐ Read *Exploring the History of Medicine* p. 4-10.

After reading the chapter listed above, turn to p. 11 of *Exploring the History of Medicine*. Write the answer to each numbered question from p. 11 on lined paper. You do not need to copy the question.

Key Idea: Imhotep was a physician in ancient Egypt. He is the most ancient physician that we know about. Hippocrates was a physician in ancient Greece. Hippocrates visited Egypt to study medicine. Many books were published in his name. Galen studied Hippocrates' writings and added his ideas. He was a physician in ancient Rome.

Reading about History | I |

Read about history in the following resource:

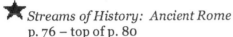 *Streams of History: Ancient Rome* p. 76 – top of p. 80

You will be writing a narration about part of the chapter *How Rome Conquered the World, but Destroyed Herself,* which is part of today's history reading.

To prepare for writing your narration, choose either to tell about Tiberius Gracchus or tell about Caius Gracchus. You may wish to look back over p. 76-80 of *Streams of History: Ancient Rome* to guide you as you write your narration.

After you have thought about which topic you will choose and how you will begin your narration, turn to Unit 26 in your *Student Notebook.* In Box 5, write a 5-8 sentence narration.

When you have finished writing, read your sentences out loud to catch any mistakes. Check for the following things: *Did you include* **who** *or* **what topic** *the reading was mainly about? Did you include* **descriptors** *of the important thing(s) that happened? Did you include a* **closing sentence**? *If not, add those things.*

Then, underline or highlight the main idea sentence in the narration. Use the *Written Narration Skills* in the Appendix as a guide for editing the narration.

Key Idea: In Rome two consuls were elected each year. This was the highest Roman office. The consuls often led the army. Tribunes were elected officials who represented the people. The Gracchi brothers were elected as tribunes.

Storytime | T |

Choose one of the following read aloud options:

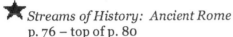 *Traveling the Way* p. 31-44

Read aloud part of the humorous book.

After the reading, have each person get a Bible and open it anywhere in Proverbs. Explain, *We will have 5 minutes to skim through the verses in Proverbs to find any connections to today's story. When a connection is found, read the verse out loud and quickly share the connection. At the end of 5 minutes, anyone who has not shared yet must read aloud one verse and make the best connection possible.*

Key Idea: Seek God's word for His guidance.

Bible Quiet Time | I |

Reading: Choose one option below.

The Illustrated Family Bible p. 298-301

Your own Bible: Luke 22:47-71

Scripture Focus: Highlight Luke 22:61-62.

Prayer Focus: Pray a prayer of supplication to make a humble and earnest request of God. Begin by reading the highlighted verses out loud as a prayer. End by praying, *Help me stand strong in my faith, especially when I am frightened. Help me to stand up for you and for what I believe.*

Scripture Memory: Copy Philippians 2:23 in your Common Place Book.
Music: *Philippians 2* CD: Track 6 (vs. 19-23)

Key Idea: Jesus was arrested and stood trial.

Independent History Study | I |

Open your *Student Notebook* to Unit 26 – Box 7. Use *Draw and Write Through History* p. 61 (step 11) as a guide to color your sketch of a Roman chariot.

Key Idea: Rome's roads connected all of her provinces. People traveled frequently and rapidly on Roman roads by chariot, on horseback, or in carriages. Messages traveled quickly as well.

Geography [T]

Have students get both the blank map and the labeled map of **Eygpt, Iraq & Saudi Arabia** that they used in Unit 22. Then, assign students the following page:

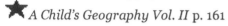 *A Child's Geography Vol. II* p. 161

Note: Do only the "Map Notes" section. Save both the blank map and the labeled map to use with the upcoming unit on Saudi Arabia.

<u>Key Idea</u>: Practice mapping locations in Iraq.

Language Arts [S]

Have students complete one dictation exercise.

Guide students to complete one reading lesson.

★ *Drawn into the Heart of Reading*

Help students complete **one** English lesson.

★ *Building with Diligence:* Lesson 49 (Half)

★ *Following the Plan:* Lesson 44

★ Your own grammar program

<u>Key Idea</u>: Practice language arts skills.

Poetry [I]

Practice reading aloud half of the poem that you chose to memorize from *Paint Like a Poet*, using the actions that you added to help you remember the words. Do this 2 times.

Then, recite half of the poem without looking at the words.

You have 2 weeks (units) to memorize the entire poem. So, you should have half of your chosen poem memorized by today.

<u>Key Idea</u>: Memorize classic poetry.

Math Exploration [S]

Choose **one** of the math options listed below.

★ *Singapore Primary Mathematics 4A/4B or 5A/5B* (see Appendix for schedules), or *Math with Confidence*, or *Apologia Math*

★ Your own math program

<u>Key Idea</u>: Use a step-by-step math program.

Science Exploration [I]

★ Read *Exploring the History of Medicine* p. 12-16. Answer the questions on p. 17 on lined paper. Then, turn to the science experiment section in your science binder or sketchbook. At the top of a blank page, write: *What is the body's natural response to bleeding?* Under the question, write: *'Guess'*. Write down your guess. In a clear glass or measuring cup, add ½ cup water and several drops of yellow food coloring. This will be plasma, which makes up half of your blood. Add ¼ tsp. salt and ¼ tsp. sugar and mix. Plasma contains sugar, salt, and hormones that your body needs. Next, measure ½ cup of cooking oil. Add several drops of red food coloring to it. The oil represents the other half of your blood, which is made of oxygen-carrying red cells and white cells. Add the colored oil to the plasma and mix. Then, to represent platelets, add 3 Tbsp. of either shredded wheat or thin fibers pulled from cotton balls or gauze. Now, place a small funnel in an empty glass. The funnel represents a blood vessel, and the thin opening represents a cut in the skin. Begin pouring the mixture through the funnel to simulate blood flowing out of a cut in the skin. A break in the skin usually cuts the wall of a blood vessel. As the blood flows out of the cut, the body's platelets form a sticky blood clot to seal the leak. Next, write: *'Procedure'*. Draw and label a picture of the experiment. Write: *'Conclusion'*. Explain what you learned.

<u>Key Idea</u>: Bloodletting, or bleeding a patient, was a common practice for centuries. This practice caused patients to bleed to death and went against the body's natural response to bleeding, which is clotting.

Learning through History
Focus: The Roman Empire

Reading about History `I`

Read about history in the following resource:

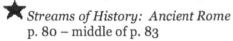 *Streams of History: Ancient Rome* p. 80 – middle of p. 83

Julius Caesar grew to be a powerful leader in Rome? Where could you look to research more about **Julius Caesar?** Use an online resource like www.wikipedia.org or a reference book.

Answer one or more of the following questions from your research: *How many years before Christ's birth was Caesar born? With whom did Caesar form a triumvirate? Describe Caesar as a general. What was the Rubicon? When the triumvirate ended, whom did Caesar battle for control of Rome? After being appointed dictator of Rome, name some of the changes Caesar made. How did Caesar die? Whom did he name as his successor?*

Key Idea: Julius Caesar was a strong leader.

History Project `S`

In this unit you will make Roman soldier's clothing to tape on a paper cutout of a soldier, an action figure, or a masculine doll. Open your *Student Notebook* to Unit 27. Read over the page titled, "What Did a Roman Soldier Wear?" Today, you will be drawing, coloring, and cutting out the tunic, the armour, and the sandals. Before beginning to draw, make sure to either draw your paper cutout of a soldier, or have your action figure or masculine doll nearby so that you know how large to make the soldier's clothing. Save the tunic, armour, and sandals in a baggie for Day 2.

Key Idea: Marius and Sulla fought each other.

Storytime `T`

Choose one of the following read aloud options:

 Traveling the Way p. 45-51

Read at least one humorous book for the next 8 days of plans.

After the reading, students will give a detailed oral narration. Select one paragraph from the story to read out loud to the students. This will be the starting point for the narration. Set a timer for 3-5 minutes. When the timer rings the narration is over, even if it isn't complete. A detailed, descriptive narration is the goal. See *Narration Tips* in the Appendix as needed.

Key Idea: Use oral narration to retell the story.

Bible Quiet Time `I`

Bible Reading: Choose one option below.

The Illustrated Family Bible p. 302-303

Your own Bible: Luke 23:1-31

Scripture Focus: Highlight Luke 23:13-15.

Prayer Focus: Pray a prayer of adoration to worship and honor God. Begin by reading the highlighted verses out loud as a prayer. End by praying, *I worship you as the King over all the earth. I know that even though you were innocent and perfect, you still chose to die to save me from my sins.*

Scripture Memory: Recite Philippians 2:24.
Music: *Philippians 2* CD: Track 6 (vs. 19-24)

Key Idea: Jesus chose death to save us!

Independent History Study `I`

Open your *Student Notebook* to Unit 16. Look at the statue from Nebuchadnezzar's dream. Note the legs of iron that Daniel prophecied in Daniel 2:33 that represent Rome in Daniel 2:40. As you look at the feet of iron and clay, what can you see happening later for the Roman Empire?

Key Idea: Daniel prophecied the coming of the Roman empire almost 500 years before Caesar's birth.

Learning the Basics
Focus: Language Arts, Math, Geography, Bible, and Science

Bible Study [T]

Read aloud and discuss with the students the following pages:

 The Radical Book for Kids p. 196-198

Key Idea: Scripture says "there is a time for everything." The Bible mentions many forms of entertainment and fun like wrestling, camping, dancing, telling stories and riddles, taking walks, chariot racing, boxing, playing music, running races, throwing parties, and more. There is a time for the fun and games mentioned in the Bible.

Language Arts [S]

Have students complete one studied dictation exercise (see Appendix for directions and passages).

Help students complete one lesson from the following reading program:

 Drawn into the Heart of Reading

Work with the students to complete **one** of the English options listed below:

 Building with Diligence: Lesson 49 (Half)

 Following the Plan: Lesson 45

 Your own grammar program

Key Idea: Practice language arts skills.

Poetry [I]

Continue memorizing the Robert Frost poem that you chose from *Paint Like a Poet* in Unit 26. You should have half of your chosen poem memorized already.

You should memorize the rest of the poem by Day 4 of this unit.

Today, read the entire poem 3 times, adding actions to the last half of the poem to help you memorize the words more easily.

Key Idea: Read and appreciate a variety of classic poetry.

Math Exploration [S]

Choose **one** of the math options listed below.

 Singapore Primary Mathematics 4A/4B or 5A/5B (see Appendix for schedules), or *Math with Confidence,* or *Apologia Math*

 Your own math program

Key Idea: Use a step-by-step math program.

Science Exploration [I]

 Read *Exploring the History of Medicine* p. 18-22.

After reading the chapter listed above, turn to p. 23 of *Exploring the History of Medicine*. Write the answer to each numbered question from p. 23 on lined paper. You do not need to copy the question.

Key Idea: Andreas Vesalius' father was an apothecary, which is like a druggist. He built Andreas a small laboratory to use as a child. By the time Andreas was 17, he was a medical student in Paris. After war broke out, he left Paris to study near Brussels in Belgium. He was fascinated with the human skeleton. While studying the human skeleton, he discovered that Galen had gained his information about the body by studying apes. As a professor of anatomy, Vesalius performed his own dissections. He found over two hundred mistakes in Galen's ancient books, which were still being taught by professors of his day.

Learning through History
Focus: The Roman Empire

Reading about History   I

Read about history in the following resource:

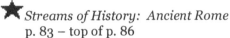 *Streams of History: Ancient Rome*
p. 83 – top of p. 86

You will be choosing a portion from today's reading that you found memorable or worthy of being reread to copy. Open your *Student Notebook* to Unit 27. In Box 4, carefully copy in cursive the portion from today's reading that you selected. Then, compare your written work to the original. Last, draw a small colorful picture in Box 4 to illustrate your sentences.

Key Idea: Julius Caesar, Pompey, and Crassus formed a triumvirate to rule Rome. Soon, Crassus was killed and Pompey became a general in the East with Caesar as a general in Gaul (or France). Eventually, Caesar and Pompey fought one another for control of Rome.

History Project   S

Today, you will continue outfitting your Roman soldier. Get the baggie with the tunic, armour, and sandals you designed on Day 2. Get your Roman soldier too. Now, open your *Student Notebook* to Unit 27. Today, you will be drawing, coloring, and cutting out the belt, the sword, and the equipment. As you're creating your soldier's outfit, make sure that it is the correct size for your Roman soldier. Save your soldier's outfit in a baggie for Day 3. If needed, you may finish making the equipment on Day 3.

Key Idea: Caesar and Pompey had a civil war for control of Rome. Caesar's soldiers battled Pompey's soldiers, until Pompey was killed.

Storytime   T

Choose one of the following read aloud options:

 Traveling the Way p. 52-58

★ Read aloud the next portion of the humorous book that you selected.

After reading, work with the students to plan a 3 minute skit with simple props to act out part of today's reading. Set a timer for 3 minutes to quickly prepare for the skit. Make sure that you participate in the skit along with the students. When the timer rings, set it again for 3 minutes and perform the skit. You do not need an audience, as the goal is the retelling.

Key Idea: Use a skit to retell part of the story.

Bible Quiet Time   I

Reading: Choose one option below.

★ *The Illustrated Family Bible* p. 304-305

★ Your own Bible: Luke 23:32-56

Scripture Focus: Highlight Luke 23:39-43.

Prayer Focus: Pray a prayer of confession to admit or acknowledge your sins to God. Begin by reading the highlighted verses out loud as a prayer. End by praying, *I confess that I deserve punishment for my sins and that I often do not fear God's judgment as I should. Yet, you died for me. Help me turn to you for forgiveness and salvation.*

Scripture Memory: Recite Philippians 2:24.
Music: *Philippians 2* CD: Track 6 (vs. 19-24)

Key Idea: We deserve death for our sins, but Jesus paid the price for us.

Independent History Study   I

★ Listen to *What in the World?* Disc 4, Track 4: "Julius Caesar and the Late Republic".

Key Idea: When Caesar became imperator of Rome, he reformed laws, changed the calendar, tried to check slavery, expanded roads, and drained marshes near Rome to make new settlements.

Learning the Basics

Focus: Language Arts, Math, Geography, Bible, and Science

Geography   [T]

Go to the website link listed on p. 6 of *A Child's Geography Vol. II.* At the link, select "History & Geography". Then, under "Knowledge Quest" select ACG2-Extra Activities". Print the "Travel Log Template" of your choice from p. 39-42. Also at the link, for older students, print and assign the "Chapter Twelve Review" on p. 79.

Assign all students the following pages:

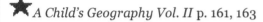*A Child's Geography Vol. II* p. 161, 163

Note: Do the "Travel Notes" section on p. 161 and the "Walk of Prayer" on p. 163. The "Food" section on p. 162 is an optional extra.

Key Idea: Share three sights from Iraq.

Poetry   [I]

Today, you will copy the last half of the Robert Frost poem from *Paint Like a Poet* that you chose to memorize this week.

Beneath the first part of the poem that you copied in the last unit, copy the rest of the poem in your *Common Place Book* in cursive.

Practice the portion of the poem that you copied today by reading it aloud.

Key Idea: Copy and memorize classic poetry.

Language Arts   [S]

Help students complete one lesson from the following reading program:

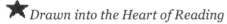*Drawn into the Heart of Reading*

Work with the students to complete **one** of the writing options listed below:

Writing & Rhetoric Book 2: Narrative I middle of p. 57-59 (Note: Guide students as needed to successfully write an amplification with dialogue.)

Your own writing program

Key Idea: Practice language arts skills.

Math Exploration   [S]

Choose **one** of the math options listed below.

Singapore Primary Mathematics 4A/4B or 5A/5B (see Appendix for schedules), or *Math with Confidence,* or *Apologia Math*

Your own math program

Key Idea: Use a step-by-step math program.

Science Exploration   [I]

Read *Exploring the History of Medicine* p. 24-30. After reading the chapter, turn to p. 31 of *Exploring the History of Medicine.* Write the answer to each numbered question from p. 31 on lined paper. You do not need to copy the question.

Key Idea: Ambroise Pare' was a barber-surgeon in France in the 1500's. He was rejected by the medical school in Paris, because he couldn't pass their tests given in Latin and Greek. So, he worked at a charity hospital and later as a war surgeon. When he ran out of oil to perform the standard treatment for gunshot wounds, he used an ointment of his own creation instead. Pare' experimented with other ways to spare soldiers from pain during surgery. He became the most skilled surgeon in France.

Reading about History | I |

Read about history in the following resource:

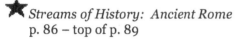 *Streams of History: Ancient Rome* p. 86 – top of p. 89

You will be adding to your timeline in your *Student Notebook* today. In Unit 27 – Box 1, draw and color two crossed swords. Label it, *Civil War in Rome (Marius vs. Sulla 107-79 B.C.).* In Box 2, draw and color chains. Label it, *Spartacus leads slave revolt (79-73 B.C.).* In Box 3, write and decorate the date March 15. Label it, *Julius Caesar is slain (44 B.C.).*

Key Idea: Caesar was assassinated in the senate by those who thought he wanted to be king. His successor was his nephew Octavius.

Storytime | T |

Choose one of the following read aloud options:

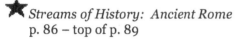 *Traveling the Way* p. 59-68

Read aloud the next portion of the humorous book that you selected.

After the reading, students will give a summary oral narration. The oral narration must be no longer than 5 sentences and should summarize the reading. As students narrate, have them hold up one finger for each sentence shared. Remind students that the focus should be on the big ideas, rather than on the details.

Key Idea: Summarize the story by narrating.

History Project | S |

Today, you will finish outfitting your Roman soldier. Get the baggie with the tunic, armour, sandals, belt, sword, and equipment that you designed on Days 1-2. Get your Roman soldier too. Now, open your *Student Notebook* to Unit 27. Today, you will be drawing, coloring, and cutting out the helmet and the javelin. As you're creating your soldier's outfit, make sure that it is the correct size for your Roman soldier. When you have completed your soldier's outfit, place it on him one piece at a time, naming each piece as you put it on him until he is fully outfitted. Now, he's ready to head into battle!

Key Idea: During the time of Julius Caesar, Roman soldiers were almost continually traveling and fighting for Rome. During the rule of Octavian (or Augustus Caesar), the Romans were mainly at peace.

Bible Quiet Time | I |

Reading: Choose one option below.

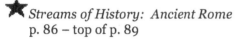 *The Illustrated Family Bible* p. 306-307

Your own Bible: Luke 24:1-12

Scripture Focus: Highlight Luke 24:6-7.

Prayer Focus: Pray a prayer of thanksgiving to express gratitude for God's divine goodness. Begin by reading the highlighted verses out loud as a prayer. End by praying, *Thank you for conquering death through your resurrection and for the promise that we will live forever with you in your kingdom!*

Scripture Memory: Recite Philippians 2:24.
Music: *Philippians 2* CD: Track 6 (vs. 19-24)

Key Idea: Jesus died and rose again on the third day, just as prophecied.

Independent History Study | I |

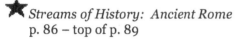 Listen to *What in the World?* Disc 4, Track 5: "Octavian vs. Mark Antony". Read Luke 2:1-4. What amazing event took place during the reign of Augustus Caesar?

Key Idea: After defeating Mark Antony, Octavian changed his name to Augustus Caesar.

Bible Study | T |

Read aloud and discuss with the students the following pages:

 The Radical Book for Kids p. 199-201

Key Idea: During Jesus' day, everyone knew Greek. The Old Testament was translated from Hebrew to Greek so that everyone could read it. God spread the Greek language across the Roman Empire so the Good News of Jesus could spread quickly. The Roman system of roads also helped the Gospel spread across the Roman Empire.

Poetry | I |

Using the actions that you added on Day 1, practice reading aloud the poem from *Paint Like a Poet* that you chose to memorize. Do this 2 times.

Then, recite the poem without looking at the words.

You should have your chosen poem memorized by Day 4 of this unit.

Key Idea: Memorize classic poetry.

Language Arts | S |

Have students complete one studied dictation exercise (see Appendix for directions and passages).

Work with the students to complete **one** of the writing options listed below:

 Writing & Rhetoric Book 2: Narrative I p. 60 (Note: Reread the Greek myth on p. 50 – top of p. 51 first. Then, guide students as needed to successfully write a monologue. Omit p. 61.)

⭐ Your own writing program

Key Idea: Practice language arts skills.

Math Exploration | S |

Choose **one** of the math options listed below.

⭐ *Singapore Primary Mathematics 4A/4B or 5A/5B* (see Appendix for schedules), or *Math with Confidence,* or *Apologia Math*

⭐ Your own math program

Key Idea: Use a step-by-step math program.

Science Exploration | I |

⭐ Read *Exploring the History of Medicine* p. 32-36.

After reading the chapter listed above, turn to p. 37 of *Exploring the History of Medicine.* Write the answer to each numbered question from p. 37 on lined paper. You do not need to copy the question.

Key Idea: William Harvey was born in England ten years after Pare's death. He went to school in Italy, where Galileo was a famous teacher. Harvey became the physician to King James I of England. For ten years, he studied the flow of blood through the heart for ten years. He finally realized that blood circulated in a closed path and was reused in the body. His book, *On the Motion of the Blood,* described his findings about circulation.

Reading about History | I

Read about history in the following resource:

 Streams of History: Ancient Rome p. 89-92

You will be writing a narration about part of the chapter *How Rome Conquered the World, but Destroyed Herself,* which is part of today's history reading.

To prepare for writing your narration, think about the important moments that you read about in Roman history. You may wish to look back over p. 89-92 of *Streams of History: Ancient Rome* to guide you as you write your narration.

After you have thought about what you will write and how you will begin your narration, turn to Unit 27 in your *Student Notebook.* In Box 5, write a 5-8 sentence narration.

When you have finished writing, read your sentences out loud to catch any mistakes.

Check for the following things: *Did you include* **who** *or* **what topic** *the reading was mainly about? Did you include* **descriptors** *of the important thing(s) that happened? Did you include a* **closing sentence**? *If not, add those things.*

Then, underline or highlight the main idea sentence in the narration. Use the *Written Narration Skills* in the Appendix as a guide for editing the narration.

Key Idea: Jesus arrived on earth at a time when the news of His resurrection could be quickly spread throughout the Roman empire. Christians found new hope in Christ, even through times of persecution.

Storytime | T

Choose one of the following read aloud options:

★ *Traveling the Way* p. 69-75

★ Read aloud part of the humorous book.

After the reading, have each person get a Bible and open it anywhere in Proverbs. Explain, *We will have 5 minutes to skim through the verses in Proverbs to find any connections to today's story. When a connection is found, read the verse out loud and quickly share the connection. At the end of 5 minutes, anyone who has not shared yet must read aloud one verse and make the best connection possible.*

Key Idea: Seek God's word for His guidance.

Bible Quiet Time | I

Reading: Choose one option below.

★ *The Illustrated Family Bible* p. 308 Optional extension: p. 208-209

★ Your own Bible: Luke 24:13-53

Scripture Focus: Highlight Luke 24:31-32.

Prayer Focus: Pray a prayer of supplication to make a humble and earnest request of God. Begin by reading the highlighted verse out loud as a prayer. End by praying, *Open my eyes and my heart to you, so I can see you at work all around me. Help me to have a deep faith in your resurrection and in the gift of eternal life.*

Scripture Memory: Copy Philippians 2:24 in your Common Place Book.
Music: *Philippians 2* CD: Track 6 (vs. 19-24)

Key Idea: Jesus walked and talked with men.

Independent History Study | I

Open your *Student Notebook* to "Prophecies About Christ". Under "Prophecy" write, *Micah 5:2.* Read the Scripture from your Bible to discover the prophecy. Under "Fulfillment" write, *Matthew 2:1-6.* Read the fulfillment Scripture. Under "Description", write a few phrases to describe the prophecy about Jesus.

Key Idea: Just as prophesied, the ruler Christ the King was born in Bethlehem. The Savior had arrived!

Learning the Basics
Focus: Language Arts, Math, Geography, Bible, and Science

Geography [T]

Read aloud to the students the following pages:

 A Child's Geography Vol. II p. 164 – second paragraph on p. 168

Discuss with the students "Field Notes" p. 167.

Key Idea: Saudi Arabia is ruled by a king. It is bordered by the Red Sea and the Persian Gulf and covers nearly all of the Arabian Peninsula. Mecca, in Saudi Arabia, is the birthplace of Mohammed and the site of the largest yearly gathering of Muslims in the world.

Language Arts [S]

Have students complete one dictation exercise.

Guide students to complete one reading lesson.

★ *Drawn into the Heart of Reading*

Help students complete **one** English lesson.

★ *Building with Diligence:* Lesson 50

★ *Following the Plan:* Lesson 46

★ Your own grammar program

Key Idea: Practice language arts skills.

Poetry [I]

Today, you will be performing a poetry recitation of the Robert Frost poem that you chose to memorize from *Paint Like a Poet*. You will recite your poem to an audience of your choosing, without looking at the words. Before reciting, practice saying the poem aloud using an expression that matches the mood of the poem. Then, stand and recite the poem aloud in front of your chosen audience.

At the end of the recitation, share the following, *I decided to choose this poem of Robert Frost's to memorize because...* Then, call on your audience to comment on what they liked about the poem that you shared.

Key Idea: Share the poetry of Robert Frost.

Math Exploration [S]

Choose **one** of the math options listed below.

★ *Singapore Primary Mathematics 4A/4B or 5A/5B* (see Appendix for schedules), or *Math with Confidence*, or *Apologia Math*

★ Your own math program

Key Idea: Use a step-by-step math program.

Science Exploration [I]

★ Read *Exploring the History of Medicine* p. 38-42. Answer the questions on p. 43 on lined paper. Then, turn to the science experiment section in your science binder or sketchbook. At the top of a blank page, write: *How do bacteria cells multiply?* Under the question, write: 'Guess'. Write down your guess. On a table, set 8 containers in a row (i.e. cups, glasses, or bowls). Place a square of masking tape on the table in front of each container. Number the squares of tape in order from '1' – '8'. Each container will represent one generation of bacteria. Place 1 counter in container '1' to represent a bacteria cell. Suggestions for counters include cereal pieces, beads, macaroni noodles, dry beans, or small building bricks. Bacteria are tiny one-celled creatures (called microorganisms) that reproduce by dividing into two cells about every 20 minutes. So, in container '2', place 2 counters to represent the bacteria cell after 20 minutes. In container '3', place 4 counters to show the division of bacteria cells that would occur after 20 more minutes. In cup '4', how many bacteria would there be? (Answer: 16) Continue the experiment, until you have reached cup 8. Approximately how much time would have passed by cup '8'? Next, write: 'Procedure'. Draw a picture of the experiment. Write: 'Conclusion'. Explain what you learned.

Key Idea: Bacteria are one-celled creatures that multiply rapidly and can only be seen under a microscope.

Reading about History   I

Read about history in the following resource:

⭐ Your own Bible: John chapter 1

John the Baptist was the promised messenger sent by God as the forerunner for Jesus. Where could you look to research more about **John the Baptist**? Read the Bible passages Luke 1 and 3:1-3, 19-20; Mark 1:4-11 and 6:14-29; and Matthew 3 and 11:1-15 as the most accurate resource on John the Baptist. Answer one or more of the following questions from your research: *Who were John the Baptist's parents? Who announced the coming birth of John to Zechariah? What did the angel Gabriel tell Zechariah about John? What happened to Zechariah after the angel departed? When and why did the baby, John, leap in Elizabeth's womb? Describe John the Baptist. What was his role? Who was ruling Rome when John began his ministry? Why did John get sent to prison? When John was in prison, what message did he send to Jesus? What was Jesus' response? How did John die?*

Key Idea: John prepared the way for Jesus.

History Project   S

In this unit you will make a disk to show the 12 men whom Jesus called to be His disciples. On white paper, trace around a dinner plate to make 2 large circles. Cut the circles out. The first circle will be like a clock face showing a different disciple for each hour on the clock. Write the hours on the clock, starting with '12' at the top. Make a dot in the center.

Key Idea: Jesus called twelve disciples.

Storytime   T

Choose one of the following read aloud options:

⭐ *Traveling the Way* p. 76-81

⭐ Read at least one humorous book for the next 4 days of plans.

After the reading, students will give a detailed oral narration. Select one paragraph from the story to read out loud to the students. This will be the starting point for the narration. Set a timer for 3-5 minutes. When the timer rings the narration is over, even if it isn't complete. A detailed, descriptive narration is the goal. See *Narration Tips* in the Appendix as needed.

Key Idea: Use oral narration to retell the story.

Bible Quiet Time   I

Bible Reading: Choose one option below.

⭐ *The Illustrated Family Bible* p. 236-237
Optional extension: p. 210

⭐ Your own Bible: John chapter 1

Scripture Focus: Highlight John 1:1-4.

Prayer Focus: Pray a prayer of adoration to worship and honor God. Begin by reading the highlighted verses out loud as a prayer. End by praying, *I praise you Jesus knowing you were with God from the beginning and that you are fully God, yet you became fully man.*

Scripture Review: Philippians 2:1-24.
Music: *Philippians 2* CD: Tracks 1-6 (all)

Key Idea: John testified Jesus is God's Son.

Independent History Study   I

⭐ Listen to *What in the World?* Disc 4, Track 6: "In the Perfect Moment of Time". Open your *Student Notebook* to "Prophecies About Christ". Under "Prophecy" write, *Isaiah 40:3-5*. Read the Scripture to discover the prophecy. Under "Fulfillment" write, *John 1:22-23*. Read the fulfillment Scripture. Under "Description", write a few phrases to describe the prophecy about Jesus.

Key Idea: 500 years before Christ, Isaiah prophecied that one would come to prepare the way for the Lord.

Learning the Basics
Focus: Language Arts, Math, Geography, Bible, and Science

Bible Study [T]

Read aloud and discuss with the students the following pages:

 The Radical Book for Kids p. 202-203

Key Idea: In the Old Testament God made a covenant with His chosen people, the Israelites. This was called the "old covenant." In the New Testament, Jesus made a covenant with His believers. This was called the "new covenant." Christians are part of the new covenant. The Lord's Supper, or Communion, is a sign and celebration of the new covenant.

Language Arts [S]

Have students complete one studied dictation exercise (see Appendix for directions and passages).

Help students complete one lesson from the following reading program:

 Drawn into the Heart of Reading

Work with the students to complete **one** of the English options listed below:

⭐ *Building with Diligence:* Lesson 51

⭐ *Following the Plan:* Lesson 47 (Half)

⭐ Your own grammar program

Key Idea: Practice language arts skills.

Poetry [I]

Open *Paint Like a Poet* to Lesson 22. Read aloud the poem *"The Vantage Point"*. On a 3 x 5 index card, neatly copy in black ink or in pencil the following highlighted lines from the poem:

And if by moon I have too much of these,
I have but to turn on my arm, and lo,
The sun-burned hillside sets my face aglow,
My breathing shakes the bluet like a breeze,
I smell the earth, I smell the bruised plant,
I look into the crater of the ant.
　　　　　　　　-Robert Frost

Check your work to make sure it is correctly copied. Then, cut around your copywork. You may choose to outline the edge of the cut-out with an orange marker. Save it for Day 3.

Key Idea: Read and appreciate a variety of classic poetry.

Math Exploration [S]

Choose **one** of the math options listed below.

⭐ *Singapore Primary Mathematics 4A/4B or 5A/5B* (see Appendix for schedules), or *Math with Confidence,* or *Apologia Math*

⭐ Your own math program

Key Idea: Use a step-by-step math program.

Science Exploration [I]

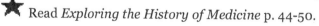

⭐ Read *Exploring the History of Medicine* p. 44-50.

After reading the chapter listed above, turn to p. 51 of *Exploring the History of Medicine*. Write the answer to each numbered question from p. 51 on lined paper. You do not need to copy the question.

Key Idea: Edward Jenner grew up in England and went to medical school in London. Captain James Cook invited Jenner to come to the South Seas as the ship's natural scientist, but Jenner chose to live quietly in Berkeley. After 20 years of study, he determined that cowpox could be used to inoculate people, so they didn't contract the more deadly smallpox disease. Exposure to cowpox built immunity to smallpox.

Reading about History   I

Read about history in the following resource:

★ Your own Bible: John chapters 2-3

You will be choosing a portion from today's reading that you found memorable or worthy of being reread to copy. Open your *Student Notebook* to Unit 28. In Box 4, carefully copy in cursive the portion from today's reading that you selected. Then, compare your written work to the original. Last, draw a small colorful picture in Box 4 to illustrate your sentences.

Key Idea: Jesus turns water to wine, and Nicodemus visits Jesus at night with questions.

History Project   S

Get the numbered circle you made on Day 1. Copy the following numbered information about the disciples like spokes on a wheel coming out from the center dot.
1. Simon Peter (Matt. 4:18-20): fisherman, wrote 1st and 2nd Peter, impulsive and bold
2. Andrew, brother to Peter (Matt. 4:18-20): fisherman, believed John the Baptist
3. James, son of Zebedee (Matt. 4:21-22): fisherman, first martyred disciple
4. John, brother to James (Matt. 4:21-22): fisherman; wrote John; 1st, 2nd, 3rd John, and Revelation; disciple whom Jesus loved
5. Philip (John 1:43-45): fisherman, told Nathanael about Jesus, questioned often
6. Bartholomew or Nathanael (John 1:46-51): honest, wasn't sure any good could come from Nazareth
7. Matthew or Levi (Matt. 9:9-13): tax collector, wrote Matthew, changed his ways

Key Idea: Before choosing the 12 apostles, Jesus spent the night praying.

Storytime   T

Choose one of the following read aloud options:

★ *Traveling the Way* p. 82-89

★ Read aloud the next portion of the humorous book that you selected.

After reading, give students a few minutes to prepare a short advertisement speech for the book. During the speech, students should hold up the book and say the book title and the name of the author. The wording of the advertisement should provide a peek into the book without giving away the ending. The goal should be for listeners to feel like they've "Got to Have This Book"!

Key Idea: Use an ad speech to share the story.

Bible Quiet Time   I

Reading: Choose one option below.

★ *The Illustrated Family Bible* p. 238-239 and p. 243; Optional extension: p. 211

★ Your own Bible: John chapters 2-3

Scripture Focus: Highlight John 2:16-17.

Prayer Focus: Pray a prayer of confession to admit or acknowledge your sins to God. Begin by reading the highlighted verses out loud as a prayer. End by praying, *I confess that I do not always focus on worship when I am at church. Help me to remember that worshiping you is the reason I go to your house.*

Scripture Review: Philippians 2:1-24.
Music: *Philippians 2* CD: Tracks 1-6 (all)

Key Idea: Jesus began His ministry on earth.

Independent History Study   I

★ Listen to *What in the World?* Disc 4, Track 7: "The Promised One". Open your *Student Notebook* to Unit 28. In Box 6, copy in cursive John 3:16.

Key Idea: Christ arrived just as God had promised Abraham He would back in Genesis.

Learning the Basics
Focus: Language Arts, Math, Geography, Bible, and Science

Geography [T]

Read aloud to the students the following pages:

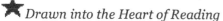 *A Child's Geography Vol. II* third paragraph on p. 168-171

Discuss with the students "Field Notes" p. 171.

Key Idea: Non-Muslims are forbidden to enter the city of Mecca. In the center of the city is Mecca's Grand Mosque. A million Muslims can stand within it at one time. They surround the *Ka'abah*, which Muslims say was built by Abraham and his son, Ishmael, over 4,000 years ago. Many Muslims also visit the Prophet's Mosque in Medina, home of Mohammed's tomb.

Language Arts [S]

Complete one lesson from the program below.

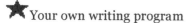 *Drawn into the Heart of Reading*

Work with the students to complete **one** of the writing options listed below:

⭐ *Writing & Rhetoric Book 2: Narrative I* p. 75 – bottom of p. 80 (Note: Omit p. 62-74. Read aloud today's text while the students follow along. Today's text includes battle violence. Then, discuss.)

⭐ Your own writing program

Key Idea: Practice language arts skills.

Poetry [I]

Open *Paint Like a Poet* to Lesson 22. Read aloud the poem *"The Vantage Point"* by Robert Frost.

Today, you will be painting a sunset backdrop. You will need painting paper, a palette, water, a large flat paintbrush, a paper towel, and blue, yellow, and red paint.

After gathering your supplies, turn to the "Step-by-Step Watercolor Tutorial" for Lesson 22 in *Paint Like a Poet*. Follow steps 1-3 to complete "Part One: Sunset Backdrop". Then, let your background dry. You will complete "Part Two" of the tutorial on Day 3.

Key Idea: Use painting to illustrate poetry.

Math Exploration [S]

Choose **one** of the math options listed below.

⭐ *Singapore Primary Mathematics 4A/4B* or *5A/5B* (see Appendix for schedules), or *Math with Confidence,* or *Apologia Math*

⭐ Your own math program

Key Idea: Use a step-by-step math program.

Science Exploration [I]

⭐ Read *Exploring the History of Medicine* p. 52-58. After reading the chapter, turn to p. 59 of *Exploring the History of Medicine.* Write the answer to each numbered question from p. 59 on lined paper. You do not need to copy the question.

Key Idea: Humphrey Davy investigated various gases for Dr. Thomas Beddoes. Humphrey breathed each gas to test it, which was a decision that almost killed him. Instead of killing him, his experiments left him physically disabled. Yet, he worked with Michael Faraday and continued his discoveries. James Simpson experimented with using ether on patients as an anesthetic. He later replaced it with chloroform.

Reading about History | I

Read about history in the following resource:

 Your own Bible: John chapter 4

You will be adding to your timeline in your *Student Notebook* today. In Unit 28 – Box 1, draw and color a laurel leaf crown. Label it, *Octavius becomes Augustus Caesar (30 B.C.).* In Box 2, draw and color a star. Label it, *Jesus is born in Bethlehem (4 B.C.).* In Box 3, draw and color the word Rome. Label it, *Tiberius Caesar becomes emperor of Rome (14 A.D.)*

Key Idea: Jesus traveled throughout Judea teaching and healing, even in Samaria!

History Project | S

Get the numbered circle you made. Copy the following information about the disciples like spokes on a wheel coming from the center dot.
8. Thomas (John 20:24-29): courageous, yet doubted Jesus' resurrection
9. James (Luke 6:14-16): son of Alphaeus
10. Judas or Thaddaeus (John 14:22): son of James, compassionate
11. Simon the Zealot (Mark 3:18): strong-willed, wanted an earthly kingdom
12. Judas Iscariot (Matt. 26:14-16, 20-25): betrayed Jesus, replaced by Matthias
Last, cut out a thin, pie-shaped slice from the blank circle from Day 1. Place the blank circle on top of the numbered circle. Attach the two circles together with a paper fastener in the center. Turn the top circle to view the names of the disciples. Write "The 12 Apostles" on the outside of the top circle.

Key Idea: Jesus' disciples traveled with Him.

Storytime | T

Choose one of the following read aloud options:

 Traveling the Way p. 90-97

Read aloud the next portion of the humorous book that you selected.

After the reading, students will give a summary oral narration. The oral narration must be no longer than 5 sentences and should summarize the reading. As students narrate, have them hold up one finger for each sentence shared. Remind students that the focus should be on the big ideas, rather than on the details.

Key Idea: Summarize the story by narrating.

Bible Quiet Time | I

Reading: Choose one option below.

The Illustrated Family Bible p. 264-265
Optional extension: p. 232

Your own Bible: John 4

Scripture Focus: Highlight John 4:13-14.

Prayer Focus: Pray a prayer of thanksgiving to express gratitude for God's divine goodness. Begin by reading the highlighted verses out loud as a prayer. End by praying, *Thank you for being the living water that we need for our thirsty souls. Help us return to you and God's word daily to quench our thirst.*

Scripture Review: Philippians 2:1-24.
Music: *Philippians 2* CD: Tracks 1-6 (all)

Key Idea: Jesus is the living water for our soul.

Independent History Study | I

Open your *Student Notebook* to "Prophecies About Christ". Under "Prophecy" write, *Psalm 40:8*. Read the Scripture to discover the prophecy. Under "Fulfillment" write, *John 4:34*. Read the fulfillment Scripture. Under "Description", write a few phrases to describe the prophecy about Jesus.

Key Idea: Jesus fulfilled the prophecy in Psalms by doing God's will and finishing His work on earth.

Learning the Basics

Focus: Language Arts, Math, Geography, Bible, and Science

Bible Study [T]

Read aloud and discuss with the students the following pages:

 The Radical Book for Kids p. 204-207

Key Idea: In Old Testament times God's people had enemies like the Egyptians, the Philistines, the Assyrians, and the Persians. When Jesus was born, the Romans were enemies of God's people. In Jesus' time, the Sadducees were rich and powerful Israelite leaders who tried not to "rock the boat" with Rome. The Pharisees tried to obey God's laws outwardly, but their hearts were unchanged. The "Zealots" thought Israel should fight the Romans. Jesus served His enemies, forgave their sins, and died for them.

Language Arts [S]

Have students complete one studied dictation exercise (see Appendix for directions and passages).

Work with the students to complete **one** of the writing options listed below:

 Writing & Rhetoric Book 2: Narrative I middle of p 81 – middle of p. 83 (Note: Omit bottom of p. 80 – top of p. 81. Guide students to complete the lesson.)

 Your own writing program

Key Idea: Practice language arts skills.

Poetry [I]

Open *Paint Like a Poet* to Lesson 22. Read aloud the poem *"The Vantage Point"* by Robert Frost.

Get the sunset backdrop that you painted on Day 2. Today, you will be adding hills and clouds. You will need a palette, water, a small flat paintbrush, and green, brown, and orange paint.

After gathering your supplies, turn to the "Step-by-Step Watercolor Tutorial" for Lesson 22 in *Paint Like a Poet*. Follow steps 4-6 to complete "Part Two: Hills and Clouds". When your painting is dry, glue your poetry copywork from Day 1 to your painting. Store your completed artwork in the place you have chosen for it.

Key Idea: Explore poetry moods with painting.

Math Exploration [S]

Choose **one** of the math options listed below.

 Singapore Primary Mathematics 4A/4B or 5A/5B (see Appendix for schedules), or *Math with Confidence,* or *Apologia Math*

 Your own math program

Key Idea: Use a step-by-step math program.

Science Exploration [I]

 Read *Exploring the History of Medicine* p. 60-66.

After reading the chapter listed above, turn to p. 67 of *Exploring the History of Medicine*. Write the answer to each numbered question from p. 67 on lined paper. You do not need to copy the question.

Key Idea: William Morton tested ether on animals, and then on himself. He used pure diethyl ether as an anesthetic. Morton went to the head of the Massachusetts General Hospital and begged to be able to use ether on a patient during surgery. Dr. Warren consented. After the successful operation, the use of ether as an anesthetic spread across Europe and the United States in two years' time.

Reading about History | I |

Read about history in the following resource:

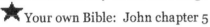 Your own Bible: John chapter 5

You will be writing a narration from the following Bible reading: *John chapter 5,* which is today's history reading.

To prepare for writing your narration, look back over what you read in John chapter 5. Think about the main idea which is the healing of the lame man by the pool of Bethesda.

After you have thought about what you will write and how you will begin your narration, turn to Unit 28 in your *Student Notebook.*

In Box 5, write a 5-8 sentence narration which tells about the healing of the lame man by the pool of Bethesda.

When you have finished writing, read your sentences out loud to catch any mistakes. Check for the following things: *Did you include* **who** *or* **what topic** *the reading was mainly about? Did you include* **descriptors** *of the important thing(s) that happened? Did you include a* **closing sentence***? If not, add those things.*

Then, underline or highlight the main idea sentence in the narration. Use the *Written Narration Skills* in the Appendix as a guide for editing the narration.

Key Idea: While Jesus was in Jerusalem for one of the Jewish feasts, He healed a man who had been lame for 38 years. Rather than rejoicing in the miracle, the Pharisees were upset that one of their rules had been broken. The Pharisees were so caught up in finding fault in Jesus through their man-made rules that they didn't recognize Him as Christ.

Storytime | T |

Choose one of the following read aloud options:

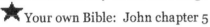 *Traveling the Way* p. 98-103

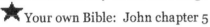 Read aloud the end of the humorous book.

After the reading, have each person get a Bible and open it anywhere in Proverbs. Explain, *We will have 5 minutes to skim through the verses in Proverbs to find any connections to today's story. When a connection is found, read the verse out loud and quickly share the connection. At the end of 5 minutes, anyone who has not shared yet must read aloud one verse and make the best connection possible.*

Key Idea: Seek God's word for His guidance.

Bible Quiet Time | I |

Reading: Choose one option below.

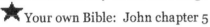 *The Illustrated Family Bible* p. 233

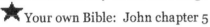 Your own Bible: John chapter 5

Scripture Focus: Highlight John 5:22-24.

Prayer Focus: Pray a prayer of supplication to make a humble and earnest request of God. Begin by reading the highlighted verses out loud as a prayer. End by praying, *I know that many religions on earth worship you, God, without worshiping Jesus. The Bible says that belief in Jesus is the only way to heaven. I ask you to keep me from false religions that miss the fact that Jesus is your Son and my Savior.*

Scripture Review: Philippians 2:1-24.
Music: *Philippians 2* CD: Tracks 1-6 (all)

Key Idea: Jesus proclaimed He is God's Son.

Independent History Study | I |

Open your *Student Notebook* to Unit 28. In the empty space above Box 7, glue in your disk of "The 12 Apostles" (from the Day 3 "History Project" Box). Then, in Box 7, copy in cursive John 1:14.

Key Idea: Although Jesus became fully man, He never ceased to be fully God. He was always with God.

Geography [T]

Get both the blank map and the labeled map of **Eygpt, Iraq & Saudi Arabia** that you saved from the study of Iraq. Or, you may print a new map from p. 48 online for each student at the link on p. 6 of *A Child's Geography Vol. II.*

Then, assign students the following page:

 ★ *A Child's Geography Vol. II* p. 172
Note: Do only the "Map Notes" section. If desired, play "Music" from the links on p. 173.

Key Idea: Practice mapping Saudi Arabia.

Language Arts [S]

Have students complete one dictation exercise.

Guide students to complete one reading lesson.

★ *Drawn into the Heart of Reading*

Help students complete **one** English lesson.

★ *Building with Diligence:* Lesson 52

★ *Following the Plan:* Lesson 47 (Last half)

★ Your own grammar program

Key Idea: Practice language arts skills.

Poetry [I]

Open *Paint Like a Poet* to Lesson 22. Today, you will be performing a poetry reading of *"The Vantage Point"*. Practice reading the poem aloud with expression that matches the mood of the poem. Then, read the poem aloud in front of your chosen audience.

At the end of the reading, share the following, *When I read this poem by Robert Frost, it made me think of...* Call on your audience to share what thoughts the poem brought to their minds. Last, say, *Did you know that for nearly 50 years, Robert Frost gave poetry readings? He gave readings up until 2 months before his death at age 88! Although these readings exhausted him, he drew a large audience and was considered to be a great performer.*

Key Idea: Share the poetry of Robert Frost.

Math Exploration [S]

Choose **one** of the math options listed below.

★ *Singapore Primary Mathematics 4A/4B or 5A/5B* (see Appendix for schedules), or *Math with Confidence,* or *Apologia Math*

★ Your own math program

Key Idea: Use a step-by-step math program.

Science Exploration [I]

★ Read *Exploring the History of Medicine* p. 68-74. Answer the questions on p. 75 on lined paper. Then, turn to the science experiment section in your science binder or sketchbook. At the top of a blank page, write: *What helps prevent germs from spreading?* Under the question, write: *'Guess'.* Write down your guess. Have a helper gently wash two apples. You should not wash the apples yourself, as you will need to have unwashed hands for the first part of this experiment. If you do not have apples, you may use 2 bananas, or 2 slices of bread. Use a clean utensil to pierce the skin of both apples by making scratches. Next, rub your unwashed hand across the scratched surface of **one** apple. Place the apple in a Ziploc bag and seal the bag. Then, wash your hands with warm soapy water for 20 seconds. Rub your clean hand across the scratched surface of the **second** apple. Then, use a cotton swab to swab rubbing alcohol across the scratches of the second apple. Place the second apple in a separate Ziploc bag and seal the bag. Store the apples in a warm, dry place and observe them for one week. Then, throw the bagged fruit away. Next, write: *'Procedure'.* Draw a picture of the experiment. Write: *'Conclusion'.* Explain what you learned.

Key Idea: Your skin provides a barrier against bacteria and infection. Alcohol is a disinfectant, which keeps germs out. Washing your hands with soap and warm water helps prevent the spread of germs.

Learning through History
Focus: Jesus, Teacher and Healer

Reading about History [I]

Read about history in the following resource:

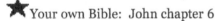 ★ Your own Bible: John chapter 6

Much of Jesus' ministry took place near the Sea of Galilee. Where could you look to research more about the **Sea of Galilee**? Use an online resource like www.wikipedia.org or a reference book. Note the Sea of Galilee is mentioned in today's reading in John 6:1.

Answer one or more of the following questions from your research: *Where is the Sea of Galilee located? What are some other names for the Sea of Galilee? Describe the lake. For what is the lake known? What river feeds the Sea of Galilee? Which thriving towns were built around the Sea of Galilee in ancient times? Which of Jesus' apostles were fisherman on the Sea of Galilee? Which of Jesus' teachings and miracles took place on or near the Sea of Galilee?*

<u>Key Idea</u>: Jesus fed 5,000 men near the Sea of Galilee. He also fed the women and children.

History Project [S]

In this unit you will make a painting of the storm the disciples faced in their boat on the Sea of Galilee. On a white piece of painting paper, paint a background of dark skies with strong winds and rough waters as described in John 6:16-19. Allow your painting to dry.

<u>Key Idea</u>: After feeding the multitudes, Jesus remained alone to pray. He sent his disciples in a boat across the Sea of Galilee. During the night, Jesus walked on the water toward the boat. He calmed the wind and the waves.

Storytime [T]

Choose one of the following read aloud options:

★ *Traveling the Way* p. 104-117

★ Read at least one realistic fiction book for the next 16 days of plans (see Appendix).

After the reading, students will give a detailed oral narration. Select one paragraph from the story to read out loud to the students. This will be the starting point for the narration. Set a timer for 3-5 minutes. When the timer rings the narration is over, even if it isn't complete. A detailed, descriptive narration is the goal. See *Narration Tips* in the Appendix as needed.

<u>Key Idea</u>: Use oral narration to retell the story.

Bible Quiet Time [I]

Bible Reading: Choose one option below.

★ *The Illustrated Family Bible* p. 258-259

★ Your own Bible: John 6

Scripture Focus: Highlight John 6:67-68.

Prayer Focus: Pray a prayer of adoration to worship and honor God. Begin by reading the highlighted verses out loud as a prayer. End by praying, *I worship you as the Christ, the Son of the living God. You alone have the words leading to eternal life.*

Scripture Memory: Recite Philippians 2:25.
Music: *Philippians 2* CD: Track 7 (verse 25)

<u>Key Idea</u>: Jesus walked on water and healed the sick. He taught the way to eternal life.

Independent History Study [I]

Open your *Student Notebook* to "Prophecies About Christ". Under "Prophecy" write, *Isaiah 35:4-6*. Read the Scripture to discover the prophecy. Under "Fulfillment" write, *Matthew 11:4-6*. Read the fulfillment Scripture. Under "Description", write a few phrases to describe the prophecy about Jesus.

<u>Key Idea</u>: Jesus fulfilled Isaiah's prophecy that the Savior would be a healer and do miracles.

Learning the Basics
Focus: Language Arts, Math, Geography, Bible, and Science

Bible Study | T |

Read aloud and discuss with the students the following pages:

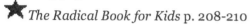 *The Radical Book for Kids* p. 208-210

Key Idea: The Bible gives facts that show Jesus rose from the dead. An empty tomb, lying guards, eyewitnesses, disciples willing to die for what they saw, and verifiable records written in the Gospels are all proof of Jesus' resurrection. People must either choose to believe Jesus is God who rose from the dead or reject Jesus and Scripture as falsehoods.

Language Arts | S |

Have students complete one studied dictation exercise (see Appendix for directions and passages).

Help students complete one lesson from the following reading program:

★ *Drawn into the Heart of Reading*

Work with the students to complete **one** of the English options listed below:

★ *Building with Diligence:* Lesson 53

★ *Following the Plan:* Lesson 48

★ Your own grammar program

Key Idea: Practice language arts skills.

Poetry | I |

Open *Paint Like a Poet* to Lesson 23. Read aloud the poem *"An Encounter"*. On a 3 x 5 index card, neatly copy in black ink or in pencil the following highlighted lines from the poem:

"You here?" I said. "Where aren't you nowadays
And what's the news you carry – if you know?
And tell me where you're off for – Montreal?
Me? I'm not off for anywhere at all.
Sometimes I wander out of beaten ways
Half looking for the orchid Calypso."
                                    -Robert Frost

Check your work to make sure it is correctly copied. Then, cut around your copywork. You may choose to outline the edge of the cut-out with a blue marker. Save it for Day 3.

Key Idea: Read and appreciate classic poetry.

Math Exploration | S |

Choose **one** of the math options listed below.

★ *Singapore Primary Mathematics 4A/4B* or *5A/5B* (see Appendix for schedules), or *Math with Confidence*, or *Apologia Math*

★ Your own math program

Key Idea: Use a step-by-step math program.

Science Exploration | I |

★ Read *Exploring the History of Medicine* p. 76-84.

After reading the chapter listed above, turn to p. 85 of *Exploring the History of Medicine*. Write the answer to each numbered question from p. 85 on lined paper. You do not need to copy the question.

Key Idea: Louis Pasteur went from a mediocre student to an avid student when he discovered his love of chemistry. It was his passion throughout his career as a scientist and teacher. His experiment with pasteurization was used to protect wine from turning sour. Pasteurization changed how food was processed and packaged. He also proved that microbes come from other microbes in the air and do not generate spontaneously as scientists had once thought.

Learning through History
Focus: Jesus, Teacher and Healer

Reading about History | I |

Read about history in the following resource:

 Your own Bible: John chapter 7

You will be choosing a portion from today's reading that you found memorable or worthy of being reread to copy. Open your *Student Notebook* to Unit 29. In Box 4, carefully copy in cursive the portion from today's reading that you selected. Then, compare your written work to the original. Last, draw a small colorful picture in Box 4 to illustrate your sentences.

Key Idea: Jesus stayed near Galilee, even though the Jews wanted to harm Him. During the Feast of the Tabernacles, Jesus taught in the Jewish temple, and the people were amazed.

Storytime | T |

Choose one of the following read aloud options:

★ *Traveling the Way* p. 118-125

★ Read aloud the next portion of the realistic fiction book that you selected.

After reading, give each person a white piece of paper or a markerboard and a marker. Set a timer for 3-5 minutes and instruct each person to do a quick outline sketch about the story. Ideas for sketches include settings, characters, actions, important objects, or symbols. When the timer rings, briefly share the sketches.

Key Idea: Use sketching to share the story.

History Project | S |

Today you will need a piece of brown paper. Cut the paper into an 8"x 8" square. Then, use a thin black marker to draw lines across the paper on both sides to make it look like pieces of wood. Next, open your *Student Notebook* to Unit 29. Follow the directions shown to fold your brown paper into an origami rowboat. Save the boat to add to your painted background on Day 3.

Key Idea: Jesus spent quite a bit of time teaching and healing people near the Sea of Galilee. His hometown of Nazareth was not far from the Sea of Galilee. The miracles of Jesus and Peter walking on the water and of Jesus stilling the storm took place on the Sea of Galilee. The feeding of the 5,000 took place near the shores of this same sea.

Bible Quiet Time | I |

Reading: Choose the option below.

★ Your own Bible: John chapter 7

Scripture Focus: Highlight John 7:16-18.

Prayer Focus: Pray a prayer of confession to admit or acknowledge your sins to God. Begin by reading the highlighted verses out loud as a prayer. End by praying, *I know that all teaching should be measured against the Bible to make sure it comes from God and not from man. I confess that I forget this sometimes. Guide me to weigh what I hear to see if it honors God or honors man.*

Scripture Memory: Recite Philippians 2:25.
Music: *Philippians 2* CD: Track 7 (verse 25)

Key Idea: Jesus explained that all His teachings came from God.

Independent History Study | I |

Open your *Student Notebook* to "Prophecies About Christ". Under "Prophecy" write, *Psalm 69:8*. Read the Scripture from the Bible to discover the prophecy. Under "Fulfillment" write, *John 7:3-5*. Read the fulfillment Scripture. Under "Description", write a few phrases to describe the prophecy about Jesus.

Key Idea: The prophecy that Jesus' own brothers would not know Him or believe in Him was fulfilled.

Geography [T]

Go to the website link listed on p. 6 of *A Child's Geography Vol. II.* At the link, select "History & Geography". Then, under "Knowledge Quest" select ACG2-Extra Activities". Print the "Travel Log Template" of your choice from p. 39-42. Also at the link, for older students, print and assign the "Chapter Thirteen Review" on p. 80.

Assign all students the following page:

★ *A Child's Geography Vol. II* p. 172
Note: Do only the "Travel Notes" section. The "Art" section of p. 173 is an optional extra.

Key Idea: Share three sights from Saudi Arabia.

Poetry [I]

Open *Paint Like a Poet* to Lesson 23. Read aloud the poem *"An Encounter"* by Robert Frost.

Today, you will be painting a roadside backdrop. You will need painting paper, a palette, water, a large flat paintbrush, a small flat paintbrush, a pencil, and blue, brown, and yellow paint.

After gathering your supplies, turn to the "Step-by-Step Watercolor Tutorial" for Lesson 23 in *Paint Like a Poet*. Follow steps 1-3 to complete "Part One: Roadside Backdrop". Then, let your background dry. You will complete "Part Two" of the tutorial on Day 3.

Key Idea: Use painting to illustrate poetry.

Language Arts [S]

Complete one lesson from the program below.

★ *Drawn into the Heart of Reading*

Work with the students to complete **one** of the writing options listed below:

★ *Writing & Rhetoric Book 2: Narrative I* middle of p. 83-85 (Note: First, as an example of how to add description, read aloud p. 62 – top of p. 64 while students follow along. Then, guide students to add description to today's lesson.)

★ Your own writing program

Key Idea: Practice language arts skills.

Math Exploration [S]

Choose **one** of the math options listed below.

★ *Singapore Primary Mathematics 4A/4B or 5A/5B* (see Appendix for schedules), or *Math with Confidence,* or *Apologia Math*

★ Your own math program

Key Idea: Use a step-by-step math program.

Science Exploration [I]

★ Read *Exploring the History of Medicine* p. 86-90. After reading the chapter, turn to p. 91 of *Exploring the History of Medicine.* Write the answer to each numbered question from p. 91 on lined paper. You do not need to copy the question.

Key Idea: During Joseph Lister's time, older doctors still thought that infection was useful as Galen had stated. Even though anesthesia was used during surgery, patients often died after surgery due to unsanitary conditions in the hospitals. Lister experimented with carbolic acid as an antiseptic. He also washed his hands before surgery and wore a clean linen apron. The results were astounding.

Learning through History
Focus: Jesus, Teacher and Healer

Reading about History | I |

Read about history in the following resource:

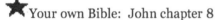 Your own Bible: John chapter 8

You will be adding to your timeline in your *Student Notebook* today. In Unit 29 – Box 1, draw and color a dove. Label it, *Jesus begins His ministry (26 A.D.)*. In Box 2, draw and color the number "12". Label it, *Jesus chooses 12 apostles (28 A.D.)*. In Box 3, draw and color 5 loaves of bread and 3 fish. Label it, *Jesus feeds 5000 (29 A.D.)*

<u>Key Idea</u>: Jesus forgave sins and warned people of the coming judgment.

Storytime | T |

Choose one of the following read aloud options:

★ *Traveling the Way* p. 126-131

★ Read aloud the next portion of the realistic fiction book that you selected.

After the reading, students will give a summary oral narration. The oral narration must be no longer than 5 sentences and should summarize the reading. As students narrate, have them hold up one finger for each sentence shared. Remind students that the focus should be on the big ideas, rather than on the details.

<u>Key Idea</u>: Summarize the story by narrating.

History Project | S |

Get the painted background of the storm that you painted on Day 1 and the origami rowboat that you folded on Day 2. Glue or tape one side of your rowboat to the background, so it appears that your boat is rolling upon the stormy waves.

Then, use a thin dark colored marker to copy Matthew 14:27, 33 onto white paper.

Next, cut around the verses and glue the paper cut-out either inside the boat or onto the stormy skies.

<u>Key Idea</u>: After Jesus' miracles many people recognized Him as a great healer and teacher. Yet, many did not see Him as the promised Savior. We need to make sure that we realize that Jesus is truly the Son of God.

Bible Quiet Time | I |

Reading: Choose the option below.

★ Your own Bible: John chapter 8

Scripture Focus: Highlight John 8:58.

Prayer Focus: Pray a prayer of thanksgiving to express gratitude for God's divine goodness. Begin by reading the highlighted verse out loud as a prayer. End by praying, *Thank you Jesus that you are clearly God and that as God you existed even before Abraham. Thank you for revealing yourself to us.*

Scripture Memory: Recite Philippians 2:25.
Music: *Philippians 2* CD: Track 7 (verse 25)

<u>Key Idea</u>: Jesus revealed to the people that He is God and that He was sent to be the light of the world.

Independent History Study | I |

Open your *Student Notebook* to Unit 29. In Box 6, copy in cursive John 8:57-58. Outline the words "I AM" in a separate color. Notice that this is the same name used by God for himself in Exodus 3:14.

<u>Key Idea</u>: Jesus was a descendent of Abraham, fulfilling the prophecy that through Abraham all nations on earth would be blessed. Jesus used God's name, "I AM" for himself, showing He is God.

Learning the Basics

Focus: Language Arts, Math, Geography, Bible, and Science

Bible Study [T]

Read aloud and discuss with the students the following pages:

 The Radical Book for Kids p. 211-213

<u>Key Idea</u>: The Gospels of Matthew, Mark, Luke, and John tell the story of Jesus. Each Gospel tells Jesus' story from a different perspective. Matthew writes like a reporter and points to Jesus as the long-awaited Messiah. Mark writes as a storyteller and shows Jesus coming down from heaven to give His life for sinners. Luke writes as a historian who shows Jesus as a loving Savior. John writes as a theologian and represents Jesus as an exalted heavenly Son who shows the glory of God.

Language Arts [S]

Have students complete one dictation exercise (see Appendix for directions and passages).

Work with the students to complete **one** of the writing options listed below:

 Writing & Rhetoric Book 2: Narrative I p. 86-90 (Note: Today's text includes Greek goddesses as part of a myth. Read aloud the text while the students follow along. Then, discuss.)

 Your own writing program

<u>Key Idea</u>: Practice language arts skills.

Poetry [I]

Open *Paint Like a Poet* to Lesson 23. Read aloud the poem *"An Encounter"* by Robert Frost.

Get the roadside backdrop that you painted on Day 2. Today, you will be adding telephone poles. You will need a palette, water, a small flat paintbrush, and brown and white paint.

After gathering your supplies, turn to the "Step-by-Step Watercolor Tutorial" for Lesson 23 in *Paint Like a Poet*. Follow steps 4-6 to complete "Part Two: Telephone Poles". When your painting is dry, glue your poetry copywork from Day 1 to your painting. Store your completed artwork in the place you have chosen for it.

<u>Key Idea</u>: Explore poetry moods with painting.

Math Exploration [S]

Choose **one** of the math options listed below.

 Singapore Primary Mathematics 4A/4B or 5A/5B (see Appendix for schedules), or *Math with Confidence,* or *Apologia Math*

 Your own math program

<u>Key Idea</u>: Use a step-by-step math program.

Science Exploration [I]

 Read *Exploring the History of Medicine* p. 92-96.

After reading the chapter listed above, turn to p. 97 of *Exploring the History of Medicine*. Write the answer to each numbered question from p. 97 on lined paper. You do not need to copy the question.

<u>Key Idea</u>: Robert Koch experimented with finding the cause of anthrax. His thorough experiments showed which bacteria caused anthrax and how it was spread. This became the germ theory of disease. When he finally presented his findings by performing the same experiments at the University of Breslau, he proved that each disease is caused by a particular bacterium.

Learning through History
Focus: Jesus, Teacher and Healer

Unit 29 - Day 4

Reading about History | I |

Read about history in the following resource:

★ Your own Bible: John chapter 9

You will be writing a narration from the following Bible reading: *John chapter 9,* which is today's history reading.

To prepare for writing your narration, look back over what you read in John chapter 9. Think about the main idea.

After you have thought about what you will write and how you will begin your narration, turn to Unit 29 in your *Student Notebook.*

In Box 5, write a 5-8 sentence narration which tells about the John chapter 9.

When you have finished writing, read your sentences out loud to catch any mistakes.

Check for the following things: *Did you include* **who** *or* **what topic** *the reading was mainly about? Did you include* **descriptors** *of the important thing(s) that happened? Did you include a* **closing sentence**? *If not, add those things.*

Then, underline or highlight the main idea sentence in the narration. Use the *Written Narration Skills* in the Appendix as a guide for editing the narration.

<u>Key Idea</u>: Jesus healed a man who had been blind since birth. He put mud on the man's eyes and sent him to wash in the Pool of Siloam. When the man did as he was told, he could see. The Pharisees questioned the blind man and then threw him out because of his answers to their questions. Jesus again spoke with the blind man and shared that He is the Son of Man.

Storytime | T |

Choose one of the following read aloud options:

★ *Traveling the Way* p. 132-138

★ Read aloud part of the realistic book.

After the reading, have each person get a Bible and open it anywhere in Proverbs. Explain, *We will have 5 minutes to skim through the verses in Proverbs to find any connections to today's story. When a connection is found, read the verse out loud and quickly share the connection. At the end of 5 minutes, anyone who has not shared yet must read aloud one verse and make the best connection possible.*

<u>Key Idea</u>: Seek God's word for His guidance.

Bible Quiet Time | I |

Reading: Choose the option below.

★ Your own Bible: John chapter 9

Scripture Focus: Highlight John 9:1-3.

Prayer Focus: Pray a prayer of supplication to make a humble and earnest request of God. Begin by reading the highlighted verses out loud as a prayer. End by praying, *Guide me to draw nearer to you when I am worried or am suffering. Help me to remember that even though we live in a fallen world filled with suffering, you give us the strength we need.*

Scripture Memory: Copy Philippians 2:25 in your Common Place Book.
Music: *Philippians 2* CD: Track 7 (verse 25)

<u>Key Idea</u>: Jesus cares for us and loves us.

Independent History Study | I |

Open your *Student Notebook* to "Prophecies About Christ". Under "Prophecy" write, *Isaiah 35:5.* Read the Scripture to discover the prophecy. Under "Fulfillment" write, *John 9:30-33.* Read the fulfillment Scripture. Under "Description", write a few phrases to describe the prophecy about Jesus.

<u>Key Idea</u>: Jesus fulfilled Isaiah's prophecy that upon Christ's coming the deaf will hear and the blind see.

Learning the Basics
Focus: Language Arts, Math, Geography, Bible, and Science

Unit 29 - Day 4

Geography [T]

Read aloud to the students the following pages:

 A Child's Geography Vol. II p. 174-179
Discuss with the students "Field Notes" p. 179.

Key Idea: The Asir highlands have heavy rains. Crops are grown on terraced mountain slopes. The Najd, which is an elevated plateau, is in the northwest region of Saudi Arabia.

Language Arts [S]

Have students complete one dictation exercise.

Guide students to complete one reading lesson.

★ *Drawn into the Heart of Reading*

Help students complete **one** English lesson.

★ *Building with Diligence:* Lesson 54

★ *Following the Plan:* Lesson 49

★ Your own grammar program

Key Idea: Practice language arts skills.

Poetry [I]

Open *Paint Like a Poet* to Lesson 23. Today, you will be performing a poetry reading of *"An Encounter"*. Read the poem aloud in front of your chosen audience. At the end of the reading, share the following, *When I read this poem by Robert Frost, it made me think of...* Call on your audience to share what thoughts the poem brought to their minds.
Last, say, *Did you know that Robert Frost had a dry sense of humor? He once remarked, "I never take my side in a quarrel." Another time he said, "I'm never serious except when I'm fooling." Can you see his humor in his poetry?*

Key Idea: Share the poetry of Robert Frost.

Math Exploration [S]

Choose **one** of the math options listed below.

★ *Singapore Primary Mathematics 4A/4B* or *5A/5B* (see Appendix for schedules), or *Math with Confidence*, or *Apologia Math*

★ Your own math program

Key Idea: Use a step-by-step math program.

Science Exploration [S]

★ Read *Exploring the History of Medicine* p. 98-106 and answer questions on p. 107. At the top of a blank page, write: *How do diseases spread?* Under the question, write: *'Guess'.* Write down your guess. **Have an adult set up the following part** of the experiment: Set out 10 cups. Add numbered masking tape to the bottom of each cup. Number two cups '1', two cups '2', and so on. Place cups with numbered pairs side by side. Add 2 Tbsp. of flour to 4 cups with different numbers. Add 2 Tbsp. of baking soda to a cup with a different number than the flour-filled cups. Remember the cup number to which you added the soda. Explain to students that one of the cups contains a disease. **Have students do the next portion:** Write *Control* on 5 pieces of masking tape, and tape one to each of the empty cups. Pour ½ of each cup's powder into its matching numbered *Control* cup. Then, transmit the disease by pouring powder from two **non-control** cups together in one cup, shaking, and dividing the powder back into two cups. Do not use any utensil to mix the powders or let the powders touch your hands. Write down the numbers of the two cups you mixed. Repeat the activity twice more, being sure to list the numbers of the cups that exchanged powder. Next, to see which cups have the disease, add 1 Tbsp. white vinegar to each cup **not** labeled *Control*. Diseased cups will foam. Try to figure out which cup had the disease first. Check your answer by adding white vinegar to each *Control* cup. The one that foams had the disease first. Look at the number taped to the bottom of that cup to see if you were correct in determining which cup had the disease first. Write, *Procedure,* and draw the experiment. Write, *Conclusion,* and explain what you learned.

Key Idea: Even after suffering a stroke, Pasteur made vaccinations for cholera, anthrax, and rabies.

Learning through History
Focus: The Shepherd and His Flock

Reading about History | I

Read about history in the following resource:

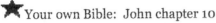 Your own Bible: John chapter 10

Jesus is often compared to a shepherd. Where could you look to research more about being a **shepherd**? Use the Bible, a reference book, or an online resource like www.wikipedia.org.

Answer one or more of the following questions from your research: *What were the duties of a shepherd? Describe a shepherd. Who were some of the Biblical heroes that were shepherds? Where were sheep gathered at night according to John 10:1? Why were sheep often gathered into a sheep pen at night? To what does Jesus compare himself in John 10:11? How is Jesus like a good shepherd? What is the difference between a hired hand and a shepherd in John 10:12-15?*

Key Idea: Jesus is like a good shepherd. He carefully watches over us like sheep and was willing to lay down His life for us.

History Project | S

In this unit you will make a mezuzah case and a mezuzah, which is a small parchment scroll. Jews attached a mezuzah to the doorpost of their home to dedicate it to God's service as in Deut. 6:9. To make dough for the case, stir together 1 cup flour and ½ cup salt. Add ½ cup hot water and stir. Knead the dough for 5 minutes, adding food coloring if desired to make colored dough. Save the dough in an airtight container.

Key Idea: In John 10:9, the Bible says that Jesus is the gate or door to salvation for us.

Storytime | T

Choose one of the following read aloud options:

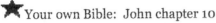 *Traveling the Way* p. 139-145

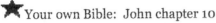 Read at least one realistic fiction book for the next 12 days of plans.

After the reading, students will give a detailed oral narration. Select one paragraph from the story to read out loud to the students. This will be the starting point for the narration. Set a timer for 3-5 minutes. When the timer rings the narration is over, even if it isn't complete. A detailed, descriptive narration is the goal. See *Narration Tips* in the Appendix as needed.

Key Idea: Use oral narration to retell the story.

Bible Quiet Time | I

Bible Reading: Choose the option below.

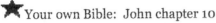 Your own Bible: John chapter 10

Scripture Focus: Highlight John 10:27-30.

Prayer Focus: Pray a prayer of adoration to worship and honor Jesus. Begin by reading the highlighted verses out loud as a prayer. End by praying, *I praise you that you are one with God and that because of that no one can snatch believers from your hand or take away eternal life.*

Scripture Memory: Recite Philippians 2:26.
Music: *Philippians 2* CD: Track 7 (vs. 25-26)

Key Idea: Jesus and God are one. We are Jesus' followers, and we know that He is our way to eternal life.

Independent History Study | I

Open your *Student Notebook* to "Prophecies About Christ". Under "Prophecy" write, *Isaiah 40:10-11*. Read the Scripture to discover the prophecy. Under "Fulfillment" write, *John 10-11*. Read the fulfillment Scripture. Under "Description", write a few phrases to describe the prophecy about Jesus.

Key Idea: Jesus fulfilled Isaiah's prophecy that the Savior would be a good shepherd who tends His flock.

Learning the Basics
Focus: Language Arts, Math, Geography, Bible, and Science

Bible Study | T |

Read aloud and discuss with the students the following pages:

 The Radical Book for Kids p. 214-216

Key Idea: As humans, we are all tied to Adam. After Adam sinned in the Garden of Eden, all mankind was born in sin after that. The only way to be saved from our sin is to be "born again" through Christ Jesus' perfect sacrfice. Those in Christ are connected to Him and loosed from the bond of Adam and sin. As Christians, we are united with Christ.

Language Arts | S |

Have students complete one studied dictation exercise (see Appendix for directions and passages).

Help students complete one lesson from the following reading program:

 Drawn into the Heart of Reading

Work with the students to complete **one** of the English options listed below:

⭐ *Building with Diligence:* Lesson 55 (Half)

⭐ *Following the Plan:* Lesson 50

⭐ Your own grammar program

Key Idea: Practice language arts skills.

Poetry | I |

Open *Paint Like a Poet* to Lesson 24. Read aloud the poem *"The Runaway"*. On a 3 x 5 index card, neatly copy in black ink or in pencil the following highlighted lines from the poem:

Once when the snow of the year was beginning to fall,
We stopped by a mountain pasture to say,
"Whose colt?"
A little Morgan had one forefoot on the wall,
The other curled at his breast. He dipped his head
And snorted to us. And then we saw him bolt.

-Robert Frost

Check your work to make sure it is correctly copied. Then, cut around your copywork. You may choose to outline the edge of the cut-out with a gray marker. Save it for Day 3.

Key Idea: Read and appreciate classic poetry.

Math Exploration | S |

Choose **one** of the math options listed below.

⭐ *Singapore Primary Mathematics 4A/4B* or *5A/5B* (see Appendix for schedules), or *Math with Confidence*, or *Apologia Math*

⭐ Your own math program

Key Idea: Use a step-by-step math program.

Science Exploration | I |

⭐ Read *Exploring the History of Medicine* p. 108-112.

After reading the chapter listed above, turn to p. 113 of *Exploring the History of Medicine*. Write the answer to each numbered question from p. 113 on lined paper. You do not need to copy the question.

Key Idea: Dr. Lind was a Scottish physician in the British Royal Navy. He studied scurvy for 10 years to determine its cause. Eventually, his studies pointed toward lack of fruits and vegetables as the cause. Captain James Cook used Lind's suggestions on his four-year voyage. He was a believer in Lind's limes! Eventually, even the admiralty ordered sailors to drink lime juice to prevent and cure scurvy.

Unit 30 - Day 2

Reading about History | I |

Read about history in the following resource:

 Your own Bible: John chapter 11

You will be choosing a portion from today's reading that you found memorable or worthy of being reread to copy. Open your *Student Notebook* to Unit 30. In Box 3, carefully copy in cursive the portion from today's reading that you selected. Then, compare your written work to the original. Last, draw a small colorful picture in Box 3 to illustrate your sentences.

Key Idea: When Mary and Martha sent Jesus word that Lazarus was sick, Jesus knew that Lazarus would die so that Jesus' power over death could be shown through a miracle.

Storytime | T |

Choose one of the following read aloud options:

 Traveling the Way p. 146-152

Read aloud the next portion of the realistic fiction book that you selected.

After reading, give each person 2 slips of paper. Each person must think of 2 questions to ask about the book and write one question on each slip of paper. Next, fold up the slips of paper and place them in a container. Each person must select at least one question from the container to answer.

Key Idea: Use questioning to share the story.

History Project | S |

Take out the air-dry dough that you saved from Day 1. To make the mezuzah case, on a piece of waxed paper roll half of the dough into a rectangle that is ¼" thick. Wrap foil around a wooden spoon handle (or anything of a similar diameter). Fold the dough around the end of the handle, flattening and smoothing it into a long narrow rectangle. Seal one end, leaving a circular opening on the other end. Add thin ribbons of dough or small flattened balls of dough to decorate the mezuzah case. Remove the foil wrapped spoon handle. Poke a hole in the top and bottom, so the case can be attached by nails to a doorframe. You may choose to use double-sided tape to attach it instead. Either allow the dough to air dry, or have an adult help you bake it at 200 degrees for 2 hours.

Key Idea: The mezuzah can remind us that we are dedicated to Jesus and that He is Lord of our home.

Bible Quiet Time | I |

Reading: Choose one option below.

The Illustrated Family Bible p. 282-283

Your own Bible: John chapter 11

Scripture Focus: Highlight John 11:32-36.

Prayer Focus: Pray a prayer of confession to admit or acknowledge your sins to Jesus. Begin by reading the highlighted verses out loud as a prayer. End by praying, *I confess that sometimes I forget how much you love me and that you know how it feels to cry and to be sad. Help me turn to you for comfort when I am sad about...*

Scripture Memory: Recite Philippians 2:26.
Music: *Philippians 2* CD: Track 7 (vs. 25-26)

Key Idea: Even though Jesus knew Lazarus would be raised from the dead, He wept. Jesus knows your needs and has compassion for you too.

Independent History Study | I |

Open your *Student Notebook* to Unit 30. In Box 5, copy in cursive John 11:25.

Key Idea: Jesus told Martha that He is the way to heaven and that He has power over life and death.

Learning the Basics
Focus: Language Arts, Math, Geography, Bible, and Science

Geography `T`

Read aloud to the students the following pages:

 A Child's Geography Vol. II p. 180 – bottom of p. 181

Discuss with the students the **first three** "Field Notes" on p. 184.

Key Idea: Saudi Arabia pumps oil, half of which is changed to gasoline. This makes Saudi Arabia a wealthy country with a flourishing economy. Many Saudis live in the Al-Hasa Oasis.

Language Arts `S`

Help students complete one lesson from the following reading program:

 Drawn into the Heart of Reading

Work with the students to complete **one** of the writing options listed below:

 Writing & Rhetoric Book 2: Narrative I p. 91 – top of p. 94 (Note: Refer back to the myth on p. 87-89 as needed for today's lesson.)

 Your own writing program

Key Idea: Practice language arts skills.

Poetry `I`

Open *Paint Like a Poet* to Lesson 24. Read aloud the poem *"The Runaway"* by Robert Frost.

Today, you will be painting a winter backdrop. You will need painting paper, a palette, water, a large flat paintbrush, and blue, red, and brown paint.

After gathering your supplies, turn to the "Step-by-Step Watercolor Tutorial" for Lesson 24 in *Paint Like a Poet*. Follow steps 1-3 to complete "Part One: Winter Backdrop". Then, let your background dry. You will complete "Part Two" of the tutorial on Day 3.

Key Idea: Use painting to illustrate poetry.

Math Exploration `S`

Choose **one** of the math options listed below.

 Singapore Primary Mathematics 4A/4B or *5A/5B* (see Appendix for schedules), or *Math with Confidence,* or *Apologia Math*

 Your own math program

Key Idea: Use a step-by-step math program.

Science Exploration `I`

 Read *Exploring the History of Medicine* p. 114-120.

After reading the chapter listed above, turn to p. 121 of *Exploring the History of Medicine*. Write the answer to each numbered question from p. 121 on lined paper. You do not need to copy the question.

Key Idea: Christiaan Eijkman looked for a germ as the cause of beriberi. Eventually, he discovered that a lack of a vitamin called thiamine, which is found in brown rice, led to patients getting the disease beriberi. Sometimes dietary deficiencies can be the cause of a disease. Eijkman won the Nobel Prize for his work.

Learning through History
Focus: The Shepherd and His Flock

Unit 30 - Day 3

Reading about History | I |

Read about history in the following resource:

★ Your own Bible: John chapter 12

You will be adding to your timeline in your *Student Notebook* today. In Unit 30 – Box 1, draw and color a golden crown of leaves. Label it, *Tiberius Caesar is Emperor of Rome (14-37 A.D.)*. In Box 2, draw and color rays of light coming down from heaven. Label it, *Jesus' ministry (26/27-30 A.D.)*.

<u>Key Idea</u>: Before the Passover, Jesus attended a dinner given in His honor in Bethany. Mary, Martha, and Lazarus were all there. Mary anointed Jesus' feet with expensive perfume.

Storytime | T |

Choose one of the following read aloud options:

★ *The Accidental Voyage* p. 9-20

★ Read aloud the next portion of the realistic fiction book that you selected.

After the reading, students will give a summary oral narration. The oral narration must be no longer than 5 sentences and should summarize the reading. As students narrate, have them hold up one finger for each sentence shared. Remind students that the focus should be on the big ideas, rather than on the details.

<u>Key Idea</u>: Summarize the story by narrating.

History Project | S |

Get the mezuzah case that you made on Day 2. If desired, use paint to carefully decorate the designs on your case. Then, open your *Student Notebook* to Unit 30 – Box 6. To make your mezuzah, use a black pen to copy **one** of the sets of Scripture from Box 6 onto a small white piece of paper. When rolled up, the paper must fit inside the circular opening in your mezuzah case. If you wish for your paper to look like parchment, you may dab the paper with a wet teabag. Once the mezuzah and its case are dry, roll up the mezuzah and slip it into the opening in the case. Then, attach the case to the right side of your doorframe at shoulder height. Use small nails, double-stick tape, or velcro.

<u>Key Idea</u>: The mezuzah also reminds us that Jesus is the Word of God who was nailed to the cross to become an open doorway to salvation for us.

Bible Quiet Time | I |

Reading: Choose one option below.

★ *The Illustrated Family Bible* p. 284-285

★ Your own Bible: John chapter 12

Scripture Focus: Highlight John 12:13.

Prayer Focus: Pray a prayer of thanksgiving to express gratitude for God's divine goodness in sending His only Son to earth. Begin by reading the highlighted verse out loud as a prayer. End by praying, *Thank you for being our promised Savior. "Hosanna! Blessed is He who comes in the name of the Lord!"*

Scripture Memory: Recite Philippians 2:26.
Music: *Philippians 2* CD: Track 7 (vs. 25-26)

<u>Key Idea</u>: Jesus was given a triumphal entry.

Independent History Study | I |

★ Listen to *What in the World?* Disc 4, **Half** of Track 8: "The Life of Jesus". After listening to half of Track 8, open your *Student Notebook* to "Prophecies About Christ". Under "Prophecy" write, *Zechariah 9:9*. Read the Scripture to discover the prophecy. Under "Fulfillment" write, *John 12:14-15*. Read the fulfillment Scripture. Under "Description", write a few phrases to describe the prophecy about Jesus.

<u>Key Idea</u>: Jesus fulfilled the prophecy made by Zechariah over 500 years earlier that the Messiah would ride into Jerusalem as king on a donkey.

Learning the Basics
Focus: Language Arts, Math, Geography, Bible, and Science

Bible Study   T

Read aloud and discuss with the students the following pages:

 The Radical Book for Kids p. 217-219

Key Idea: Approximately one-third of the chapters in the Gospels are devoted to the last eight days in Jesus' life. This last week of Christ's life is known as "Passion Week." While Jesus was a teacher and healer, His ultimate role was to die for mankind in fulfillment of God's promise. Jeus came "to serve, and to give His life as a ransom for many." (Mark 10:45)

Language Arts   S

Have students complete one studied dictation exercise (see Appendix for directions and passages).

Work with the students to complete **one** of the writing options listed below:

 Writing & Rhetoric Book 2: Narrative I p. 97-100 (Note: Omit p. 94-96. Read aloud today's text, while the students follow along. Then, guide students to write an amplification with dialogue and description.)

 Your own writing program

Key Idea: Practice language arts skills.

Poetry   I

Open *Paint Like a Poet* to Lesson 24. Read aloud the poem *"The Runaway"* by Robert Frost.

Get the winter backdrop that you painted on Day 2. Today, you will be adding clouds and snow. You will need a palette, water, a small flat paintbrush, a pencil, and blue, grey, and white paint.

After gathering your supplies, turn to the "Step-by-Step Watercolor Tutorial" for Lesson 24 in *Paint Like a Poet*. Follow steps 4-5 to complete "Part Two: Clouds and Snow". When your painting is dry, glue your poetry copywork from Day 1 to your painting. Store your completed artwork in the place you have chosen for it.

Key Idea: Explore poetry moods with painting.

Math Exploration   S

Choose **one** of the math options listed below.

 Singapore Primary Mathematics 4A/4B or 5A/5B (see Appendix for schedules), or *Math with Confidence*, or *Apologia Math*

 Your own math program

Key Idea: Use a step-by-step math program.

Science Exploration   I

 Read *Exploring the History of Medicine* p. 122-128.

After reading the chapter listed above, turn to p. 129 of *Exploring the History of Medicine*. Write the answer to each numbered question from p. 129 on lined paper. You do not need to copy the question.

Key Idea: William Crookes experimented with cathode rays. Eventually, scientists realized that cathode rays were streams of high-speed electrons. Atoms were made of electrons! Wilhelm Roentgen experimented with a Crookes tube and discovered a second invisible type of ray that could see through human flesh. The x-ray became a practical new tool to help doctors treat their patients.

Reading about History [I]

Read about history in the following resource:

 Your own Bible: John chapter 13

You will be writing a narration from the following Bible reading: *John chapter 13,* which is today's history reading.

To prepare for writing your narration, look back over what you read in John chapter 13. Think about the main idea.

After you have thought about what you will write and how you will begin your narration, turn to Unit 30 in your *Student Notebook.*

In Box 4, write a 5-8 sentence narration which tells about the John chapter 13.

When you have finished writing, read your sentences out loud to catch any mistakes.

Check for the following things: *Did you include **who** or **what topic** the reading was mainly about? Did you include **descriptors** of the important thing(s) that happened? Did you include a **closing sentence**? If not, add those things.*

Then, underline or highlight the main idea sentence in the narration. Use the *Written Narration Skills* in the Appendix as a guide for editing the narration.

Key Idea: Before the Passover meal, Jesus acted as a servant, washing each of His disciples' feet. Through this act, He taught the disciples to serve one another, to serve God, and to serve others. Then, Jesus gave a piece of bread dipped in wine to Judas to signify that he would betray Jesus. Jesus also predicted Peter would deny Him three times.

Storytime [T]

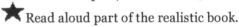

Choose one of the following read aloud options:

 The Accidental Voyage p. 21-35 (Warning: The content on p. 24-26 is violent.)

 Read aloud part of the realistic book.

After the reading, have each person get a Bible and open it anywhere in Proverbs. Explain, *We will have 5 minutes to skim through the verses in Proverbs to find any connections to today's story. When a connection is found, read the verse out loud and quickly share the connection. At the end of 5 minutes, anyone who has not shared yet must read aloud one verse and make the best connection possible.*

Key Idea: Seek God's word for His guidance.

Bible Quiet Time [I]

Reading: Choose the option below.

 Your own Bible: John chapter 13

Scripture Focus: Highlight John 13:34-35.

Prayer Focus: Pray a prayer of supplication to make a humble and earnest request of Jesus. Begin by reading the highlighted verses out loud as a prayer. End by praying, *Help me to love others as you love me. Guide me to follow your example so that others can see you in me. Help me to overcome arguing, jealousy, and...*

Scripture Memory: Copy Philippians 2:26 in your Common Place Book.
Music: *Philippians 2* CD: Track 7 (vs. 25-26)

Key Idea: Jesus asks us to love one another.

Independent History Study [I]

 Listen to *What in the World?* Disc 4, **Last Half** of Track 8: "The Life of Jesus".

Key Idea: Jesus didn't do the things the people expected a king to do. The people were expecting an earthly king to overthrow Roman rule, but Jesus was a heavenly King who will one day return to earth.

Learning the Basics
Focus: Language Arts, Math, Geography, Bible, and Science

Unit 30 - Day 4

Geography [T]

Read aloud to the students the following pages:

★ *A Child's Geography Vol. II* bottom of p. 181 – 184

Discuss the **last three** "Field Notes" on p. 184.

Key Idea: Farmers in Saudi Arabia use water from underground aquifers for their cattle and their crops. Rub Al Khali, or the Sands, is in the northwest region of Saudi Arabia This region has extreme heat and endless dunes.

Language Arts [S]

Have students complete one dictation exercise.

Guide students to complete one reading lesson.

★ *Drawn into the Heart of Reading*

Help students complete **one** English lesson.

★ *Building with Diligence:* Lesson 55 (Half)

★ *Following the Plan:* Lesson 51

★ Your own grammar program

Key Idea: Practice language arts skills.

Poetry [I]

Open *Paint Like a Poet* to Lesson 24. Today, you will be performing a poetry reading of *"The Runaway"*. Practice reading the poem with expression that matches the poem's mood. Then, read the poem aloud in front of your chosen audience. At the end of the reading, share the following, *When I read this poem by Robert Frost, it made me think of...* Call on your audience to share what thoughts the poem brought to their minds.

Last, say, *Did you know that Robert Frost won the Pulitzer Prize four times for poetry? The Pulitzer Prize is given yearly in the U.S. in a variety of categories. Frost won as the most distinguished author of original verse.*

Key Idea: Share the poetry of Robert Frost.

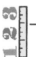

Math Exploration [S]

Choose **one** of the math options listed below.

★ *Singapore Primary Mathematics 4A/4B or 5A/5B* (see Appendix for schedules), or *Math with Confidence*, or *Apologia Math*

★ Your own math program

Key Idea: Use a step-by-step math program.

Science Exploration [I]

★ Read *Exploring the History of Medicine* p. 130-134. Answer the questions on p. 135 on lined paper. Then, turn to the science experiment section in your science binder or sketchbook. At the top of a blank page, write: *What is a half-life of a radioactive element?* Under the question, write: *'Guess'*. Write down your guess. Energy is locked inside an atom. The energy is stored inside the nucleus, which is why it is called nuclear energy. Every time a nucleus breaks apart, energy is released. Unstable atoms disintegrate at predictable rates. The rate of radioactive decay is a half-life, which is the time it takes half of the atoms in a radioactive element to decay. You will need 60 counters to represent radioactive nuclei (i.e. pennies, dry cereal pieces, dry beans, macaroni noodles, beads, or candies). Place the counters in a glass. Label the glass *Radioactive Nuclei*. Label a bowl, *Decayed Nuclei*. Cover and shake the glass. Pour the nuclei onto a paper towel. Place half of the counters into the *Decayed Nuclei* bowl. Write down the number of radioactive nuclei remaining under the heading "One half-life". Place only the radioactive nuclei back in the glass. Repeat the activity, halving the counters at the end of each toss and writing down each half-life. If there is an extra counter, place it back in the glass. Stop when only 1 counter remains. Next, write: *'Procedure'*. Make a list or diagram to show your results. Write: *'Conclusion'*. Explain what you learned.

Key Idea: The Curies experimented with radioactive elements. Radium was the most radioactive element that they discovered.

Learning through History
Focus: Jesus Lays Down His Life

Reading about History $\boxed{\text{I}}$

Read about history in the following resource:

★ Your own Bible: John chapters 14-15

Caiaphas was the Jewish high priest appointed by the Romans at the time of Jesus' death. Where could you look to research more about **Caiaphas**? Use a Bible or an online resource like www.wikipedia.org. Answer one or more of the following questions from your research: *In John 11:45-54 what did Caiaphas prophecy about Jesus? In John 18:12-14, who did Jesus have a hearing with after His arrest? After Annas, who did Jesus see next in Matthew 26:57-68? After Jesus' resurrection in Matthew 28:12-15, what did Caiaphas do? In Acts 4:5-21, what role does Caiaphas have in trying to silence Peter and John?*

Key Idea: As high priest, Caiaphas should have recognized Jesus as the Promised Savior.

History Project $\boxed{\text{S}}$

In this unit you will use a map to review the locations of the main events in the life of Christ. Open your *Student Notebook* to the map on Unit 31. Each event from the life of Jesus is numbered on the map in the order that the event occurred. Begin with event 1, *Born to virgin Mary,* and find its location at Bethlehem. Continue on with event 2, *Simeon and Anna recognize the Messiah,* and find its location at Jerusalem. Go on to event 3, *Flight to Egypt,* and find its location heading toward Egypt. Continue on in this manner until you have found the locations of the first 15 events.

Key Idea: Jesus traveled in Judea, Samaria, and Galilee.

Storytime $\boxed{\text{T}}$

Choose one of the following read aloud options:

★ *The Accidental Voyage* p. 36-43

★ Read at least one realistic fiction book for the next 8 days of plans.

After the reading, students will give a detailed oral narration. Select one paragraph from the story to read out loud to the students. This will be the starting point for the narration. Set a timer for 3-5 minutes. When the timer rings the narration is over, even if it isn't complete. A detailed, descriptive narration is the goal. See *Narration Tips* in the Appendix as needed.

Key Idea: Use oral narration to retell the story.

Bible Quiet Time $\boxed{\text{I}}$

Bible Reading: Choose the option below.

★ Your own Bible: John chapters 14-15

Scripture Focus: Highlight John 14:1-3.

Prayer Focus: Pray a prayer of adoration to worship and honor Jesus. Begin by reading the highlighted verses out loud as a prayer. End by praying, *I praise you for the promise you've given me that you are preparing a place for me in heaven, so I can share my life with you if I believe in you.*

Scripture Memory: Recite Philippians 2:27.
Music: *Philippians 2* CD: Track 7 (vs. 25-27)

Key Idea: Jesus promised His disciples that He was going to prepare a place for them and that one day they would live in heaven with Him.

Independent History Study $\boxed{\text{I}}$

Open your *Student Notebook* to "Prophecies About Christ". Under "Prophecy" write, *Psalm 69:4.* Read the Scripture from your Bible to discover the prophecy. Under "Fulfillment" write, *John 15:24-25.* Read the fulfillment Scripture. Under "Description", write a few phrases to describe the prophecy about Jesus.

Key Idea: Just as prophecied, Jesus was hated without reason.

Bible Study | T |

Read aloud and discuss with the students the following pages:

 The Radical Book for Kids p. 220-222

Key Idea: Jesus' followers wrote letters to tell others the Good News of Jesus. Many of the New Testament books are letters. The apostles also sent letters to help guide and encourage their fellow believers. The letters addressed problems Christians faced like temptation, erroneous teaching, and persecution.

Language Arts | S |

Have students complete one studied dictation exercise (see Appendix for directions and passages).

Help students complete one lesson from the following reading program:

 Drawn into the Heart of Reading

Work with the students to complete **one** of the English options listed below:

 Building with Diligence: Lesson 56

 Following the Plan: Lesson 52 (Half)

 Your own grammar program

Key Idea: Practice language arts skills.

Poetry | I |

Open *Paint Like a Poet* to Lesson 25. Read aloud the poem *"Nothing Gold Can Stay"*. On a 3 x 5 index card, neatly copy in ink or pencil the following highlighted lines from the poem:

Nature's first green is gold,
Her hardest hue to hold.
Her early leaf's a flower;
But only so an hour.
Then leaf subsides to leaf.
So Eden sank to grief,
So dawn goes down to day.
Nothing gold can stay.
                                    -Robert Frost

Check your work to make sure it is correctly copied. Then, cut around your copywork. You may choose to outline the edge of the cut-out with a gold marker. Save it for Day 3.

Key Idea: Read and appreciate classic poetry.

Math Exploration | S |

Choose **one** of the math options listed below.

 Singapore Primary Mathematics 4A/4B or *5A/5B* (see Appendix for schedules), or *Math with Confidence*, or *Apologia Math*

 Your own math program

Key Idea: Use a step-by-step math program.

Science Exploration | I |

 Read *Exploring the History of Medicine* p. 136-140.

After reading the chapter listed above, turn to p. 141 of *Exploring the History of Medicine*. Write the answer to each numbered question from p. 141 on lined paper. You do not need to copy the question.

Key Idea: Gerhard Domagk served as a medic in WWI and later earned his medical degree. After the war, he worked for I.G. Farben, a German chemical company. His job was to study new dyes for possible uses as medicine. The dye Prontosil contained the drug, Sulfanilamide, from which came a whole family of sulfa drugs. Sulfa kills one-celled bacteria, without hurting the cells of human tissue. It was a "wonder drug".

Reading about History | I |

Read about history in the following resource:

 Your own Bible: John chapter 16

You will be choosing a portion from today's reading that you found memorable or worthy of being reread to copy. Open your *Student Notebook* to Unit 31. In Box 3, carefully copy in cursive the portion from today's reading that you selected. Then, compare your written work to the original. Last, draw a small colorful picture in Box 3 to illustrate your sentences.

Key Idea: Jesus taught the disciples that He would always be with them through the Holy Spirit. He told the disciples that He would be leaving the world soon and returning to His Father in heaven.

Storytime | T |

Choose one of the following read aloud options:

★ *The Accidental Voyage* p. 44-49

★ Read aloud the next portion of the realistic fiction book that you selected.

After reading, work with the students to plan a 3 minute skit with simple props to act out part of today's reading. Set a timer for 3 minutes to quickly prepare for the skit. Make sure that you participate in the skit along with the students. When the timer rings, set it again for 3 minutes and perform the skit. You do not need an audience, as the goal is the retelling.

Key Idea: Use a skit to retell part of the story.

History Project | S |

Open your *Student Notebook* to the map on Unit 31. Each event from the life of Jesus is numbered on the map in the order that the event occurred. Begin with event 16, *Heals centurion's servant,* and find its location at Capernaum. Continue on with event 17, *Raises widow's son,* and find its location at Nain. Go on to event 18, *Pharisees' opposition,* and find its location at Capernaum. Continue on in this manner until you have found the location of event 31. Which event came before and which event came after the death of John the Baptist? Which locations have the most events from Jesus' life?

Key Idea: Jesus had returned to Jerusalem for the Passover knowing that His time on earth was short and that He would soon be betrayed. He was preparing His disciples for this event.

Bible Quiet Time | I |

Reading: Choose the option below.

★ Your own Bible: John chapter 16

Scripture Focus: Highlight John 16:33.

Prayer Focus: Pray a prayer of confession to admit or acknowledge your sins to God. Begin by reading the highlighted verse out loud as a prayer. End by praying, *Help me to be courageous in times of trouble. Forgive me for being surprised by troubles and guide me to have peace knowing you are with me.*

Scripture Memory: Recite Philippians 2:27.
Music: *Philippians 2* CD: Track 7 (vs. 25-27)

Key Idea: Jesus tells us that in this world we will have troubles, but He also says that He has overcome the world.

Independent History Study | I |

Open your *Student Notebook* to Unit 31. In Box 5, copy in cursive John 16:33.

Key Idea: We should not be surprised by troubles, as this sinful world is filled with them! However, Jesus encourages us that we can have peace in Him in spite of our troubles, because He is far greater.

Learning the Basics
Focus: Language Arts, Math, Geography, Bible, and Science

Geography   [T]

Have students get both the blank map and the labeled map of **Egypt, Iraq & Saudi Arabia** that they used in Unit 28.

Then, assign students the following page:

 A Child's Geography Vol. II p. 185

Note: Do only the "Map Notes" section. The "Books" and "Poetry" on p. 186 are optional.

Key Idea: Practice finding and recording the locations of various places on a map of Saudi Arabia.

Language Arts   [S]

Help students complete one lesson from the following reading program:

 Drawn into the Heart of Reading

Work with the students to complete **one** of the writing options listed below:

 Writing & Rhetoric Book 2: Narrative I p. 101 – middle of p. 107 (Note: Read aloud the text, while the students follow along. Then, discuss.)

 Your own writing program

Key Idea: Practice language arts skills.

Poetry   [I]

Open *Paint Like a Poet* to Lesson 25. Read aloud the poem *"Nothing Gold Can Stay"* by Robert Frost.

Today, you will be painting a meadow backdrop. You will need painting paper, a palette, water, a large flat paintbrush, a paper towel, and light blue, yellow, and green paint.

After gathering your supplies, turn to the "Step-by-Step Watercolor Tutorial" for Lesson 25 in *Paint Like a Poet*. Follow steps 1-3 to complete "Part One: Meadow Backdrop". Then, let your background dry. You will complete "Part Two" of the tutorial on Day 3.

Key Idea: Use painting to illustrate poetry.

Math Exploration   [S]

Choose **one** of the math options listed below.

 Singapore Primary Mathematics 4A/4B or 5A/5B (see Appendix for schedules), or *Math with Confidence,* or *Apologia Math*

 Your own math program

Key Idea: Use a step-by-step math program.

Science Exploration   [I]

 Read *Exploring the History of Medicine* p. 142-146. After reading the chapter, turn to p. 147 of *Exploring the History of Medicine.* Read the review.

Key Idea: As sulfa began its general use as an antibiotic, Alexander Fleming was discovering penicillin. He discovered that penicillium mold released a chemical that he named penicillin. The chemical prevented bacteria from forming a cell wall and weakened the germs. Two chemists, Florey and Chain, visited Fleming 10 years after his initial discovery of penicillin. They worked to make penicillin a usable antibiotic. Eventually, penicillin was mass-produced in the United States.

Learning through History
Focus: Jesus Lays Down His Life

Unit 31 - Day 3

Reading about History $\boxed{I}$

Read about history in the following resource:

⭐ Your own Bible: John chapter 17

You will be adding to your timeline in your *Student Notebook* today. In Unit 31 – Box 1, draw and color a blue star with 6 points to represent the Jews. Label it, *Caiaphas is High Priest (18-36 A.D.)*. In Box 2, draw and color a crown of thorns. Label it, *Pontius Pilate is Governor of Judea (26-36 A.D.)*.

Key Idea: Jesus prayed for Himself, for His disciples, and for future believers like you and me. He prayed for the disciples to be unified and to be protected from the evil one.

Storytime $\boxed{T}$

Choose one of the following read aloud options:

⭐ *The Accidental Voyage* p. 50-57

⭐ Read aloud the next portion of the realistic fiction book that you selected.

After the reading, students will give a summary oral narration. The oral narration must be no longer than 5 sentences and should summarize the reading. As students narrate, have them hold up one finger for each sentence shared. Remind students that the focus should be on the big ideas, rather than on the details.

Key Idea: Summarize the story by narrating.

History Project $\boxed{S}$

Open your *Student Notebook* to the map on Unit 31. Each event from the life of Jesus is numbered on the map in the order that the event occurred. Begin with event 32, *Jews demand a sign,* and find its location at Dalmanutha. Continue on with event 33, *Heals blind man,* and find its location at Bethsaida. Continue on in this manner until you have found the location of event 47. Why did Jesus stay away from Jerusalem between events 14 and 37, only returning to Jerusalem near the end of His ministry? Where was Jesus for much of that time? After Jesus raised Lazarus from the dead, the Pharisees were even more eager to kill Jesus. Where do the final events of Jesus' life take place? Where did Jesus appear to His disciples after His resurrection in events 45, 46, and 47?

Key Idea: Jesus' life is recorded in the Gospels.

Bible Quiet Time $\boxed{I}$

Reading: Choose the option below.

⭐ Your own Bible: John chapter 17

Scripture Focus: Highlight John 17:4-5.

Prayer Focus: Pray a prayer of thanksgiving to express gratitude for Jesus' divine goodness. Begin by reading the highlighted verses out loud as a prayer. End by praying, *Thank you for completing your work on earth. I know you are in heaven with your Father once again, just as you were before the world began.*

Scripture Memory: Recite Philippians 2:27.
Music: *Philippians 2* CD: Track 7 (vs. 25-27)

Key Idea: Jesus was ready to complete His work on earth and return to His Father in heaven.

Independent History Study $\boxed{I}$

Open your *Student Notebook* to Unit 31 – Box 6. Use a light colored marker such as yellow, orange, pink, blue, or green to color in the number next to any events on the map that were miracles that Jesus performed during His time on earth. In what region did most of Jesus' miracles take place?

Key Idea: Jesus did many miracles during His time on earth. Only some of them are recorded in the Bible.

Learning the Basics

Focus: Language Arts, Math, Geography, Bible, and Science

Bible Study [T]

Read aloud and discuss with the students the following pages:

 The Radical Book for Kids p. 223-225

Key Idea: We know from Scripture that the New Testament churches read and taught God's Word. They sang and prayed and gave testimonies. The early church celebrated the Lord's Supper. They also collected offerings and used their gifts to serve others. Love was to guide all the early church did. Next Sunday, look for ways you can encourage someone at your church!

Language Arts [S]

Have students complete one studied dictation exercise (see Appendix for directions and passages).

Work with the students to complete **one** of the writing options listed below:

 Writing & Rhetoric Book 2: Narrative I middle of p. 108 – top of p. 111 (Note: Omit bottom of p. 107 – middle of p. 108. Guide students through the lesson as needed.)

 Your own writing program

Key Idea: Practice language arts skills.

Poetry [I]

Open *Paint Like a Poet* to Lesson 25. Read aloud the poem *"Nothing Gold Can Stay"* by Robert Frost.

Get the meadow backdrop that you painted on Day 2. Today, you will be adding trees and golden grass. You will need a palette, water, a small round paintbrush, and green, yellow, and white paint.

After gathering your supplies, turn to the "Step-by-Step Watercolor Tutorial" for Lesson 25 in *Paint Like a Poet*. Follow steps 4-6 to complete "Part Two: Trees and Golden Grass". When your painting is dry, glue your poetry copywork from Day 1 to your painting. Store your completed artwork in the place you have chosen for it.

Key Idea: Explore poetry moods with painting.

Math Exploration [S]

Choose **one** of the math options listed below.

 Singapore Primary Mathematics 4A/4B or *5A/5B* (see Appendix for schedules), or *Math with Confidence,* or *Apologia Math*

 Your own math program

Key Idea: Use a step-by-step math program.

Science Exploration [I]

 Read *Exploring the History of Medicine* p. 148-152.

After reading the chapter listed above, turn to p. 153 of *Exploring the History of Medicine*. Read the review on p. 153. There are no questions to answer today.

Key Idea: In the 1900's, doctors made advancements in blood-typing for more successful transfusions. They also made advancements in two new areas, organ transplants and artificial organs. In 1954 the first organ transplant was a kidney transplanted from one twin brother to another. In 1967, the first heart transplant took place in South Africa. Who knows what advancements in medicine the 2000's will bring?

Learning through History
Focus: Jesus Lays Down His Life

Reading about History | I |

Read about history in the following resource:

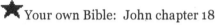 Your own Bible: John chapter 18

You will be writing a narration from the following Bible reading: *John chapter 18,* which is today's history reading.

To prepare for writing your narration, look back over what you read in John chapter 18. Think about the main idea.

After you have thought about what you will write and how you will begin your narration, turn to Unit 31 in your *Student Notebook.*

In Box 4, write a 5-8 sentence narration which tells about the John chapter 18.

When you have finished writing, read your sentences out loud to catch any mistakes.

Check for the following things: *Did you include **who** or **what topic** the reading was mainly about? Did you include **descriptors** of the important thing(s) that happened? Did you include a **closing sentence**? If not, add those things.*

Then, underline or highlight the main idea sentence in the narration. Use the *Written Narration Skills* in the Appendix as a guide for editing the narration.

Key Idea: Judas betrayed Jesus by handing Him over to the soldiers and officials of the chief priests and Pharisees. Simon Peter defended Jesus by drawing a sword and cutting off the right ear of the high priest's servant. Jesus healed the ear and admonished Peter. Jesus knew that He must die in order for God's plan of redemption to be fulfilled.

Storytime | T |

Choose one of the following read aloud options:

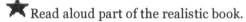 *The Accidental Voyage* p. 58-67

Read aloud part of the realistic book.

After the reading, have each person get a Bible and open it anywhere in Proverbs. Explain, *We will have 5 minutes to skim through the verses in Proverbs to find any connections to today's story. When a connection is found, read the verse out loud and quickly share the connection. At the end of 5 minutes, anyone who has not shared yet must read aloud one verse and make the best connection possible.*

Key Idea: Seek God's word for His guidance.

Bible Quiet Time | I |

Reading: Choose the option below.

Your own Bible: John chapter 18

Scripture Focus: Highlight John 18:37.

Prayer Focus: Pray a prayer of supplication to make a humble and earnest request of God. Begin by reading the highlighted verse out loud as a prayer. End by praying, *Strengthen me to follow Jesus' example and trust in your plan for my life. Help me to know the truth and accept it. Guide me to follow your example and be truthful too.*

Scripture Memory: Copy Philippians 2:27 in your Common Place Book.
Music: *Philippians 2* CD: Track 7 (vs. 25-27)

Key Idea: Jesus did what He was born to do.

Independent History Study | I |

Open your *Student Notebook* to "Prophecies About Christ". Under "Prophecy" write, *Psalm 41:9.* Read the Scripture to discover the prophecy. Under "Fulfillment" write, *John 13:18.* Read the fulfillment Scripture. Under "Description", write a few phrases to describe the prophecy about Jesus.

Key Idea: Just as prophecied, Jesus was betrayed by one with whom He shared His bread. Judas "lifted his heel" against Jesus in exchange for money.

Learning the Basics
Focus: Language Arts, Math, Geography, Bible, and Science

Geography | T

Go to the website link listed on p. 6 of *A Child's Geography Vol. II*. At the link, select "History & Geography". Then, under "Knowledge Quest" select ACG2-Extra Activities". Print the "Travel Log Template" of your choice from p. 39-42. Also at the link, for older students, print and assign the "Chapter Fourteen Review" on p. 81. Assign all students the following page:

★ *A Child's Geography Vol. II* p. 185, 188
Note: Do the "Travel Notes" section on p. 185 and the "Walk of Prayer" on p. 188. The "Food" section on p. 187 is an optional extra.

<u>Key Idea:</u> Share 3 sights from Saudi Arabia.

Language Arts | S

Have students complete one dictation exercise.

Guide students to complete one reading lesson.

★ *Drawn into the Heart of Reading*

Help students complete **one** English lesson.

★ *Building with Diligence:* Lesson 57

★ *Following the Plan:* Lesson 52 (Last half)

★ Your own grammar program

<u>Key Idea:</u> Practice language arts skills.

Poetry | I

Open *Paint Like a Poet* to Lesson 25. Today, you will be performing a poetry reading of *"Nothing Gold Can Stay"*. Practice reading the poem aloud with expression that matches the mood of the poem. Then, read the poem aloud in front of your chosen audience.

At the end of the reading, share the following, *When I read this poem by Robert Frost, it made me think of...* Call on your audience to share what thoughts the poem brought to their minds. Last, say, *Did you know that Robert Frost's poems were mainly inspired by a deep appreciation of nature and images from everyday life in New England? Frost himself said his rural surroundings were a source for insight and wisdom. He also said, "Literature begins with geography".*

<u>Key Idea:</u> Share the poetry of Robert Frost.

Math Exploration | S

Choose **one** of the math options listed below.

★ *Singapore Primary Mathematics 4A/4B or 5A/5B* (see Appendix for schedules), or *Math with Confidence,* or *Apologia Math*

★ Your own math program

<u>Key Idea:</u> Use a step-by-step math program.

Science Exploration | I

★ Read *An Illustrated Adventure in Human Anatomy* p. 1-5. Then, turn to the science experiment section in your science binder or sketchbook. At the top of a blank page, write: *How do different types of joints move?* Under the question, write: *'Guess'.* Write down your guess. Look at the joints noted with a pointing finger on p. 2 of *An Illustrated Adventure in Human Anatomy*. Next, write: *'Procedure'.* In a column under *'Procedure'*, list the joints shown on p. 2. Next to each joint, write whether its motion is like a hinge, a ball and socket, a swivel, a glider, or whether it's immovable. To test each joint's motion, find an object that performs the same motion. For example, a door opening and closing on its hinge is like a hinge joint. A wheel on the bottom of a rolling chair is like a ball and socket joint. A swing or a pendulum on a clock is like a gliding joint. A chair that swivels or the motion used when twisting off a jar lid is like a swivel joint. An immovable joint does not move. Write: *'Conclusion'.* Explain what you learned.

<u>Key Idea:</u> The elbow, finger, knee, toe, and jaw are hinge joints. The shoulder and hip are ball and socket joints. The neck is a swivel joint. The wrist and ankle are gliding joints. The skull is an immovable joint.

Learning through History
Focus: The Way, the Truth, and the Life

Unit 32 - Day 1

Reading about History — I

Read about history in the following resource:

⭐ Your own Bible: John chapter 19

Pontius Pilate was governor of the province of Judea at the time of Christ's death. Pilate is mentioned in all 4 of the Gospels. Where could you look to research more about **Pontius Pilate**? Answer one or more of the following questions: *In John 18:28, when did Jesus come before Pilate? What did Pilate ask Jesus in John 18:33? How did Jesus respond in John 18:36? What is Pilate's reaction to Jesus in Mark 15:5? What is Pilate's first judgment of Jesus in John 18:38? In Luke 23:7-12 who did Pilate send Jesus to see next? What is Herod's judgment in Luke 23:13-16? In John 19:6, what did Pilate say a second time? In John 19:7-11, what caused Pilate to be afraid? How did Pilate try to release Jesus in Matthew 27:15-18? What message did Pilate's wife send him in Matt. 27:19? After the people continued to ask for Jesus' crucifixion, what did Pilate do in Matthew 27:24? What sign did Pilate place above Jesus on the cross in John 19:19-22?*

<u>Key Idea</u>: Pilate crucified an innocent man.

History Project — S

In this unit you will make an etched cross to remind you of Christ's death and resurrection. On heavy white paper, draw and cut out a cross. Color the cross in sections, using a different colored crayon for each section until no white space remains. Press hard when coloring to get a deep, rich color. Last, use a black or a dark purple crayon to color a heavy layer over top of the multi-colors.

<u>Key Idea</u>: Jesus died for you and for me!

Storytime — T

Choose one of the following read aloud options:

⭐ *The Accidental Voyage* p. 68-81

⭐ Read at least one realistic fiction book for the next 4 days of plans.

After the reading, students will give a detailed oral narration. Select one paragraph from the story to read out loud to the students. This will be the starting point for the narration. Set a timer for 3-5 minutes. When the timer rings the narration is over, even if it isn't complete. A detailed, descriptive narration is the goal. See *Narration Tips* in the Appendix as needed.

<u>Key Idea</u>: Use oral narration to retell the story.

Bible Quiet Time — I

Bible Reading: Choose the option below.

⭐ Your own Bible: John chapter 19

Scripture Focus: Highlight John 19:30.

Prayer Focus: Pray a prayer of adoration to worship and honor God. Begin by reading the highlighted verse out loud as a prayer. End by praying, *Through reading the Scripture, I can glimpse your death on the cross. I worship you for finishing God's work of salvation and for paying for my sins in full.*

Scripture Memory: Recite Philippians 2:28.
Music: *Philippians 2* CD: Track 7 (vs. 25-28)

<u>Key Idea</u>: Knowing Jesus was innocent, Pilate still condemned Him to die. Jesus died to fulfill the Old Testament promise of a Savior.

Independent History Study — I

Open your *Student Notebook* to "Prophecies About Christ". Under "Prophecy" write, *Numbers 9:12*. Read the Scripture to discover the prophecy. Under "Fulfillment" write, *John 19:31-36*. Read the fulfillment Scripture. Under "Description", write a few phrases to describe the prophecy about Jesus.

<u>Key Idea</u>: Jesus became the Old Testament fulfillment of the Passover lamb without one bone broken.

Learning the Basics
Focus: Language Arts, Math, Geography, Bible, and Science

Bible Study | T

Read aloud and discuss with the students the following pages:

 The Radical Book for Kids p. 226-227

Key Idea: God reveals Himself to us through Scripture. He inspired people through the Holy Spirit to write the Scriptures. Then, God guided poeple to accept His inspired Word. He preserved and protected His Word, so it was not lost. God gave people the ability to translate His Word into many languages. As you read His Word, God illuminates it for you.

Language Arts | S

Have students complete one studied dictation exercise (see Appendix for directions and passages).

Help students complete one lesson from the following reading program:

★ *Drawn into the Heart of Reading*

Work with the students to complete **one** of the English options listed below:

★ *Building with Diligence:* Lesson 58

★ *Following the Plan:* Lesson 53

★ Your own grammar program

Key Idea: Practice language arts skills.

Poetry | I

Open *Paint Like a Poet* to Lesson 26. Read aloud the poem *"Blueberries"*. On a 3 x 5 index card, neatly copy in black ink or in pencil the following highlighted lines from the poem:

"You ought to have seen what I saw on my way
To the village, through Mortenson's pasture to-day:
Blueberries as big as the end of your thumb,
Real sky-blue, and heavy, and ready to drum
In the cavernous pail of the first one to come!
And all ripe together, not some of them green
And some of them ripe! You ought to have seen!"

-Robert Frost

Check your work to be sure it is correctly copied. Then, cut around your copywork, and outline the edge of it with a blue marker.

Key Idea: Read and appreciate classic poetry.

Math Exploration | S

Choose **one** of the math options listed below.

★ *Singapore Primary Mathematics 4A/4B* or *5A/5B* (see Appendix for schedules), or *Math with Confidence*, or *Apologia Math*

★ Your own math program

Key Idea: Use a step-by-step math program.

Science Exploration | I

★ Read *An Illustrated Adventure in Human Anatomy* p. 10-11. You will read p. 7-9 on Day 2. Today, you will add to your science notebook. At the top of an unlined paper, copy Job 10:11-12 in cursive. Beneath the verse, sketch and label the three kinds of muscles shown at the top of p. 10 of *An Illustrated Adventure in Human Anatomy*. Below your sketches, draw an arrow to each kind of muscle and either copy the text from p. 10 to describe each kind of muscle or write a description of each kind of muscle in your own words. Last, lightly color each muscle.

Key Idea: God made skeletal muscles to connect your bones and help you move. He made smooth muscles inside your organs to work all the time. He made cardiac muscles in your heart to contract faster when you exercise and to slow down when you are asleep.

Reading about History [I]

Read about history in the following resource:

★ Your own Bible: John chapters 20-21

You will be choosing a portion from today's reading that you found memorable or worthy of being reread to copy. Open your *Student Notebook* to Unit 32. In Box 4, carefully copy in cursive the portion from today's reading that you selected. Then, compare your written work to the original. Last, draw a small colorful picture in Box 4 to illustrate your sentences.

Key Idea: When Mary Magdalene and the women arrived at the tomb, Jesus' body wasn't there! She ran to tell Peter and John. When Peter and John came to the tomb, they saw the grave clothes still lying there. Jesus had risen!

Storytime [T]

Choose one of the following read aloud options:

★ *The Accidental Voyage* p. 82-92 (Note: If you are Catholic, omit or rephrase p. 90.)

★ Read aloud the next portion of the realistic fiction book that you selected.

After reading, give students a few minutes to prepare a short advertisement speech for the book. During the speech, students should hold up the book and say the book title and the name of the author. The wording of the advertisement should provide a peek into the book without giving away the ending. The goal should be for listeners to feel like they've "Got to Have This Book"!

Key Idea: Use an ad speech to share the story.

History Project [S]

Today you will do a baking project to represent Jesus' resurrection. You will finish your cross etching on Day 3. Either use 1 can of crescent rolls or 1 can of refrigerator biscuits. Lay out one roll or biscuit to be the tomb of Jesus. Take one large marshmallow to represent Christ's body. Dip it in melted butter and roll it in cinnamon and sugar to represent the spices Jesus' body was wrapped in upon His burial. Lay the marshmallow on the dough and carefully wrap it around the marshmallow. Pinch all seams together well to seal the tomb. Repeat the steps with the remaining rolls or biscuits. Bake according to the package directions. Then, cool on a wire rack. When you break open each tomb, the body of Christ is no longer there! He has risen!

Key Idea: Jesus rose from the dead! He's alive!

Bible Quiet Time [I]

Reading: Choose one option below.

★ *The Illustrated Family Bible* p. 309-311

★ Your own Bible: John chapters 20-21

Scripture Focus: Highlight John 20:27.

Prayer Focus: Pray a prayer of confession to admit or acknowledge your sins to God. Begin by reading the highlighted verse out loud as a prayer. End by praying, *I confess that sometimes I have doubts about my faith. Please forgive my doubting and help me to believe as you commanded us to do.*

Scripture Memory: Recite Philippians 2:28.
Music: *Philippians 2* CD: Track 7 (vs. 25-28)

Key Idea: Are you a doubting Thomas? What would Jesus say to you?

Independent History Study [I]

Open your *Student Notebook* to "Prophecies About Christ". Under "Prophecy" write, *Zechariah 12:10.* Read the Scripture to discover the prophecy. Under "Fulfillment" write, *John 20:25-29.* Read the fulfillment Scripture. Under "Description", write a few phrases to describe the prophecy about Jesus.

Key Idea: Jesus' hands, feet, and side were pierced as prophecied by Zechariah in the Old Testament.

Geography [T]

Read aloud to the students the following pages:

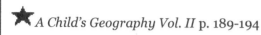 *A Child's Geography Vol. II* p. 189-194

Discuss with the students "Field Notes" p. 195.

Key Idea: The King's Highway that Moses mentioned in Numbers can be be seen in Jordan today. People still use Jordan as a highway through the desert. In Scripture, the Ammonites were the ancient inhabitants of Ammon, which is found in Jordan. A mosaic tile floor map at a Greek Orthodox Church in Madaba shows the Holy Land.

Language Arts [S]

Help students complete one lesson from the following reading program:

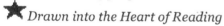 *Drawn into the Heart of Reading*

Work with the students to complete **one** of the writing options listed below:

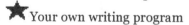 *Writing & Rhetoric Book 2: Narrative I* top of p. 111 – bottom of p. 113 (Note: Read aloud the text while the students follow along. Then, guide the students to write a new middle part to the story.)

⭐ Your own writing program

Key Idea: Practice language arts skills.

Poetry [I]

Open *Paint Like a Poet* to Lesson 26. Read aloud the poem *"Blueberries"* by Robert Frost.

Today, you will be painting a table backdrop. You will need painting paper, a palette, water, a large flat paintbrush, a pencil, a paper towel, and yellow, white, and brown paint.

After gathering your supplies, turn to the "Step-by-Step Watercolor Tutorial" for Lesson 26 in *Paint Like a Poet*. Follow steps 1-3 to complete "Part One: Table Backdrop". Then, let your background dry. You will complete "Part Two" of the tutorial on Day 3.

Key Idea: Use painting to illustrate poetry.

Math Exploration [S]

Choose **one** of the math options listed below.

⭐ *Singapore Primary Mathematics 4A/4B* or *5A/5B* (see Appendix for schedules), or *Math with Confidence,* or *Apologia Math*

⭐ Your own math program

Key Idea: Use a step-by-step math program.

Science Exploration [I]

⭐ Read *An Illustrated Adventure in Human Anatomy* p. 7-9. Orally retell or narrate to an adult the portion of text that you read today. Use the *Narration Tips* in the Appendix for help as needed.

Key Idea: There are more than 600 muscles in your body. Muscles are made of protein and water. They contract, or shorten, to move bones. Muscles and bones are joined together by tendons, which allow your muscles to move your bones. Tendons are even stronger than bones!

Reading about History | I

Read about history in the following resource:

★ Your own Bible: Acts chapters 1-2

You will be adding to your timeline in your *Student Notebook* today. In Unit 32 – Box 1, draw and color a cross. Label it, *Christ's Crucifixion and Resurrection (30 A.D.)*. In Box 2, draw and color clouds. Label it, *Christ's Ascension (40 days later - 30 A.D.)*. In Box 3, draw and color a flame. Label it, *Pentecost (10 days after the Ascension - 30 A.D)*.

Key Idea: Acts is a continuation of the story told in the Gospel of Luke. Both were written by Luke, a Greek and a Gentile physician. Luke was also a close friend and companion to Paul.

Storytime | T

Choose one of the following read aloud options:

★ *The Accidental Voyage* p. 93-101

★ Read aloud the next portion of the realistic fiction book that you selected.

After the reading, students will give a summary oral narration. The oral narration must be no longer than 5 sentences and should summarize the reading. As students narrate, have them hold up one finger for each sentence shared. Remind students that the focus should be on the big ideas, rather than on the details.

Key Idea: Summarize the story by narrating.

History Project | S

Get the cross that you colored on Day 1. Use the pointed end of a paper clip or the sharpened tip of a pencil to etch designs and patterns through the top layer of crayon on your cross. Make sure that your etchings are beautiful and that they honor Jesus' sacrifice on the cross. When you are done etching, punch a small hole in the top of your cross. Thread a piece of yarn or ribbon through the hole and tie it to make a hanger. Hang your cross in a place where it will remind you of Christ's deep love for you and of His death on the cross so that you can have eternal life.

Key Idea: After Jesus' resurrection, He appeared to the women at the tomb, the travelers on the road to Emmaus, the disciples, His brother James, and to a crowd of 500.

Bible Quiet Time | I

Reading: Choose one option below.

★ *The Illustrated Family Bible* p. 312-313 and p. 316-317

★ Your own Bible: Acts chapters 1-2

Scripture Focus: Highlight Acts 2:36-38.

Prayer Focus: Pray a prayer of thanksgiving to express gratitude for God's divine goodness. Begin by reading the highlighted verses out loud as a prayer. End by praying, *Thank you for the gift of the Holy Spirit as our Counselor and our helper. Thank you for sending a part of you to always be with us.*

Scripture Memory: Recite Philippians 2:28.
Music: *Philippians 2* CD: Track 7 (vs. 25-28)

Key Idea: After Jesus' ascension into heaven, He sent the gift of the Holy Spirit at Pentecost.

Independent History Study | I

Open your *Student Notebook* to "Prophecies About Christ". Under "Prophecy" write, *Psalm 16:8-11*. Read the Scripture to discover the prophecy. Under "Fulfillment" write, *Acts 2:24-36*. Read the fulfillment Scripture. Under "Description", write a few phrases to describe the prophecy about Jesus.

Key Idea: Just as David had prophecied over 800 years earlier, Jesus conquered death through His resurrection and is seated at God's right hand.

Learning the Basics
Focus: Language Arts, Math, Geography, Bible, and Science

Bible Study · T

Read aloud and discuss with the students the following pages:

 The Radical Book for Kids p. 228-229

Key Idea: It is good for you to hear God's Word, because hearing God's Word strengthens your faith. This is why it is good to go to church and listen to sermons. Before the sermon, ask God to help you listen well and hear His Word. Pray for the Holy Spirit to teach you. During the sermon, follow the speaker's outline or plan. Write things down as you listen. Look for actions you can take to respond to what you heard. Then, think about or discuss what you heard.

Language Arts · S

Have students complete one dictation exercise.

Work with the students to complete **one** of the writing options listed below:

 Writing & Rhetoric Book 2: Narrative I bottom of p. 113 – bottom of p. 115 (Note: Reread the story on p. 103-104 first. Then, guide students to rewrite the story from Alexander's, Philip's, or Bucephalus' point of view. Omit "Speak It" p. 115-116.)

★ Your own writing program

Key Idea: Practice language arts skills.

Poetry · I

Open *Paint Like a Poet* to Lesson 26. Read aloud the poem *"Blueberries"* by Robert Frost.

Get the table backdrop that you painted on Day 2. Today, you will be adding blueberries. You will need a palette, water, a small round paintbrush, a toothpick, and green, brown, blue, grey, and red paint.

After gathering your supplies, turn to the "Step-by-Step Watercolor Tutorial" for Lesson 26 in *Paint Like a Poet*. Follow steps 4-6 to complete "Part Two: Blueberries". When your painting is dry, glue your poetry copywork from Day 1 to your painting. Store your completed artwork in the place you have chosen for it.

Key Idea: Explore poetry moods with painting.

Math Exploration · S

Choose **one** of the math options listed below.

★ *Singapore Primary Mathematics 4A/4B or 5A/5B* (see Appendix for schedules), or *Math with Confidence*, or *Apologia Math*

★ Your own math program

Key Idea: Use a step-by-step math program.

Science Exploration · I

★ Read *An Illustrated Adventure in Human Anatomy* p. 13-15. Write the answer to each numbered question on lined paper. You do not need to copy the question. Use the listed page to help you answer each question.
1. What is the nervous system? (p. 14)
2. Write the words *autonomic system* and *somatic system* and give their definitions. (p. 14)
3. Draw and label the lobes of the brain and the activities controlled by each lobe. (p. 14)
4. List the parts of the brain and tell what each part does. (p. 15)
5. According to Romans 1:20, what should we see when we examine the wonders of Creation?

Key Idea: The brain and nerves work together to form the main communication system of the body.

Reading about History | I |

Read about history in the following resource:

⭐ Your own Bible: Acts chapters 3-4

You will be writing a narration from the following Bible reading: *Acts chapter 3*, which is part of today's history reading.

To prepare for writing your narration, look back over what you read in Acts chapter 3. Think about the main idea.

After you have thought about what you will write and how you will begin your narration, turn to Unit 32 in your *Student Notebook*.

In Box 5, write a 5-8 sentence narration which tells about the Acts chapter 3.

When you have finished writing, read your sentences out loud to catch any mistakes.

Check for the following things: *Did you include **who** or **what topic** the reading was mainly about? Did you include **descriptors** of the important thing(s) that happened? Did you include a **closing sentence**? If not, add those things.*

Then, underline or highlight the main idea sentence in the narration. Use the *Written Narration Skills* in the Appendix as a guide for editing the narration.

Key Idea: At the temple, Peter and John healed a man in Jesus' name who had been crippled since birth. The people were amazed by the miracle, and Peter boldly shared about Jesus with them. Peter and John were brought before the Jewish ruling council, the Sanhedrin. Both Annas and Caiaphas, who had tried Jesus and found Him guilty were there. The priests wanted to punish Peter and John but could not find any grounds to do so.

Storytime | T |

Choose one of the following read aloud options:

⭐ *The Accidental Voyage* p. 102-111

⭐ Read aloud the next portion of the realistic fiction book that you selected.

After the reading, have each person get a Bible and open it anywhere in Proverbs. Explain, *We will have 5 minutes to skim through the verses in Proverbs to find any connections to today's story. When a connection is found, read the verse out loud and quickly share the connection. At the end of 5 minutes, anyone who has not shared yet must read aloud one verse and make the best connection possible.*

Key Idea: Seek God's word for His guidance.

Bible Quiet Time | I |

Reading: Choose one option below.

⭐ *The Illustrated Family Bible* p. 318-320

⭐ Your own Bible: Acts chapters 3-4

Scripture Focus: Highlight Acts 3:19-20.

Prayer Focus: Pray a prayer of supplication to make a humble and earnest request of God. Begin by reading the highlighted verses out loud as a prayer. End by praying, *At times when I must choose between obeying God and obeying men, help me to choose wisely and obey you, Lord.*

Scripture Memory: Copy Philippians 2:28 in your Common Place Book.
Music: *Philippians 2* CD: Track 7 (vs. 25-28)

Key Idea: It is more important to follow God than to follow men.

Independent History Study | I |

⭐ Open your *Student Notebook* to Unit 32 – Box 6. Look at the map showing the New Testament churches that were planted during the disciples' and Paul's ministry. Find Jerusalem where it all began.

Key Idea: The Romans controlled Judea at this time. The news of Jesus spread across the Roman Empire.

Learning the Basics
Focus: Language Arts, Math, Geography, Bible, and Science

Geography [T]

Read aloud to the students the following pages:

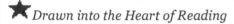 ★ *A Child's Geography Vol. II* p. 195 (first column) - 198

Discuss with the students "Field Notes" p. 198.

Key Idea: Mt. Nebo (where God buried Moses) is in Jordan, overlooking the Jordan Valley and the Dead Sea. King Herod's Machaerus fortress once stood near Mount Nebo and was the site of John the Baptist's death.

Language Arts [S]

Have students complete one dictation exercise.

Guide students to complete one reading lesson.

★ *Drawn into the Heart of Reading*

Help students complete **one** English lesson.

★ *Building with Diligence:* Lesson 59
★ *Following the Plan:* Lesson 54
★ Your own grammar program

Key Idea: Practice language arts skills.

Poetry [I]

Open *Paint Like a Poet* to Lesson 26. Today, you will be performing a poetry reading of *"Blueberries"*. Practice reading the poem aloud with expression to match the mood of the poem. Then, read the poem aloud in front of your chosen audience. At the end of the reading, share the following, *When I read this poem by Robert Frost, it made me think of...* Call on your audience to share what thoughts the poem brought to their minds. Last, say, *Did you know that when T.S. Eliot, the great English poet, gave a toast at a dinner held in Frost's honor, he said that Frost wrote about the whole world, and feelings and ideas that everyone, everywhere, understood? Later, Frost would tell his students, "There ought to be in everything you write some sign that you come from almost anywhere."*

Key Idea: Share the poetry of Robert Frost.

Math Exploration [S]

Choose **one** of the math options listed below.

★ *Singapore Primary Mathematics 4A/4B or 5A/5B* (see Appendix for schedules), or *Math with Confidence*, or *Apologia Math*
★ Your own math program

Key Idea: Use a step-by-step math program.

Science Exploration [I]

★ Read *An Illustrated Adventure in Human Anatomy* p. 16. Then, choose one of the experiments on p. 17 of *An Illustrated Adventure in Human Anatomy* to perform. Next, turn to the science experiment section in your science binder or sketchbook. At the top of a blank page, write a question that the experiment you've chosen brings to mind. Under the question, write: *'Guess'*. Write down a guess to answer the question.

Perform your chosen experiment as outlined on p. 17. Next, write: *'Procedure'*. Draw a picture of the experiment. Write: *'Conclusion'*. Explain what you learned. If time allows, perform more than one experiment from those provided on p. 17.

Key Idea: Nerves carry electricity and can send messages instantly throughout the body. Your body has sensory nerve cells, integration nerve cells, and motor nerve cells. Which kinds of nerve cells did you use during your experiment?

Learning through History
Focus: The Church Is Persecuted and Scattered

Reading about History | I

Read about history in the following resource:

★ Your own Bible: Acts chapters 5-6

Herod Antipas was ruler over Galilee and Perea at the time of John the Baptist, Jesus, and the apostles. Where could you look to research more about **Herod Antipas**? Use the Bible and a reference book or an online resource like www.wikipedia.org. Answer one or more of the following questions: *Herod Antipas was the son of whom? When did he rule Galilee and Judea? Where did he build his capitol city, and what was it named? According to Luke 3:1, who was Caesar at this time? According to Mark 6:17-29, why did Herod have John the Baptist put in prison and later beheaded? What did Herod think about Jesus according Luke 9:7-9? In Luke 23:6-12, when did Herod finally see Jesus? What was Herod's reaction? What does Acts 4:27 say about Herod?*

Key Idea: Peter and John continued to preach.

History Project | S

In this unit you will make rocks that symbolize Peter as the rock upon which the early church was built. Read Matthew 16:13-19 to see how Peter's life fulfilled Jesus' words. To make the rocks, mix ¼ cup plain flour and ¼ cup salt. Have an adult stir in ¼ cup boiling water. If you desire scented rocks, mix in **either** 1/8 tsp. essential oil **or** a small bit of perfume or cologne. Divide the dough into 10 parts to make different colored rocks. Shape into flat rocks. Add flour if the dough is too sticky. To color the rocks, drop food coloring one drop at a time on each rock and rub with a paper towel. To dry rocks, bake at 200 degrees 10-15 min.

Key Idea: Jesus changed Simon into Peter.

Storytime | T

Choose one of the following read aloud options:

★ *The Accidental Voyage* p. 112-121

★ Read at least one folk tale for the next 12 days of plans (see Appendix for suggestions).

After the reading, students will give a detailed oral narration. Select one paragraph from the story to read out loud to the students. This will be the starting point for the narration. Set a timer for 3-5 minutes. When the timer rings the narration is over, even if it isn't complete. A detailed, descriptive narration is the goal. See *Narration Tips* in the Appendix as needed.

Key Idea: Use oral narration to retell the story.

Bible Quiet Time | I

Bible Reading: Choose one option below.

★ *The Illustrated Family Bible* p. 321-324
Optional extension: p. 315

★ Your own Bible: Acts chapters 5-6

Scripture Focus: Highlight Acts 5:29-32.

Prayer Focus: Pray a prayer of adoration to worship and honor God. Begin by reading the highlighted verses out loud as a prayer. End by praying, *I exalt you as my Prince and Savior, who has conquered death!*

Scripture Memory: Recite Philippians 2:29.
Music: *Philippians 2* CD: Track 7 (vs. 25-29)

Key Idea: Jesus is our Savior. He has conquered death.

Independent History Study | I

★ Open your *Student Notebook* to Unit 33 – Box 7. Follow the directions from *Draw and Write Through History* p. 45-48 (through step 6) to draw the Colosseum. You will finish drawing on Day 2.

Key Idea: Many Jews had wanted Jesus to be an earthly Messiah to save them from Roman oppression.

Learning the Basics
Focus: Language Arts, Math, Geography, Bible, and Science

Bible Study   [T]

Read aloud and discuss with the students the following pages:

 The Radical Book for Kids p. 230-232
(Note: Making the sundial on p. 231-323 is **optional.**)

Key Idea: In Old Testament times, sundials were often used to tell time. A sundial used a straight stick to cast a shadow that highlighted a number revealing the time of day. The sundial worked because God's universe runs on a precise schedule. The rising and setting sun follows the pattern He set.

Language Arts   [S]

Have students complete one studied dictation exercise (see Appendix for directions and passages).

Help students complete one lesson from the following reading program:

 Drawn into the Heart of Reading

Work with the students to complete **one** of the English options listed below:

 Building with Diligence: Lesson 60

 Following the Plan: Lesson 55

 Your own grammar program

Key Idea: Practice language arts skills.

Poetry   [I]

Open *Paint Like a Poet* to Lesson 27. Read aloud the poem *"A Time to Talk"*. On a 3 x 5 index card, neatly copy in black ink or in pencil the following highlighted lines from the poem:

When a friend calls to me from the road
And slows his horse to a meaning walk,
I don't stand still and look around
On all the hills I haven't hoed,
And shout from where I am, What is it?
No, not as there is a time to talk.
                                  -Robert Frost

Check your work to make sure it is correctly copied. Then, cut around your copywork. You may choose to outline the edge of the cut-out with a gray marker. Save it for Day 3.

Key Idea: Read and appreciate a variety of classic poetry.

Math Exploration   [S]

Choose **one** of the math options listed below.

 Singapore Primary Mathematics 4A/4B or *5A/5B* (see Appendix for schedules), or *Math with Confidence*, or *Apologia Math*

 Your own math program

Key Idea: Use a step-by-step math program.

Science Exploration   [I]

 Read *An Illustrated Adventure in Human Anatomy* p. 19-21. Today, you will add to your science notebook. At the top of an unlined paper, copy Leviticus 17:11 in cursive. Beneath the verse, write the heading "Contents of Blood". Then, sketch and label *red blood cells, platelets, white blood cells,* and *plasma* as shown at the bottom of p. 21 of *An Illustrated Adventure in Human Anatomy*. Then, draw an arrow to each sketch, and either copy the text from p. 21 to describe each part of the blood, or write a description of each part in your own words. Last, lightly color the sketches.

Key Idea: Your circulatory system includes your heart, blood, and blood vessels. Each part of the circulatory system is responsible for delivering what your body and cells need to survive.

Unit 33 - Day 2

Reading about History | I |

Read about history in the following resource:

⭐ Your own Bible: Acts chapters 7-8

You will be choosing a portion from today's reading that you found memorable or worthy of being reread to copy. Open your *Student Notebook* to Unit 33. In Box 4, carefully copy in cursive the portion from today's reading that you selected. Then, compare your written work to the original. Last, draw a small colorful picture in Box 4 to illustrate your sentences.

Key Idea: Stephen was arrested and brought before the Sanhedrin, the Jewish council. Stephen summarized the teachings about Jesus by retelling Israel's history. Stephen was stoned for his speech, and upon his death he saw heaven opened and Jesus sitting at the right hand of God the Father.

History Project | S |

Follow the directions in the *Student Notebook* – Unit 15 to fold two colored paper boxes, using one box as the base and one as the lid. This lidded box will hold your rocks once they are dry. On the box lid, write, *... on this rock I will build my church. Matthew 16:18.* Use a fine-tipped permanent marker to write the following bolded words, one per rock, to describe Peter: **Family Member** (Mark 1:16, Mark 1:30, 1 Corinthians 9:5 – Cephas is Peter); **Worker** (Luke 5:4-7); **Disciple** (Matthew 4:18-20); **Believer** (Matthew 16:16). Then, use your Bible to look up the references for Peter. Finish labeling the rocks on Day 3.

Key Idea: Stephen believed in Jesus.

Storytime | T |

Choose one of the following read aloud options:

⭐ *The Accidental Voyage* p. 122-131

⭐ Read aloud the next portion of the folk tale that you selected.

After reading, give each person a white piece of paper or a markerboard and a marker. Set a timer for 3-5 minutes and instruct each person to do a quick outline sketch about the story. Ideas for sketches include settings, characters, actions, important objects, or symbols. When the timer rings, briefly share the sketches.

Key Idea: Use sketching to share the story.

Bible Quiet Time | I |

Reading: Choose one option below.

⭐ *The Illustrated Family Bible* p. 325 and p. 328-239

⭐ Your own Bible: Acts chapters 7-8

Scripture Focus: Highlight Acts 7:60.

Prayer Focus: Pray a prayer of confession to admit or acknowledge your sins to God. Begin by reading the highlighted verse out loud as a prayer. End by praying, *I confess that it is hard to forgive those who have hurt me. Help me to be like Stephen and learn to forgive those who have hurt me, such as...*

Scripture Memory: Recite Philippians 2:29.
Music: *Philippians 2* CD: Track 7 (vs. 25-29)

Key Idea: Stephen forgave those who hurt him.

Independent History Study | I |

⭐ Open your *Student Notebook* to Unit 33 – Box 7. Follow the directions from *Draw and Write Through History* p. 49 (steps 7-9) to finish drawing the Colosseum. You will color your drawing on Day 3.

Key Idea: After the death of Stephen, open persecution of Christians began forcing them out of Jerusalem and into Judea and Samaria. This fulfilled Jesus' command in Acts 1:8.

Learning the Basics

Focus: Language Arts, Math, Geography, Bible, and Science

Geography [T]

Get both the blank map and the labeled map of **Israel & Jordan** that you saved from the study of Israel. Or, you may print a new map online for each student at the link on p. 6 of *A Child's Geography Vol. II*. At the link, select "History & Geography". Then, under "Knowledge Quest" select ACG2-Extra Activities". Print p. 46.

Then, assign students the following page:

 A Child's Geography Vol. II p. 199
Note: Do only the "Map Notes" section. If desired, play "Music" from the links on p. 200.

<u>Key Idea</u>: Practice finding and recording the locations of various places on a map of Jordan.

Poetry [I]

Open *Paint Like a Poet* to Lesson 27. Read aloud the poem *"A Time to Talk"* by Robert Frost.

Today, you will be painting an outdoor backdrop. You will need painting paper, a palette, water, a large flat paintbrush, a pencil, a paper towel, and blue, grey, and green paint.

After gathering your supplies, turn to the "Step-by-Step Watercolor Tutorial" for Lesson 27 in *Paint Like a Poet*. Follow steps 1-3 to complete "Part One: Outdoor Backdrop". Then, let your background dry. You will complete "Part Two" of the tutorial on Day 3.

<u>Key Idea</u>: Use painting to illustrate poetry.

Language Arts [S]

Help students complete one lesson from the following reading program:

 Drawn into the Heart of Reading

Work with the students to complete **one** of the writing options listed below:

 Writing & Rhetoric Book 2: Narrative I p. 117-121 (Note: Read aloud the text while the students follow along. Then, brainstorm ideas with students for today's lesson.)

 Your own writing program

<u>Key Idea</u>: Practice language arts skills.

Math Exploration [S]

Choose **one** of the math options listed below.

 Singapore Primary Mathematics 4A/4B or 5A/5B (see Appendix for schedules), or *Math with Confidence*, or *Apologia Math*

 Your own math program

<u>Key Idea</u>: Use a step-by-step math program.

Science Exploration [I]

 Read *An Illustrated Adventure in Human Anatomy* p. 22-23. Choose one or more of the experiments on p. 23 to do as an optional extra. Orally retell or narrate to an adult the portion of text that you read today. Use the *Narration Tips* in the Appendix for help as needed.

<u>Key Idea</u>: The heart pumps blood through the arteries. The thick muscular walls of the arteries help squeeze blood out to the cells. Capillaries are the smallest vessels. They attach to arteries and veins to reach every cell. The capillaries drop off food energy, water, and oxygen to your blood cells and pick up waste products. Veins are larger vessels that are thin-walled, with few muscles. They have valves to move blood back to the heart.

Reading about History   I

Read about history in the following resource:

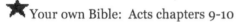 Your own Bible: Acts chapters 9-10

You will be adding to your timeline in your *Student Notebook* today. In Unit 33 – Box 1, draw and color a rock. Label it, *Disciples' ministry in Jerusalem – led by Peter (30 A.D.).* In Box 2, draw and color a blinding light. Label it, *Stephen martyred/Saul's conversion (35 A.D.).* In Box 3, draw and color arrows going out from the center. Label it, *Gospel spreads to Judea and Samaria (35 A.D.).*

Key Idea: Saul began a zealous campaign to persecute Christians, until Jesus spoke to him on the road to Damascus.

Storytime   T

Choose one of the following read aloud options:

★ *The Accidental Voyage* p. 132-141

★ Read aloud the next portion of the folk tale that you selected.

After the reading, students will give a summary oral narration. The oral narration must be no longer than 5 sentences and should summarize the reading. As students narrate, have them hold up one finger for each sentence shared. Remind students that the focus should be on the big ideas, rather than on the details.

Key Idea: Summarize the story by narrating.

History Project   S

Get the rocks you made on Day 1. Use a fine-tipped permanent marker to continue writing the following bolded words, one per rock, to describe Peter: **Witness** (John 20:6-9); **Leader** (Matthew 16:15-18); **Preacher** (Acts 2:14, 38); **Missionary** (Acts 9:32, 42; Acts 11:11); **Writer** (Author of 1 Peter and 2 Peter); **Martyr** (tradition claims Peter was crucified in Rome). Then, use your Bible to look up the references about Peter.

When your rocks are completely dry, place them in the box that you made on Day 2. By reading the inscriptions on the ten rocks, you will be reminded of what the early church was founded upon and what continues to be the church's foundation today.

Key Idea: What will you do to help the church be strengthened and grow?

Bible Quiet Time   I

Reading: Choose one option below.

★ *The Illustrated Family Bible* p. 330-333
Optional extension: p. 314

★ Your own Bible: Acts chapters 9-10

Scripture Focus: Highlight Acts 9:31.

Prayer Focus: Pray a prayer of thanksgiving to express gratitude for God's divine goodness. Begin by reading the highlighted verse out loud as a prayer. End by praying, *Thank you for the time of growth you planned for your churches. Help my church to be strengthened and to grow in numbers too. Guide us to be encouraged by your Spirit.*

Scripture Memory: Recite Philippians 2:29.
Music: *Philippians 2* CD: Track 7 (vs. 25-29)

Key Idea: The Christian churches grew.

Independent History Study   I

★ Open your *Student Notebook* to Unit 33 – Box 7. Use *Draw and Write Through History* p. 50 as a guide to color your sketch of the Colosseum. You will finish coloring your sketch on Day 4.

Key Idea: After Saul's conversion to Christianity, the persecution of the early church lessened for a time.

Learning the Basics

Focus: Language Arts, Math, Geography, Bible, and Science

Bible Study   [T]

Read aloud and discuss with the students the following pages:

 The Radical Book for Kids p. 233-237

<u>Key Idea</u>: Sarah Edwards was the wife of famous pastor and theologian Jonathan Edwards. As a pastor of a large congregation, Jonathan spent 14 hours a day in his work. This left Sarah to run the daily business of their household and their family of eleven children. Sarah's life was filled with hard work, homemaking, and child training. Yet, she purposefully pursued a relationship with Christ and found joy in God.

Language Arts   [S]

Have students complete one studied dictation exercise (see Appendix for directions and passages).

Work with the students to complete **one** of the writing options listed below:

 Writing & Rhetoric Book 2: Narrative I p. 118-121 (Note: Have students read their stories aloud to you. Then, help the students correct and edit their stories.)

 Your own writing program

<u>Key Idea</u>: Practice language arts skills.

Poetry   [I]

Open *Paint Like a Poet* to Lesson 27. Read aloud the poem *"A Time to Talk"* by Robert Frost.

Get the outdoor backdrop that you painted on Day 2. Today, you will be adding a tree and a stone wall. You will need a palette, water, a small flat paintbrush, paper towels (or a sponge), and brown, grey, orange, and green paint.

After gathering your supplies, turn to the "Step-by-Step Watercolor Tutorial" for Lesson 27 in *Paint Like a Poet*. Follow steps 4-6 to complete "Part Two: Tree and Stone Wall". When your painting is dry, glue your poetry copywork from Day 1 to your painting. Store your completed artwork in the place you have chosen for it.

<u>Key Idea</u>: Explore poetry moods with painting.

Math Exploration   [S]

Choose **one** of the math options listed below.

 Singapore Primary Mathematics 4A/4B or 5A/5B (see Appendix for schedules), or *Math with Confidence*, or *Apologia Math*

 Your own math program

<u>Key Idea</u>: Use a step-by-step math program.

Science Exploration   [I]

 Read *An Illustrated Adventure in Human Anatomy* p. 25-27. Write the answer to each numbered question on lined paper. You do not need to copy the question. Use the listed page numbers for reference.

1. How do you breathe? (p. 26)
2. Write the words *pharynx* and *trachea* and give their definitions. (p. 26)
3. Draw (or trace) and label the lower respiratory system as shown on p. 27.
4. How many ribs do you have on each side? (p. 27)
5. What does Psalm 150:6 say that we should do as long as we have breath?

<u>Key Idea</u>: The brain, nose, throat, larynx, vocal chord, trachea, lungs, diaphragm, and blood vessels form the respiratory system.

Learning through History
Focus: The Church Is Persecuted and Scattered

Reading about History | I |

Read about history in the following resource:

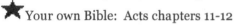 Your own Bible: Acts chapters 11-12

You will be writing a narration from the following Bible reading: *Acts chapter 12,* which is part of today's history reading.

To prepare for writing your narration, look back over what you read in Acts chapter 12. Think about the main idea.

After you have thought about what you will write and how you will begin your narration, turn to Unit 33 in your *Student Notebook.*

In Box 5, write a 5-8 sentence narration which tells about the Acts chapter 12. When you have finished writing, read your sentences out loud to catch any mistakes.

Check for the following things: *Did you include* **who** *or* **what topic** *the reading was mainly about? Did you include* **descriptors** *of the important thing(s) that happened? Did you include a* **closing sentence**? *If not, add those things.*

Then, underline or highlight the main idea sentence in the narration. Use the *Written Narration Skills* in the Appendix as a guide for editing the narration.

Key Idea: Peter explained the vision the Lord had given him that Gentiles were included in God's plan of salvation. Around this time, Herod Agrippa had James, the brother of John, put to death and Peter arrested. While the church was praying for Peter, an angel of the Lord miraculously freed Peter from prison. When Peter arrived at the place where the Christians were praying, they could hardly believe it was him. God later struck Herod Agrippa down with death.

Storytime | T |

Choose one of the following read aloud options:

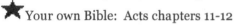 *The Accidental Voyage* p. 142-152

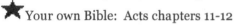 Read aloud the next portion of the folk tale that you selected.

After the reading, have each person get a Bible and open it anywhere in Proverbs. Explain, *We will have 5 minutes to skim through the verses in Proverbs to find any connections to today's story. When a connection is found, read the verse out loud and quickly share the connection. At the end of 5 minutes, anyone who has not shared yet must read aloud one verse and make the best connection possible.*

Key Idea: Seek God's word for His guidance.

Bible Quiet Time | I |

Reading: Choose one option below.

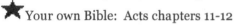 *The Illustrated Family Bible* p. 334-337

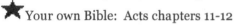 Your own Bible: Acts chapters 11-12

Scripture Focus: Highlight Acts 12:5.

Prayer Focus: Pray a prayer of supplication to make a humble and earnest request of God. Begin by reading the highlighted verse out loud as a prayer. End by praying, *Help me remember that you always hear my prayers. Fill me with the desire to pray earnestly and often, believing you will answer. I pray...*

Scripture Memory: Copy Philippians 2:29 in your Common Place Book.
Music: *Philippians 2* CD: Track 7 (vs. 25-29)

Key Idea: The church prayed for Peter.

Independent History Study | I |

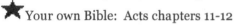 Open your *Student Notebook* to Unit 33 - Box 7. Finish coloring your drawing from Day 3, if needed. Then, in Box 6, copy in cursive the **second paragraph** of *Draw and Write Through History* p. 62.

Key Idea: The early church continued to spread in spite of persecution.

Learning the Basics
Focus: Language Arts, Math, Geography, Bible, and Science

Geography [T]

Go to the website link listed on p. 6 of *A Child's Geography Vol. II*. At the link, select "History & Geography". Then, under "Knowledge Quest" select ACG2-Extra Activities". Print the "Travel Log Template" of your choice from p. 39-42. Also at the link, for older students, print and assign the "Chapter Fifteen Review" on p. 82. Assign all students the page below.

★ *A Child's Geography Vol. II* p. 199
Note: Do only the "Travel Notes" section on p. 199. The "Music" and "Poetry" sections on p. 200-201 are optional extras.

<u>Key Idea</u>: Share three sights from Jordan.

Language Arts [S]

Have students complete one dictation exercise.

Guide students to complete one reading lesson.

★ *Drawn into the Heart of Reading*

Help students complete **one** English lesson.

★ *Building with Diligence:* Lesson 61 (Half)
★ *Following the Plan:* Lesson 56 (Half)
★ Your own grammar program

<u>Key Idea</u>: Practice language arts skills.

Poetry [I]

Open *Paint Like a Poet* to Lesson 27. Today, you will perform a poetry reading of *"A Time to Talk"*. Practice the poem with expression. Then, read it for your chosen audience. At the end of the reading, share the following, *When I read this poem by Robert Frost, it made me think of...* Call on your audience to share what thoughts the poem brought to their minds. Last, say, *Did you know that it's been said that Robert Frost was a paradox? He was a loner who liked company. As a poet he liked isolation, yet sought a mass audience. He was a man who preferred to stay at home, yet traveled more than any poet of his generation. He spoke and lectured often, yet remained terrified of public speaking to the end. Frost once said, "On my stone I'd have written of me: I had a lover's quarrel with the world."*

<u>Key Idea</u>: Share the poetry of Robert Frost.

Math Exploration [S]

Choose **one** of the math options listed below.

★ *Singapore Primary Mathematics 4A/4B or 5A/5B* (see Appendix for schedules), or *Math with Confidence*, or *Apologia Math*
★ Your own math program

<u>Key Idea</u>: Use a step-by-step math program.

Science Exploration [I]

★ Read *An Illustrated Adventure in Human Anatomy* p. 28-29. Turn to the science experiment section in your science binder or sketchbook. At the top of a blank page, write: *How do your lungs work?* Under the question, write: *'Guess'*. Write down your guess. Perform the experiment as outlined on p. 29 of *An Illustrated Adventure in Human Anatomy*. If you do not have the needed supplies for the experiment, then view the internet links below instead. Next, write: *'Procedure'*. Draw a picture of the experiment. Which part of the respiratory system does each part of the model represent? Label the *trachea, lung,* and *diaphragm*. Write: *'Conclusion'*. Explain what you learned.

If you have access to the internet, go to the following link to participate in a virtual respiratory journey online. At the link, interactively go on a journey through the respiratory system.
https://biomanbio.com/HTML5GamesandLabs/Physiologygames/respiratory_journeyhtml5page.html

<u>Key Idea</u>: The respiratory system carries needed oxygen from the nose to the lungs and out to the blood.

Reading about History [I]

Read about history in the following resource:

⭐ Your own Bible: Acts chapters 13-14
After Jesus' death and resurrection, James (one of Jesus' brothers), became an important leader in the Jerusalem church. Where could you look to research more about **James the Just**? Read the Biblical account for the most accurate resource. Answer one or more of the following questions: *When did Jesus appear to James in 1 Corin. 15:3-8? In Acts 12:17, what did Peter want James to know? What does Acts 15:12-19 show us about James' leadership? How does Paul describe James in Galatians 2:8-9? What does Paul do upon returning to Jerusalem in Acts 21:17-18? In James 1:1, who does it say wrote that book?*

Key Idea: James became a believer in Jesus.

History Project [S]

In this unit you will make a map of Apostle Paul's three missionary journeys and of his trip to Rome. Use the website at the following link to view the route Paul and Barnabas took on the **first** missionary journey. Link: http://www.apostlepaulthefilm.com/paul/journeys.htm

If the above link does not work, use this link: https://viz.bible/journeys/

Open your *Student Notebook* to Unit 32 – Box 6. Use a pencil to neatly mark Paul's **first** journey on the map in Box 6. Trace over the pencil line with a green fine-tipped marker.

Key Idea: This was the first missionary trip.

Storytime [T]

Choose one of the following read aloud options:

⭐ *The Accidental Voyage* p. 153-163

⭐ Read at least one folk tale for the next 8 days of plans.

After the reading, students will give a detailed oral narration. Select one paragraph from the story to read out loud to the students. This will be the starting point for the narration. Set a timer for 3-5 minutes. When the timer rings the narration is over, even if it isn't complete. A detailed, descriptive narration is the goal. See *Narration Tips* in the Appendix as needed.

Key Idea: Use oral narration to retell the story.

Bible Quiet Time [I]

Bible Reading: Choose one option below.

⭐ *The Illustrated Family Bible* p. 340-343
   Optional extension: p. 338

⭐ Your own Bible: Acts 13-14

Scripture Focus: Highlight Acts 14:15.

Prayer Focus: Pray a prayer of adoration to worship and honor God. Begin by reading the highlighted verse out loud as a prayer. End by praying, *I praise you as the living God, maker of heaven and earth and sea. You alone should be worshiped!*

Scripture Memory: Recite Philippians 2:30.
Music: *Philippians 2* CD: Track 7 (vs. 25-30)

Key Idea: At Lystra, the Greeks wanted to offer sacrifices to Paul and Barnabas as if they were gods.

Independent History Study [I]

Open your *Student Notebook* to "Prophecies About Christ". Under "Prophecy" write, *Isaiah 49:6*. Read the Scripture to discover the prophecy. Under "Fulfillment" write, *Acts 26:22-23*. Read the fulfillment Scripture. Under "Description", write a few phrases to describe the prophecy about Jesus.

Key Idea: Jesus fulfilled Isaiah's prophecy of a Savior for the Jews and also became a light for the Gentiles.

Learning the Basics
Focus: Language Arts, Math, Geography, Bible, and Science

Bible Study ⟨T⟩

Read aloud and discuss with the students the following pages:

 The Radical Book for Kids p. 238-241

Key Idea: Hanna Faust was a servant of Christ among German Christians. She spent her life helping those in need and spreading Christ's love. She nursed the poor and the sick through cholera, smallpox, and typhus. She visited prisons and helped those on the street. Her life was far from easy, and she suffered much herself. Yet, she remained steadfast in her commitment to serve others as Jesus did.

Language Arts ⟨S⟩

Have students complete one studied dictation exercise (see Appendix for directions and passages).

Help students complete one lesson from the following reading program:

 Drawn into the Heart of Reading

Work with the students to complete **one** of the English options listed below:

★ *Building with Diligence:* Lesson 61 (Half)

★ *Following the Plan:* Lesson 56 (Last half)

★ Your own grammar program

Key Idea: Practice language arts skills.

Poetry ⟨I⟩

Choose one of Robert Frost's poems from Lessons 28-33 in *Paint Like a Poet* to memorize.

You will have 2 weeks (units) to memorize the entire poem. So, you should have half of your chosen poem memorized by Day 4 of this unit.

After you have chosen your poem to memorize, read it three times, adding actions to help you remember the words.

Key Idea: Read and appreciate classic poetry.

Math Exploration ⟨S⟩

Choose **one** of the math options listed below.

 Singapore Primary Mathematics 4A/4B or 5A/5B (see Appendix for schedules), or *Math with Confidence*, or *Apologia Math*

 Your own math program

Key Idea: Use a step-by-step math program.

Science Exploration ⟨I⟩

★ Read *An Illustrated Adventure in Human Anatomy* p. 31-34. Today, you will add to your science notebook. At the top of an unlined paper, copy Job 12:11 in cursive. Beneath the verse, write the heading "The Digestive System". Then, draw a diagram of the twelve parts of the digestive system as shown on p. 31-34 of *An Illustrated Adventure in Human Anatomy*. Draw an arrow to each part of the diagram and label each part. Younger students may print a diagram of the digestive system to label, cut-out and glue in the notebook instead: http://www.tipztime.com/minicharts/digestivesystemb.html

Key Idea: The digestive system works to digest the food that you eat and turn it into fuel for your cells.

Reading about History | I

Read about history in the following resource:

★ Your own Bible: Acts chapters 15-16

You will be choosing a portion from today's reading that you found memorable or worthy of being reread to copy. Open your *Student Notebook* to Unit 34. In Box 4, carefully copy in cursive the portion from today's reading that you selected. Then, compare your written work to the original. Last, draw a small colorful picture in Box 4 to illustrate your sentences.

Key Idea: The council of apostles and elders met in Jerusalem to discuss what should be required of Gentile Christians.

Storytime | T

Choose one of the following read aloud options:

★ *The Accidental Voyage* p. 164-173 (Note: If you are Catholic, omit or screen p. 172.)

★ Read aloud the next portion of the folk tale that you selected.

After reading, give each person 2 slips of paper. Each person must think of 2 questions to ask about the book and write one question on each slip of paper. Next, fold up the slips of paper and place them in a container. Each person must select at least one question from the container to answer.

Key Idea: Use questioning to share the story.

History Project | S

Open your *Student Notebook* to Unit 32 – Box 6. In the "Key: Paul's Missionary Journeys" Box, draw a green line next to "First Journey", a purple line next to "Second Journey", a red line next to "Third Journey", and a blue line next to "Trip to Rome".

Use the internet link in the "History Project" Box on Unit 34 - Day 1 to view the route Paul and Silas took on the **second** missionary journey.

Then, use a pencil to neatly mark Paul's **second** journey on the map in Box 6. Trace over the pencil line with a purple fine-tipped marker.

Key Idea: Paul and Barnabas disagreed about taking John Mark on the journey. So, Paul went with Silas, and Barnabas went with Mark.

Bible Quiet Time | I

Reading: Choose one option below.

★ *The Illustrated Family Bible* p. 344-347 Optional extension: p. 339

★ Your own Bible: Acts chapters 15-16

Scripture Focus: Highlight Acts 16:25.

Prayer Focus: Pray a prayer of confession to admit or acknowledge your sins to God. Begin by reading the highlighted verse out loud as a prayer. End by praying, *I confess that in times of trouble I sometimes get caught up in feeling sorry for myself. Help me to sing and pray instead, knowing others are listening to see if Christ is living within me.*

Scripture Memory: Recite Philippians 2:30.
Music: *Philippians 2* CD: Track 7 (vs. 25-30)

Key Idea: Paul and Silas prayed and sang.

Independent History Study | I

★ Open your *Student Notebook* to Unit 34 – Box 7. Follow the directions from *Draw and Write Through History* p. 51-52 (through step 5) to draw a gladiator. You will finish drawing on Day 2.

Key Idea: As the early church spread throughout the Roman Empire, gladiator games were very popular.

Learning the Basics
Focus: Language Arts, Math, Geography, Bible, and Science

Geography [T]

Read aloud to the students the following pages:

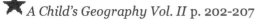 *A Child's Geography Vol. II* p. 202-207

Discuss with the students "Field Notes" p. 207.

<u>Key Idea</u>: The city of Karak in Jordan was the ancient capital of Moab. Jordan receives little rain each year and is one of the ten most water-deprived countries in the world. Weddings in Jordan are arranged, and often first cousins marry one another! In modern times, the lost city of Petra was known only to the Bedouins until 1812. It was once the home of the Edomites.

Language Arts [S]

Help students complete one lesson from the following reading program:

 Drawn into the Heart of Reading

Work with the students to complete **one** of the writing options listed below:

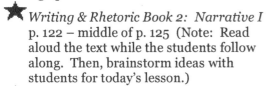 *Writing & Rhetoric Book 2: Narrative I* p. 122 – middle of p. 125 (Note: Read aloud the text while the students follow along. Then, brainstorm ideas with students for today's lesson.)

 Your own writing program

<u>Key Idea</u>: Practice language arts skills.

Poetry [I]

Today, you will copy half of the Robert Frost poem from *Paint Like a Poet* that you chose to memorize this week.

At the top of a clean page in your *Common Place Book,* copy the title and the author of the poem. Then, copy half of the poem in cursive, leaving the rest of the page blank.

You will copy the remaining half of the poem during the next unit.

Practice the portion of the poem that you copied today by reading it aloud.

<u>Key Idea</u>: Copy and memorize classic poetry.

Math Exploration [S]

Choose **one** of the math options listed below.

 Singapore Primary Mathematics 4A/4B or *5A/5B* (see Appendix for schedules), or *Math with Confidence,* or *Apologia Math*

 Your own math program

<u>Key Idea</u>: Use a step-by-step math program.

Science Exploration [I]

 Read *An Illustrated Adventure in Human Anatomy* p. 35. Orally retell or narrate to an adult the portion of text that you read today. Use the *Narration Tips* in the Appendix for help as needed.

<u>Key Idea</u>: A healthy balance of food is important for getting your body the nutrients that it needs. Choosing the right food can be aided by thinking of a food pyramid and by counting the number of servings of each part of the pyramid that you eat daily. Brushing your teeth is another important part of maintaining a healthy digestive system.

Reading about History $\boxed{\text{I}}$

Read about history in the following resource:

⭐ Your own Bible: Acts chapters 17-18

You will be adding to your timeline in your *Student Notebook* today. In Unit 34 – Box 1, draw and color a path. Label it, *Paul's First Missionary Journey (with Barnabas 46-48 A.D.)*. In Box 2, draw and color a path. Label it, *Paul's Second Missionary Journey (with Silas 50-52 A.D.)*. In Box 3, draw and color a path. Label it, *Paul's Third Missionary Journey (to Ephesus 53-57 A.D.)*.

Key Idea: In Athens, Paul was distressed by the number of idols in the city.

Storytime $\boxed{\text{T}}$

Choose one of the following read aloud options:

⭐ *The Accidental Voyage* p. 174-183

⭐ Read aloud the next portion of the folk tale that you selected.

After the reading, students will give a summary oral narration. The oral narration must be no longer than 5 sentences and should summarize the reading. As students narrate, have them hold up one finger for each sentence shared. Remind students that the focus should be on the big ideas, rather than on the details.

Key Idea: Summarize the story by narrating.

History Project $\boxed{\text{S}}$

Use the internet link in the "History Project" Box on Unit 34 - Day 1 to view the route Paul took on his **third** missionary journey.

Then, use a pencil to neatly mark Paul's **third** journey on the map on Unit 32 – Box 6. Trace over the pencil line with a red fine-tipped marker.

Next, use the internet link in the "History Project" Box on Unit 34 - Day 1 to view the route Paul took on his **trip to Rome**.

Then, use a pencil to neatly mark Paul's **trip to Rome** on the map on Unit 32 – Box 6. Trace over the line with a blue fine-tipped marker.

Key Idea: Paul debated the Epicurean and Stoic philosophers at the Acropolis in Athens. In Acts 17:22-31, he warned the Greeks against worshiping gods made by human hands.

Bible Quiet Time $\boxed{\text{I}}$

Reading: Choose one option below.

⭐ *The Illustrated Family Bible* p. 348-349

⭐ Your own Bible: Acts chapters 17-18

Scripture Focus: Highlight Acts 17:24-25.

Prayer Focus: Pray a prayer of thanksgiving to express gratitude for God's divine goodness. Begin by reading the highlighted verses out loud as a prayer. End by praying, *Thank you for making the world and for giving us breath that we may live to glorify you. Help me seek you and know you more each day.*

Scripture Memory: Recite Philippians 2:30.
Music: *Philippians 2* CD: Track 7 (vs. 25-30)

Key Idea: Paul warned against worshiping idols, as many of the Greeks in Athens did.

Independent History Study $\boxed{\text{I}}$

⭐ Open your *Student Notebook* to Unit 34 – Box 7. Follow the directions from *Draw and Write Through History* p. 53-54 (steps 6-8) to finish drawing a gladiator. You will color your drawing on Day 4.

Key Idea: From the time of Augustus Caesar, the Romans had loved watching gladiators fight one another and fight wild animals. The Romans built huge arenas to house the games.

Learning the Basics
Focus: Language Arts, Math, Geography, Bible, and Science

Bible Study [T]

Read aloud and discuss with the students the following pages:

 The Radical Book for Kids p. 242-245 (Note: Making the catapult on p. 245 is **optional**.)

Key Idea: The Bible includes many stories of warfare. After sin entered the world, the world became filled with conflict and fighting. The Bible speaks of both physical warfare and spiritual warfare. As followers of Christ, we are often engaged in spiritual warfare. Through His death and resurrection, Christ has won this fight. He has defeated sin, death, and Satan.

Poetry [I]

Practice reading aloud half of the poem that you chose to memorize from *Paint Like a Poet*, using the actions that you added to help you remember the words. Do this 2 times.

Then, recite half of the poem without looking at the words.

You have 2 weeks (units) to memorize the entire poem. So, you should have half of your chosen poem memorized by Day 4 of this unit.

Key Idea: Memorize classic poetry.

Language Arts [S]

Have students complete one studied dictation exercise (see Appendix for directions and passages).

Work with the students to complete **one** of the writing options listed below:

 Writing & Rhetoric Book 2: Narrative I p. 122 – middle of p. 125 (Note: Have students read their stories aloud to you. Then, help the students correct and edit their stories.)

Your own writing program

Key Idea: Practice language arts skills.

Math Exploration [S]

Choose **one** of the math options listed below.

 Singapore Primary Mathematics 4A/4B or 5A/5B (see Appendix for schedules), or *Math with Confidence,* or *Apologia Math*

Your own math program

Key Idea: Use a step-by-step math program.

Science Exploration [I]

Read *An Illustrated Adventure in Human Anatomy* p. 37-39. Write the answer to each numbered question on lined paper. You do not need to copy the question. Use the listed page numbers for reference.
1. How are your eyes protected? (p. 38)
2. Draw the way the iris and pupil look in bright light and in dim light. (p. 38)
3. Draw (or trace) and label the anatomy of an eye as shown on p. 39.
4. Write the words *rods* and *cones* and give their definitions. (p. 39)
5. What does Proverbs 20:12 teach you about your eyes and ears?

Key Idea: The eyes collect information about the world around you and send it to your brain. The brain decodes and makes sense of the information that your eyes see.

Unit 34 - Day 4

Reading about History | I

Read about history in the following resource:

★ Your own Bible: Acts chapters 19-20

You will be writing a narration from the following Bible reading: *Acts chapter 19,* which is part of today's history reading.

To prepare for writing your narration, look back over what you read in Acts chapter 19. Think about the main idea.

After you have thought about what you will write and how you will begin your narration, turn to Unit 34 in your *Student Notebook.*

In Box 5, write a 5-8 sentence narration which tells about the Acts chapter 19. When you have finished writing, read your sentences out loud to catch any mistakes.

Check for the following things: *Did you include **who** or **what topic** the reading was mainly about? Did you include **descriptors** of the important thing(s) that happened? Did you include a **closing sentence**? If not, add those things.*

Then, underline or highlight the main idea sentence in the narration.

Use the *Written Narration Skills* in the Appendix as a guide for editing the narration.

Key Idea: Ephesus was one of the great Roman cities on the Mediterranean Sea. It was the capital of the Roman province of Asia. Paul stayed in Ephesus for over two years on his third missionary journey so that all living in the province of Asia could hear the Gospel of Jesus. Paul did many miracles in Ephesus. He was there when the people rioted over worshiping the god Artemis, rather than Jesus.

Storytime | T

Choose one of the following read aloud options:

★ *The Accidental Voyage* p. 184-191

★ Read aloud the next part of the folk tale.

After the reading, have each person get a Bible and open it anywhere in Proverbs. Explain, *We will have 5 minutes to skim through the verses in Proverbs to find any connections to today's story. When a connection is found, read the verse out loud and quickly share the connection. At the end of 5 minutes, anyone who has not shared yet must read aloud one verse and make the best connection possible.*

Key Idea: Seek God's word for His guidance.

Bible Quiet Time | I

Reading: Choose one option below.

★ *The Illustrated Family Bible* p. 350-351

★ Your own Bible: Acts chapters 19-20

Scripture Focus: Highlight Acts 20:23-24.

Prayer Focus: Pray a prayer of supplication to make a humble and earnest request of God. Begin by reading the highlighted verse out loud as a prayer. End by praying, *Help me complete the tasks you have for me, even if I am facing hardships. Help me to know what you want me to do. Strengthen me to do your will.*

Scripture Memory: Copy Philippians 2:30 in your Common Place Book.
Music: *Philippians 2* CD: Track 7 (vs. 25-30)

Key Idea: Paul knew hardships awaited him.

Independent History Study | I

★ Open your *Student Notebook* to Unit 34 – Box 7. Use *Draw and Write Through History* p. 54 (step 9) as a guide to color your sketch of the gladiator.

Key Idea: The Roman fascination with death and bloodshed led to more persecution of Christians.

Learning the Basics
Focus: Language Arts, Math, Geography, Bible, and Science

Unit 34 - Day 4

Geography [T]

Read aloud to the students the following pages:

 A Child's Geography Vol. II p. 208-212

Discuss with the students "Field Notes" p. 211.

Key Idea: Petra is hidden behind the mountains with an entrance through the Siq, or shaft. Wadi Rum is a high plateau with pillars of rock. The Bedouins are the only inhabitants of Wadi Rum.

Language Arts [S]

Have students complete one dictation exercise.

Guide students to complete one reading lesson.

★ *Drawn into the Heart of Reading*

Help students complete **one** English lesson.

★ *Building with Diligence:* Lesson 62

★ *Following the Plan:* Lesson 57

★ Your own grammar program

Key Idea: Practice language arts skills.

Poetry [I]

Practice reading aloud half of the poem that you chose to memorize from *Paint Like a Poet*, using the actions that you added to help you remember the words. Do this 2 times.

Then, recite half of the poem without looking at the words.

You have 2 weeks (units) to memorize the entire poem. So, you should have half of your chosen poem memorized by today.

Key Idea: Memorize classic poetry.

Math Exploration [S]

Choose **one** of the math options listed below.

★ *Singapore Primary Mathematics 4A/4B or 5A/5B* (see Appendix for schedules), or *Math with Confidence*, or *Apologia Math*

★ Your own math program

Key Idea: Use a step-by-step math program.

Science Exploration [I]

★ Read *An Illustrated Adventure in Human Anatomy* p. 40-41. Turn to the science experiment section in your science binder or sketchbook. At the top of a blank page, write: *How does the lens of your eye help you see?* Under the question, write: 'Guess'. Write down your guess. Fill a sandwich bag with water and zip it closed. Then, shine a flashlight on a blank wall in a darkened room. It should make a spot on the wall. This is the focal point. Slowly place the bag of water in front of the flashlight. The spot of light will be dimmer. This is because the focal point of the light has changed. The spot of light will be brightest when the beam is in focus. Now, look at your eye in a mirror. The lens is below the outer covering of the eye. Notice how the lens is convex shaped, or curved inward. Hold up the water-filled bag in front of one eye and look at an object across the room. Now, place the bag in front of your eye again, but this time stretch the bag to make it thinner. Then, squeeze the bag to make it thicker. What happens to the object that you are looking at through the bag? Your eye has a flexible lens like the bag of water. Based on your experiment, how does the lens of your eye change its focus from objects nearby to objects far away. How did the bag change its focus? Next, write: 'Procedure'. Draw a picture of the experiment. Write: 'Conclusion'. Explain what you learned.

Key Idea: The eye's lens is convex-shaped. It bends light rays toward a common point called the *focal point*.

Learning through History
Focus: To the Ends of the Earth

Unit 35 - Day 1

Reading about History   I

Read about history in the following resource:

★ Your own Bible: Acts chapters 21-22

Paul was a Roman citizen. Where could you look to research more about being a **Roman citizen**? Use a reference book or an online resource like www.wikipedia.org.

Answer one or more of the following questions from your research: *How did a person become a Roman citizen? What were some of the rights of a Roman citizen? In Acts 22:23-29, why did it make a difference that Paul was a Roman citizen? What was the difference between a person born as a Roman citizen and one who purchased his citizenship? Even though the Bible does not say how Paul died, why is it likely that Paul was not crucified?*

Key Idea: Paul was born a Roman citizen.

History Project   S

In this unit you will make a small wordless book, which has often been used to share the gospel of Jesus all over the world. You will have 3 options for making the wordless book. **Option 1:** Make it out of paper, stapling the binding. **Option 2:** Make it out of felt, stitching the binding. **Option 3:** Make it as a bracelet, using colored beads on yarn or rawhide. Choose one of the 3 options for Day 2.

The wordless book has 5 different colored blank pages, felt, or beads in the following order: gold, black, red, white, green.

Key Idea: Jesus died, so we can be forgiven.

Storytime   T

Choose one of the following read aloud options:

★ *The Accidental Voyage* p. 192-205

★ Read at least one folk tale for the next 4 days of plans.

After the reading, students will give a detailed oral narration. Select one paragraph from the story to read out loud to the students. This will be the starting point for the narration. Set a timer for 3-5 minutes. When the timer rings the narration is over, even if it isn't complete. A detailed, descriptive narration is the goal. See *Narration Tips* in the Appendix as needed.

Key Idea: Use oral narration to retell the story.

Bible Quiet Time   I

Bible Reading: Choose one option below.

★ *The Illustrated Family Bible* p. 352-353
Optional extension: p. 327

★ Your own Bible: Acts chapters 21-22

Scripture Focus: Highlight Acts 22:21.

Prayer Focus: Pray a prayer of adoration to worship and honor God. Begin by reading the highlighted verse out loud as a prayer. End by praying, *I worship you Lord for bringing salvation to the Gentiles, as well as the Jews. I praise you for the opportunity to be saved and know that you are the one, true God.*

Scripture Review: Philippians 2:1-30.
Music: *Philippians 2* CD: Tracks 1-7 (all)

Key Idea: The Lord sent Paul to the Gentiles.

Independent History Study   I

★ Open your *Student Notebook* to Unit 35 – Box 7. Follow the directions from *Draw and Write Through History* p. 55-57 (through step 6) to draw a lion. You will color your drawing on Day 2.

Key Idea: As a Roman citizen Paul could not be punished without being proven guilty of a crime.

Learning the Basics
Focus: Language Arts, Math, Geography, Bible, and Science

Bible Study [T]

Read aloud and discuss with the students the following pages:

 The Radical Book for Kids p. 246-248

Key Idea: The cross is the universal symbol for Christianity. It points to Jesus' death on the cross for our sins and represents the Good News of His sacrifice for sinners. Other Christian symbols include the *alpha* and *omega,* an anchor, a dove, the *chi* and *rho,* the *ichthus,* and the triangle.

Language Arts [S]

Have students complete one studied dictation exercise (see Appendix for directions and passages).

Help students complete one lesson from the following reading program:

 Drawn into the Heart of Reading

Work with the students to complete **one** of the English options listed below:

★ *Building with Diligence:* Lesson 63 (Half)

★ *Following the Plan:* Lesson 58 (Half)

★ Your own grammar program

Key Idea: Practice language arts skills.

Poetry [I]

You will continue memorizing the Robert Frost poem that you chose from *Paint Like a Poet* in Unit 34. You should have half of your chosen poem memorized already.

You should memorize the rest of the poem by Day 4 of this unit.

Today, read the entire poem 3 times, adding actions to the last half of the poem to help you memorize the words more easily.

Key Idea: Read and appreciate a variety of classic poetry.

Math Exploration [S]

Choose **one** of the math options listed below.

 Singapore Primary Mathematics 4A/4B or *5A/5B* (see Appendix for schedules), or *Math with Confidence,* or *Apologia Math*

 Your own math program

Key Idea: Use a step-by-step math program.

Science Exploration [I]

★ Read *An Illustrated Adventure in Human Anatomy* p. 43-45. Today, you will add to your science notebook. At the top of an unlined paper, copy Mark 4:23-24 in cursive. Beneath the verse, write the heading "Inside Your Ears". Then, draw or trace the diagram of the parts of the ear as shown on p. 45 of *An Illustrated Adventure in Human Anatomy.* Draw an arrow to each part of the diagram and label each part. Younger students may choose to print a diagram of the ear from an internet site instead to label, cut out, and glue in the notebook. An unlabeled image can be found at the following link: http://etc.usf.edu/clipart/50600/50621/50621_ear.htm

Key Idea: Your ear has 3 main parts of the outer ear, the middle ear, and the inner ear. Each of these parts of the ear is further divided into smaller parts.

Reading about History [I]

Read about history in the following resource:

★ Your own Bible: Acts chapters 23-24

You will be choosing a portion from today's reading that you found memorable or worthy of being reread to copy. Open your *Student Notebook* to Unit 35. In Box 4, carefully copy in cursive the portion from today's reading that you selected. Then, compare your written work to the original. Last, draw a small colorful picture in Box 4 to illustrate your sentences.

Key Idea: The Roman commander brought Paul to the Sanhedrin to find out why the Jews were accusing him. When Paul shared that he was a Pharisee and believed in the resurrection of the dead, the Pharisees and Sadducees began to argue amongst themselves. The Roman commander had to take Paul away by force.

History Project [S]

Prepare to make whichever option of the wordless book that you chose on Day 1. If you chose to make a paper or a felt book, neatly measure and cut rectangular pages that are each 4" x 3". Then, stack the pages in the following order: gold, black, red, white, green. If you chose to make a paper book, neatly staple the binding. If you chose to make a felt book, use a needle and thread to stitch the binding.

If you chose to make a bracelet, knot the end of your string or rawhide. Slide the beads onto the bracelet in the following order: gold, black, red, white, green. Tie a knot on the other end.

Key Idea: Paul courageously shared the gospel.

Storytime [T]

Choose one of the following read aloud options:

★ *The Accidental Voyage* p. 206-215

★ Read aloud the next portion of the folk tale that you selected.

After reading, work with the students to plan a 3 minute skit with simple props to act out part of today's reading. Set a timer for 3 minutes to quickly prepare for the skit. Make sure that you participate in the skit along with the students. When the timer rings, set it again for 3 minutes and perform the skit. You do not need an audience, as the goal is the retelling.

Key Idea: Use a skit to retell part of the story.

Bible Quiet Time [I]

Reading: Choose one option below.

★ *The Illustrated Family Bible* p. 354-355

★ Your own Bible: Acts chapters 23-24

Scripture Focus: Highlight Acts 23:11.

Prayer Focus: Pray a prayer of confession to admit or acknowledge your sins to God. Begin by reading the highlighted verse out loud as a prayer. End by praying, *I confess that I spend much time thinking about my plans and what I want to do, but I often fail to think of your plans for my life. Help me to take courage in your will for me and to follow it.*

Scripture Review: Philippians 2:1-30.
Music: *Philippians 2* CD: Tracks 1-7 (all)

Key Idea: The Lord spoke to Paul and guided his actions. Paul trusted the Lord.

Independent History Study [I]

★ Open your *Student Notebook* to Unit 35 – Box 7. Use *Draw and Write Through History* p. 57 (step 7) as a guide to color your sketch of the lion.

Key Idea: The Lord told Paul that he would also have to testify in Rome, just as he had in Jerusalem.

Learning the Basics

Focus: Language Arts, Math, Geography, Bible, and Science

Geography [T]

Have students get both the blank map and the labeled map of **Israel & Jordan** that they used in Unit 33.

Then, assign students the following page:

 A Child's Geography Vol. II p. 213

Note: Do only the "Map Notes" section on p. 213. The "Books," "Poetry," and "Food" on p. 214-215 are optional.

<u>Key Idea</u>: Practice finding and recording the locations of various places on a map of Jordan.

Poetry [I]

Today, you will copy the last half of the Robert Frost poem from *Paint Like a Poet* that you chose to memorize this week.

Beneath the first part of the poem that you copied in the last unit, copy the rest of the poem in your *Common Place Book* in cursive.

Practice the portion of the poem that you copied today by reading it aloud.

<u>Key Idea</u>: Copy and memorize classic poetry.

Language Arts [S]

Help students complete one lesson from the following reading program:

 Drawn into the Heart of Reading

Work with the students to complete **one** of the writing options listed below:

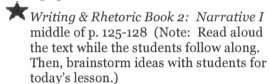 *Writing & Rhetoric Book 2: Narrative I* middle of p. 125-128 (Note: Read aloud the text while the students follow along. Then, brainstorm ideas with students for today's lesson.)

 Your own writing program

<u>Key Idea</u>: Practice language arts skills.

Math Exploration [S]

Choose **one** of the math options listed below.

 Singapore Primary Mathematics 4A/4B or 5A/5B (see Appendix for schedules), or *Math with Confidence,* or *Apologia Math*

 Your own math program

<u>Key Idea</u>: Use a step-by-step math program.

Science Exploration [I]

 Read *An Illustrated Adventure in Human Anatomy* p. 46-47. Choose to perform one or more of the experiments found on p. 47. Orally retell or narrate to an adult the portion of text that you read today. Use the *Narration Tips* in the Appendix for help as needed.

<u>Key Idea</u>: Sound waves are vibrations in the air that move down the ear canal, making the eardrum move. As the eardrum moves the malleus bone, a chain reaction of movement is set off within the middle ear. The middle ear bones magnify tiny vibrations from the eardrum, moving the fluid in the cochlea. Tiny hairs touch the cochlea's membrane and send nerve impulses to the brain.

Reading about History | I |

Read about history in the following resource:

★ Your own Bible: Acts chapters 25-26

You will be adding to your timeline in your *Student Notebook* today. In Unit 35 – Box 1, draw and color a fire. Label it, *Nero becomes Emperor of Rome (54 A.D.).* In Box 2, draw and color a sword. Label it, *Peter and Paul killed, Christians persecuted (64-68 A.D.).* In Box 3, draw and color a broken stone wall. Label it, *Rome and Titus destroy Jerusalem (70 A.D.).*

Key Idea: After standing trial before Felix and Festus, Paul appealed to Caesar. While waiting to go to Rome, Paul spoke to Herod Agrippa II.

Storytime | T |

Choose one of the following read aloud options:

★ *The Accidental Voyage* p. 216-224

★ Read aloud the next portion of the folk tale that you selected.

After the reading, students will give a summary oral narration. The oral narration must be no longer than 5 sentences and should summarize the reading. As students narrate, have them hold up one finger for each sentence shared. Remind students that the focus should be on the big ideas, rather than on the details.

Key Idea: Summarize the story by narrating.

History Project | S |

Get your version of the wordless book that you made on Day 2. Practice using it to share the Gospel as outlined below. The **gold** color is for God, our perfect Creator who wants us to be in heaven with Him one day (share John 3:16). The **dark** color is for the darkness of sin that separates us from God (share Romans 3:23). The **red** color is for the blood that Jesus shed to take the punishment for your sin and mine (share Romans 6:23). The **clean** white color is for the washing away of our sin when we **a**dmit to God that we have sinned, we **b**elieve that Jesus is God's Son, and we **c**hoose to follow Him. It's easy to remember as "a, b, c" (share John 1:12). The **green** page is to remind us to grow in Christ (share 2 Peter 3:18). Remember to grow: **G**o to church. **R**ead your Bible. **O**bey God's word. **W**itness to others.

Key Idea: Be willing to share about Jesus.

Bible Quiet Time | I |

Reading: Choose the option below.

★ Your own Bible: Acts chapters 25-26

Scripture Focus: Highlight Acts 26:22-23.

Prayer Focus: Pray a prayer of thanksgiving to express gratitude for God's divine goodness. Begin by reading the highlighted verses out loud as a prayer. End by praying, *Thank you for the fulfillment of your prophecies to Moses through Christ Jesus. Thank you for Christ's light to all Christians who believe in Him.*

Scripture Review: Philippians 2:1-30.
Music: *Philippians 2* CD: Tracks 1-7 (all)

Key Idea: Paul testified that Christ is the risen Savior of Jews and Gentiles alike.

Independent History Study | I |

★ Open your *Student Notebook* to Unit 35 - Box 7. Finish coloring your drawing from Day 2, if needed. Then, in Box 6, copy in cursive the **first paragraph** of *Draw and Write Through History* p. 62.

Key Idea: When Paul headed to Rome as a prisoner to be tried by Caesar, Nero was emperor of Rome.

Learning the Basics
Focus: Language Arts, Math, Geography, Bible, and Science

Bible Study |T|

Read aloud and discuss with the students the following pages:

 The Radical Book for Kids p. 249-253

Key Idea: During His years on earth, Jesus experienced pain and suffering and death. We should not be surprised when bad things happen. Ever since sin entered the world, everyone faces hard times. God promises that one day there will be a new creation without sin or suffering or pain. Until then, when bad things happen we should take our troubles to our Father in heaven who cares for us. Then, we should trust in God's good plan for our lives.

Poetry |I|

Using the actions that you added on Day 1, practice reading aloud the poem from *Paint Like a Poet* that you chose to memorize. Do this 2 times.

Then, recite the poem without looking at the words.

You should have your chosen poem memorized by Day 4 of this unit.

Key Idea: Memorize classic poetry.

Language Arts |S|

Have students complete one dictation exercise (see Appendix for directions and passages).

Work with the students to complete **one** of the writing options listed below:

 Writing & Rhetoric Book 2: Narrative I middle of p. 125-128 (Note: Have students read their stories aloud to you. Then, help the students correct and edit their stories.)

★ Your own writing program

Key Idea: Practice language arts skills.

Math Exploration |S|

Choose **one** of the math options listed below.

 Singapore Primary Mathematics 4A/4B or 5A/5B (see Appendix for schedules), or *Math with Confidence,* or *Apologia Math*

 Your own math program

Key Idea: Use a step-by-step math program.

Science Exploration |I|

★ Read *An Illustrated Adventure in Human Anatomy* p. 49-52. Write the answer to each numbered question on lined paper. You do not need to copy the question. Use the listed page numbers for reference.
1. Name the two parts of your nervous system called the "chemical senses". (p. 50)
2. What makes the olfactory smell receptor cells unique? (p. 50)
3. Describe the 6 steps of how you smell things. (p. 50-51)
4. Write the words *papillae* and *taste buds* and give their definitions. (p. 52)
5. What does Psalm 119:103 say about God's words?

Key Idea: The senses of taste and smell work together. The brain processes signals from the olfactory cells and the taste receptor cells to help you taste and smell.

Reading about History   I

Read about history in the following resource:

 Your own Bible: Acts chapters 27-28

You will be writing a narration from the following Bible reading: *Acts chapter 27,* which is part of today's history reading.

To prepare for writing your narration, look back over what you read in Acts chapter 27. Think about the main idea.

After you have thought about what you will write and how you will begin your narration, turn to Unit 35 in your *Student Notebook.*

In Box 5, write a 5-8 sentence narration which tells about the Acts chapter 27. When you have finished writing, read your sentences out loud to catch any mistakes.

Check for the following things: *Did you include **who** or **what topic** the reading was mainly about? Did you include **descriptors** of the important thing(s) that happened? Did you include a **closing sentence**? If not, add those things.*

Then, underline or highlight the main idea sentence in the narration. Use the *Written Narration Skills* in the Appendix as a guide for editing the narration.

Key Idea: Paul sailed for Rome along with Luke and Aristarchus, a Macedonian. A Roman centurion named Julius was assigned to guard Paul. At Crete, Paul warned the pilot of the ship not to set sail, but he did anyway. When a deadly storm arose, Paul shared that God had given him the lives of all on the ship in order that Paul could stand trial before Caesar. Though the ship was destroyed, not a man was lost. The prisoners and crew reached Malta.

Storytime   T

Choose one of the following read aloud options:

 The Accidental Voyage p. 225-235

 Read aloud the next part of the folk tale.

After the reading, have each person get a Bible and open it anywhere in Proverbs. Explain, *We will have 5 minutes to skim through the verses in Proverbs to find any connections to today's story. When a connection is found, read the verse out loud and quickly share the connection. At the end of 5 minutes, anyone who has not shared yet must read aloud one verse and make the best connection possible.*

Key Idea: Seek God's word for His guidance.

Bible Quiet Time   I

Reading: Choose one option below.

 The Illustrated Family Bible p. 356-359

 Your own Bible: Acts chapters 27-28

Scripture Focus: Highlight Acts 28:27-28.

Prayer Focus: Pray a prayer of supplication to make a humble and earnest request of God. Begin by reading the highlighted verses out loud as a prayer. End by praying, *Open my eyes, let me hear with my ears, and help me understand with my heart that Jesus is your Son and my only way to heaven. Help me to be filled with your Spirit and believe more.*

Scripture Review: Philippians 2:1-30.
Music: *Philippians 2* CD: Tracks 1-7 (all)

Key Idea: Paul preached in Rome to the Jews.

Independent History Study   I

Open your *Student Notebook* to "Prophecies About Christ". Under "Prophecy" write, *Isaiah 6:9-10.* Read the Scripture to discover the prophecy. Under "Fulfillment" write, *Acts 28:24-28.* Read the fulfillment Scripture. Under "Description", write a few phrases to describe the prophecy about Jesus.

Key Idea: As prophecied, the Jews' hearts were hardened. Christ's message was brought to the Gentiles.

Learning the Basics
Focus: Language Arts, Math, Geography, Bible, and Science

Geography [T]

Go to the website link listed on p. 6 of *A Child's Geography Vol. II*. At the link, select "History & Geography". Then, under "Knowledge Quest" select ACG2-Extra Activities". Print the "Travel Log Template" of your choice from p. 39-42. Also at the link, for older students, print and assign the "Chapter Sixteen Review" on p. 83. Assign all students the page below.

⭐ *A Child's Geography Vol. II* p. 213, 216
Note: Do the "Travel Notes" section on p. 213 and the "Walk of Prayer" on p. 216.

<u>Key Idea</u>: Share three sights from Jordan.

Language Arts [S]

Have students complete one dictation exercise.

Guide students to complete one reading lesson.
⭐ *Drawn into the Heart of Reading*

Help students complete **one** English lesson.
⭐ *Building with Diligence:* Lesson 63 (Half)
⭐ *Following the Plan:* Lesson 58 (Last half)
⭐ Your own grammar program

<u>Key Idea</u>: Practice language arts skills.

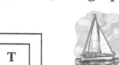

Poetry [I]

Today, you will be performing a poetry recitation of the Robert Frost poem that you chose to memorize from *Paint Like a Poet*. You will recite your poem to an audience of your choosing, without looking at the words.

Before reciting, practice saying the poem aloud using an expression that matches the mood of the poem. Then, stand and recite the poem aloud in front of your chosen audience.

At the end of the recitation, share the following, *I decided to choose this poem of Robert Frost's to memorize because...*
Then, call on your audience to comment on what they liked about the poem that you shared.

<u>Key Idea</u>: Share the poetry of Robert Frost.

Math Exploration [S]

Choose **one** of the math options listed below.
⭐ *Singapore Primary Mathematics 4A/4B* or *5A/5B* (see Appendix for schedules), or *Math with Confidence*, or *Apologia Math*
⭐ Your own math program

<u>Key Idea</u>: Use a step-by-step math program.

Science Exploration [I]

⭐ Read *An Illustrated Adventure in Human Anatomy* p. 53. Then, choose one of the experiments on p. 53 of *An Illustrated Adventure in Human Anatomy* to perform. Next, turn to the science experiment section in your science binder or sketchbook. At the top of a blank page, write a question that the experiment you've chosen brings to mind. Under the question, write: *'Guess'*. Write down a guess to answer the question.

Perform your chosen experiment as outlined on p. 53. Next, write: *'Procedure'*. Draw a picture of the experiment. Write: *'Conclusion'*. Explain what you learned. If time allows, perform more than one experiment from those provided on p. 53.

<u>Key Idea</u>: The tongue senses the following 4 basic tastes: sweet, salty, bitter, and sour. Each flavor is a combination of the 4 basic tastes. Bitter has the most sensitive taste receptors.

Appendix

Bibliography: Storytime Titles

There are 3 book set options for the Storytime plans of *Hearts for Him Through Time: Creation to Christ.* The sets are the following: History Interest Set, Boy Interest Set, and Girl Interest Set. If you desire to read aloud books that coordinate with the historical time period being studied, you will want to choose the History Interest Set. In keeping with the ancient time period, the History Interest Set does contain some violent content. If you wish to avoid this, choose the Boy Interest Set or Girl Interest Set instead; these sets do not match the history, but were instead selected to provide excellent read-alouds from 9 different genres. Sixth and seventh graders should either listen to the History Interest Set read aloud, or read the Extension Package books (as scheduled in the Appendix), or do both of these options in order to extend their learning. If you are a family that enjoys reading aloud, you may choose to read aloud more than one set of books from the Basic Package. The Basic Package is highly recommended, unless you need to economize or are short on time. Whether you choose 1, 2, or 3 of these sets – you cannot possibly make a mistake because all of these books are simply excellent!

For your convenience, these resources may be purchased from Heart of Dakota either as an entire set or as individual titles. The packages are called the *Hearts for Him Through Time: Creation to Christ* **Basic Package Option 1: History Interest Set, Basic Package Option 2: Boy Interest Set,** and **Basic Package Option 3: Girl Interest Set.** View packages on the website www.heartofdakota.com or call (605) 428-4068 for more information. The following book descriptions are taken from the book or card catalog listing.

Basic Package Option 1: History Interest Set:

Units 1-2: *Dinosaurs of Eden* by Ken Ham, 2015, Revised Edition 2022, Master Books
  Two teenagers travel through time and discover facts about dinosaurs in many eras. Who were the dinosaurs? Are they mentioned in the Bible? How long ago did they live? Did they ever share the earth with mankind... and are any of these "terrible lizards" still living? On their journey, the teens also witness the fall of man, discover the need for a Savior, and travel into the future to see the judgment. Scripture and historical information intertwine to present a factual account of history from creation to judgment by way of salvation through Jesus Christ. This fascinating, lavishly illustrated resource is sure to please!

Units 2-5: *The Golden Bull* by Marjorie Cowley, 2008 Charlesbridge Publishing
  In ancient Mesopotamia during a terrible drought, Jomar and Zefa's father must send his children away to the city of Ur because he can no longer feed them. At 14, Jomar is old enough to apprentice with Sidah, a master goldsmith for the temple of the moongod, but there is no place for Zefa in Sidah's household. Zefa, a talented but untrained musician, is forced to play her music and sing for alms on the streets of Ur. The author vividly imagines life in ancient Ur, and also shows the harsh struggle for survival in ancient Mesopotamia.

Units 5-7: *Boy of the Pyramids: A Mystery of Ancient Egypt* by Ruth Fosdick Jones, 2007 Simply Charlotte Mason, LLC
  Kaffe, a 10 year-old Egyptian boy, his slave girl Sari, and his father set out to solve the mystery of the pyramid's missing jewels and catch the thief. This gentle, yet exciting mystery masterfully weaves many aspects of Ancient Egypt into the storyline: homes, meals, feasts, slaves, architecture, Nile River, transportation, trades, geography, climate, clothing, social classes, temple, palace, pharaoh, entertainment, annual flood, and more!

Unit 8: Your own Bible – the book of Ruth

<u>Units 9-11</u>: *Jashub's Journal: An Old Testament Law Story* by Rebekah Shafer, Ruth Shafer, Sonya Shafer; 2006 Simply Charlotte Mason
Join Jashub, his family, and friends as they settle into an abandoned Canaanite village during the final days of Joshua. Help them learn to resolve their everyday disputes and situations according to God's good Law, as given in Exodus, Leviticus, and Numbers. When the Bible Study pauses the story, use the given Bible passages to determine what God's Law says the townspeople should do. Then, return to the story to see if you made the right choice.

<u>Units 12-15</u>: *God King: A Story in the Days of King Hezekiah* by Joanne Williamson, 2002 Bethlehem Books
Around 701 B.C. young Prince Taharka, succeeds unexpectedly to the throne of Ancient Egypt. He begins to find his way until a treacherous plot pushes him into exile and into the hands of Amos, an emissary of King Hezekiah. Far from home, near Jerusalem, Taharka encounters two kings in conflict. One is the mighty Assyrian, Sennacherib, promising alliance; the other is Hezekiah, the Jew who trusts in Yahweh. Taharka must choose with whom to live or die. In keeping with the ancient time period, there is some violent content. King Taharka is also called "god" by the Egyptians, since they believed Pharaoh was a god.

<u>Units 15-16</u>: Your own Bible – the book of Jonah

<u>Units 16-18</u>: Your own Bible – the Book of Esther

<u>Units 18-22</u>: *Archimedes and the Door of Science* by Jeanne Bendick, 1995 Bethlehem Books
Archimedes was one of the greatest minds of the ancient world because he had a passion for ideas and learning. This captivating book tells the story of Archimedes' life and gives vivid imagery into his accomplishments using simple, effective text and delightful line-drawn illustrations. It's a biography, a study of mathematical and scientific concepts, and an overview of the culture of ancient Greece – all rolled into one!

<u>Units 22-23</u>: *Cleopatra* by Diane Stanley & Peter Vennema, 1997 HarperTrophy
"It is traditionally believed that Cleopatra dazzled Caesar with her great beauty. Instead, it was the power of her intelligence and personality that drew him to her." In this biography, Stanley and Vennema reveal a vital, warm, and politically adroit ruler. Stanley's stunning full-color artwork is lovely in its large, well-composed images in flat Greek style. The figures of Cleopatra, Julius Caesar, and Mark Antony stride powerfully across Egypt and Rome, and Cleopatra emerges as a savvy, astute, and complex leader who followed her heart and mind.

<u>Units 23-25</u>: *City: A Story of Roman Planning and Construction* by David Macaulay, 1974 Houghton Mifflin Company
David Macaulay expertly describes and illustrates the construction of the imaginary Roman city of Verbonia, based on hundreds of real ancient Roman cities built. A multitude of black and white line drawings illustrate the story of Roman urban planners as they design and construct a new city. Every stage is explained using text, illustrations, charts, and cross-sections. This is a terrific book for learning about Roman cities in this time period and for studying the way the cities were put together to provide for all the needs of the inhabitants.

<u>Units 26-30</u>: *Traveling the Way* by Drusilla McGowan, Reprint 1977 Rod & Staff Publishers
Life for Cleon as the slave of Marcus Vitruvius was no joke. Marcus Vitruvius was noted for his terrible temper, so Cleon escaped. Running away did not turn out quite as Cleon had expected at first. A home is not a home unless one is loved and accepted there. Could Cleon find a home? And if he could, would he win the love of the family he found? Along with the racial prejudices that Cleon experienced, he also had the choice of a religion. Pagan, Jew, Christian – they were all mixed up. So, who was right?

<u>Units 30-35</u>: *The Accidental Voyage: Discovering Hymns of the Early Centuries* by Douglas Bond, 2005 P & R Publishing

Get ready for a great story about two American teens traveling in Rome with an English organist known in his parish as Mr. Pipes. Follow Mr. Pipes, Annie, and Drew on an exciting adventure through mysterious lands and seas. Ride a moped with Drew through the streets of Rome, explore dark catacombs with Annie, and listen as Mr. Pipes celebrates the hymns of the early centuries. During a series of hair-raising adventures across Europe, Mr. Pipes introduces Annie and Drew to sixteen hymns from the early centuries, and to hymnists as well. Readers are sure to come away with a new knowledge and appreciation of the hymns.

Basic Package Option 2: Boy Interest Set:

Biography: (Units 1-4)

Carry On, Mr. Bowditch by Jean Lee Latham, 1983 Clarion Books

Nathaniel Bowditch grew up in a sailor's world, with masted-ships from foreign ports crowding the wharves. Nat seemed to be too physically small, but no one guessed that he had the persistence and determination to master sea navigation in the days when men sailed only by "log, lead, and lookout." Nat's long hours of study and observation, collected in his famous work, *The American Practical Navigator* (also known as the "*Sailors' Bible*"), stunned the sailing community and made him a New England hero.

Adventure: (Units 5-8)

Summer of the Monkeys by Wilson Rawls, 2004 Yearling

The last thing a 14 year-old boy expects to find along an old Ozark river bottom is a tree full of monkeys. Jay Berry Lee's grandpa had an explanation though – as he did for most things. The monkeys had escaped from a traveling circus, and there was a handsome reward for anyone who could catch them. Grandpa said there wasn't any animal that couldn't be caught somehow, and Jay Berry started out believing him. But by the end of the summer, Jay Berry Lee had learned a lot more than he ever bargained for – and not just about monkeys. He learned about faith, and wishes coming true, and knowing what it is you really want.

Historical Fiction: (Units 9-12)

Mr. Revere and I by Robert Lawson, 1981 Little Brown

This engaging tale tells the story of the early days of the American Revolution through the eyes of a single horse, who goes from being the steed of a British officer to the mount of Paul Revere (and the adored pet of his children). Through her ears we eavesdrop on the conversations that planted the seeds of the Declaration of Independence and the Constitution. An incredible transformation took place slowly but surely after Sam Adams talked her out of the glue cart into the home of a patriot, and soon the mare knew all about the Revere family, the trade of the silversmith, and even the doings of The Sons of Liberty.

Fantasy: (Units 13-16)

The Twenty -One Balloons by William Pene du Bois, 1986 Puffin

Professor William Waterman Sherman intends to fly across the Pacific Ocean. But through a twist of fate, he lands on Krakatoa, and discovers a world of unimaginable wealth, eccentric inhabitants, and incredible balloon inventions. Winner of the 1948 Newbery Medal, this classic fantasy-adventure is now available in a new edition. The author combines his rich imagination, scientific tastes, and brilliant artistry to tell a story that has no age limit.

Bibliography: Storytime Titles
(continued)

Mystery: (17-20)

Brighty: Of the Grand Canyon by Marguerite Henry, 1981 Aladdin
Long ago, a lone little burro roamed the high cliffs of the Grand Canyon and touched the hearts of all who knew him: a grizzled old miner, a big-game hunter, even President Teddy Roosevelt. Named Brighty by the prospector who befriended him, he remained a free spirit at heart. But when a ruthless claim-jumper murdered the prospector, loyal Brighty risked everything to bring the killer to justice. Brighty's adventures have delighted generations of readers, and he has become the symbol of a joyous way of life. Come along for the ride as Brighty finds the mysterious killer and solves the crime.

Nonfiction: (21-24)

Diary of an Early American Boy: Noah Blake 1805 by Eric Sloane, 2004 Dover Publications
This reprint of an actual early 19th century diary provides today's readers with an engaging rarity: a 15 year old farm boy's brief, concise notebook and author Eric Sloane's delightful drawings and explanatory narrative of the daily entries. A bygone era, preserved in its simplicity, is revealed in text that tells of life on a New England farm and such common tasks as nail making, bridge building, shingle splitting, and spring plowing.

Humor: (25-28)

Henry Reed, Inc. by Keith Robertson, 1986 Puffin Books
Henry Reed has arrived in Grover's Corner, and the town will never be the same. While spending the summer with his aunt and uncle, Henry comes up with a sure-fire money-making project: Henry Reed, Inc. Research. Henry's neighbor, Midge Glass, has an even more sure-fire hit: Reed and Glass, Inc. Now with Henry's ingenious mind and Midge's practical reasoning, Reed and Glass Inc. turns into a huge success, while creating more bewildering and outrageous schemes than the townsfolk could have ever imagined!

Realistic Fiction: (29-32)

Swallows and Amazons by Arthur Ransome, 1985 David R. Godine
First published in 1930, *Swallows and Amazons* is about six children who sail and camp, and find timeless adventure during a holiday in England's Lake District. It is a book full of excitement, a little danger, and a quality of thinking, planning, and fun that is delightful. The many characters are distinct individuals – from the Australian mom to a neighboring farm wife, to serious older siblings and the head-over-heels enthusiastic younger kids. The pace quickens when the sailboat battles occur and relaxes when the children collapse around the fire. Reading it, we lose ourselves in the golden days.

Folk Tales: (33-35)

The Shining Sword: Book I by Charles G. Coleman, 1984 Zeezok Publishing
"For the King!" is the battle cry of the royal army as soldiers in the service of the King of kings and Lord of lords set out to wage war against the forces of evil. Lanus, a new recruit, finds he has much to learn about obedience, failure, victory, and the vital importance of putting on the full armor of the King. In this fascinating tale of spiritual warfare, the story of Lanus vividly illustrates the Christian's conflict with Satan. With Lanus, learn to wield the ultimate weapon of righteousness, the Sword of the Word of God and see how battles, armory, castle, and swords represent our Christian walk. (While this title is more allegorical, it has been placed in the folk tale category since it has elements of fairy tales).

Basic Package Option 3: Girl Interest Set:

Biography: (Units 1-4)

Laura Ingalls Wilder: A Biography by William Anderson, 1992 Collins
From her pioneer days on the prairie to her golden years with her husband, Almanzo, and their daughter, Rose, Laura Ingalls Wilder has become a friend to all who have read about her adventures. This behind-the-scenes account chronicles the real events in Laura's life that inspired her to write her stories and also describes her life after the last Little House book ends. Many more people and events from Wilder's childhood and mature years appear here than in other accounts, and quotations from her works are woven into the text.

Adventure: (Units 5-8)

The Good Master by Kate Seredy, 1986 Puffin
Jancsi is overjoyed to hear that his cousin from Budapest is coming to spend the summer on his father's ranch on the Hungarian plains, but their summer proves more adventurous than he had hoped when headstrong Kate arrives. Together they share horseback races across the plains, country fairs and festivals, and a dangerous run-in with the gypsies. In vividly detailed scenes, this Newbery Award winning author presents an unforgettable world and characters that will be remembered forever.

Historical Fiction: (Units 9-12)

Caddie Woodlawn by Carol Ryrie Brink, 2006 Aladdin
Caddie Woodlawn is a real adventurer. She'd rather hunt than sew and plow than bake, and she tries to beat her brother's dares every chance she gets. Caddie is a friend with the Indians, who scare most of the neighbors who, like her mother and sisters, don't understand her at all. Caddie is brave, and her story is special because it's based on the life and memories of Carol Ryrie Brink's grandmother, the real Caddie Woodlawn. Her spirit and sense of fun have made this book a classic that readers have enjoyed for more than 70 years.

Fantasy: (Units 13-16)

Hitty: Her First Hundred Years by Rachel Field, 1998 Aladdin
On a cold Maine night in 1829, a peddler carved a small doll out of a piece of wood and named her Hitty. Phoebe Preble takes Hitty from Boston to India. From the hands of Phoebe, Hitty travels on with a snake charmer, a Civil War soldier, a captain's daughter, and a former slave. Along the way she meets presidents and painters, relating each adventure in vivid detail. Rachel Field's masterful novel *Hitty: Her First Hundred Years* was first published in 1929. It was awarded the Newbery Medal in 1930. While not always politically correct in its word choice, the charm of this original version still makes it worth reading.

Mystery: (Units 17-20)

Gone-Away Lake by Elizabeth Enright, 1985 Odyssey Classics
When Portia sets out for a visit with her cousin Julian, she expects fun and adventure of the usual kind, but this summer is different. On their first day exploring, Portia and Julian discover an enormous boulder with a mysterious message, a swamp choked with reeds and quicksand, and on the far side of the swamp... a ghost town. Once upon a time the swamp was a splendid lake, and the fallen houses along its shore an elegant resort community. But though the lake is long gone and the resort faded away, the houses still hold a secret life: two people who have never left Gone-Away... and who can tell the story of what happened there.

Bibliography: Storytime Titles
(continued)

Nonfiction: (Units 21-24)

Bound for Oregon by Jean Van Leeuwen, 1996 Puffin Books
This is an account of Mary Ellen Todd's 2000-mile trek from Arkansas to Oregon in the 1850's, as it was written down by Todd's daughter. Details about events and people have been added to create a fact-based novel engagingly told in the voice of a 10 year-old. The story begins with the preparations and difficulty of leaving home. It chronicles the hardships the family encountered: raging rivers, bad weather, sickness and death, limited food, and the constant push to beat the first snows. There are also small pleasures, including the birth of a brother. Readers will see how choices made often make the difference between success or failure, life or death. This is a convincing picture of a pioneer journey that does a good job of showing the tremendous sacrifices people made to follow their dream of a better life.

Humor: (Units 25-28)

Anne of Green Gables by Lucy Maud Montgomery, 2015 Puffin Books; Reprint Edition
This is the tale of an orphan girl, mistakenly adopted by the Cuthberts. Anne Shirley, age eleven, is bright, talkative, imaginative, sometimes hot-tempered, and always optimistic. She instantly loves the farmhouse called Green Gables and all of Avonlea, Prince Edward Island. But will the Cuthberts send her back to the asylum? They wanted a boy. One thing's for certain, no house that Anne's in will ever be dull! Anne always looks at the bright side of things, through thick and thin, and readers can learn a lot from her as they enjoy seeing Anne grow up, adjust to life, and make new friends in an unfamiliar place.

Realistic Fiction: (Units 29-32)

Ballet Shoes by Noel Streatfeild and Diane Goode, 1965 Yearling Books for Young Readers
Pauline, Petrova, and Posie start life off as carefree children, but when their adopted Great Uncle Max (a.k.a. Gum) disappears on a fossil hunting expedition, the young girls find themselves becoming the breadwinners of the family. As stage performers they are able to give back to the only family they have ever known, and they have their own adventures while they're at it. Pauline falls in love with acting, Posy is a natural dancer, and poor Petrova would rather fix cars and learn to fly planes than be on stage. This charming and often humorous story stands the test of time. The strong female characters solve many conflicts on their own. In the end, each girl is also able to choose her own path in life.

Folk Tales: (33-35)

The Little Lame Prince (and the Traveling Cloak) by Miss Mulock, 2017 Yesterday's Classics
The Prince's christening was to be a grand affair. By six in the morning all off the royal household had dressed itself in its very best. The little Prince was dressed in his best – his magnificent christening-robe, but as his nurse carried him to the chapel she stumbled and let him fall. She picked him up right away, and the accident was so slight it seemed hardly worth speaking of, so no one did. This is a touching story of a young prince who becomes lame on the way to his christening. Later, the death of his parents leaves him at the mercy of his cruel uncle who keeps him hidden in a tower. However, a strange turn of events brings hope and love to the lonely boy. This enchanting tale is a sure treat for your listeners!

Bibliography: Self-Study Extension Package for Older Students

When to use this Extension Package Schedule: Adding this optional package to the Economy Package extends the area of history to include more advanced, independent reading material. This allows your 6th and 7th grade students to learn along with your younger students. Due to the more mature content of the books set during the ancient time period, both in the violence that was prevalent during this period and in the depravity of worship of pagan gods, this extension package is best suited for mature 6th and 7th graders who are strong, independent readers. For very sensitive 6th or 7th graders, or for those who are not yet strong readers, we recommend the Storytime History Set for the parent to read aloud instead.

Books for the Extension Package Schedule:

Note: The books listed below are required in order to use the Extension Package Schedule. For ease of use, Heart of Dakota Publishing sells the books listed below as a set called **Self-Study Extension Package for Older Students** on the website www.heartofdakota.com or by telephone at (605) 428-4068. Book descriptions are from the publisher or book reviewer.

Units 1-2: *Dinosaurs by Design* by Duane T. Gish, Ph. D., 1992, 2022 Master Books
Everyone wants to know about dinosaurs! *Dinosaurs by Design* takes you into the exciting world of dinosaurs to find out what they were really like. Discover how fossils are formed, dug up, and assembled for museums. Travel with the dinosaurs as they board Noah's Ark and then enter the strange new world after the Flood. Find out what happened to the dinosaurs and if there are any alive today. Join us on an exciting adventure to learn more about these magnificent creatures that God designed and created.

Units 3-7: *A Cry from Egypt* by Hope Auer, 2013 Great Waters Press
Set in the time of the ten plagues, *A Cry from Egypt* focuses on the lives of a Hebrew slave, Jarah, and her family. As slaves in Egypt, the work is hard. To make life harder, Jarah's family is split between the God of Abraham, Isaac, and Jacob and the Egyptian gods. When a possible marriage enters the picture, Jarah's life becomes even more complicated. Now, she needs God more than ever! Adventure, excitement, love, and faith come together when Jarah and her family find themselves at the culmination of four hundred years of history.

Units 8-12: *Hittite Warrior* by Joanne Williamson, 1999 Bethlehem Books
When Uriah's Hittite home is destroyed by Greeks, his dying father tells him to go south to seek a Canaanite named Sisera. There he saves a young boy from being sacrificed to the pagan god Moloch, and he is given succor for a time by the Hebrews. Later, he joins Sisera in war against these same people. When the Canaanites are defeated, Uriah has the opportunity to come to a peace with himself, the Hebrew people, and their God. This well-researched novel is set in the time of Judges, and incorporates Biblical facts with a gripping story. While this novel has violence befitting the time period, it does not go into a graphic amount of detail and does bring an important period in the Hebrew people's history to life.

Units 13-18: *Within the Palace Gates* by Anna Pierpoint Siviter, 1992 AB Publishing
The rich tapestry of the ancient Persian court is woven into the intriguing story of Nehemiah, King Artaxerxes's noble cup bearer. The story allows us to grasp the deep significance of Nehemiah's devotion to God, to Jerusalem, and to his people. Readers are also given a breathtaking glimpse of life in Babylon, the king's court, and the difficulty of life for the Hebrew people who were left behind in a crumbling Jerusalem. This story gradually builds until it's hard to put down; but far beyond its plot, is the story's sacred focus.

Bibliography: Self-Study Extension Package for Older Students
(continued)

Units 18-20: *Peeps at Many Lands: Ancient Greece* by James Baikie, 2008 Yesterdays Classics
Through the eyes of a traveler to ancient Greece, we see how, by reason of geography, Greece became a land of city-states. After examining several different city-states and their land and naval forces, we watch all Greece come together for the Olympic games. Turning our attention to Athens, we marvel at the theatre, architecture, and sculpture of the age of Pericles. This book, which was written by a pastor in 1920, provides a thorough, narrative look at ancient Greece, placing the Greek civilization in its proper perspective.

Units 21-23: *Alexander the Great* by John Gunther, 2007 Sterling Publishing
Some say Alexander the Great was the mightiest warrior in history. He built an empire that extended from Europe to Africa, and from India to Central Asia. In a stirring narrative, famed historian John Gunther tells the story of Alexander the Great who, at only age 21, became King of Macedonia and set off on a 12-year journey to conquer the known world and extend the boundaries of Greek civilization. Gunther takes us from Alexander's boyhood to his victory over the Persian Empire. Alexander's battles are described in vivid detail, as well as his travels and his lifestyle.

Units 23-28; 34-35: *Famous Men of Rome* by John H. Haaren & A.B. Poland, 2006 Memoria Press
Famous Men of Rome offers 30 stories, covering the history of Rome from its founding under Romulus to the last emperor in the West. Your children will see the rise and fall of history's greatest civilization through the lives of Horatius, Camillus, Caesar, Cicero, Marcus Aurelius, and many other larger-than-life figures. While the Roman culture was primarily pagan, an understanding of modern political history is impossible without a thorough understanding of Rome. Thus, its study provides a foundation for all other history study. This reprinting includes 30 beautiful oil paintings of the significant events.

Units 28-30: *Ben-Hur* Audio Drama by Lew Wallace, Paul McCusker, and Focus on the Family Radio Theatre; 2007 Tyndale Entertainment (2 CD Set, 2 hours, abridged addition)
Ben-Hur is the powerful story of two friends who share a love for learning and a passion to be soldiers. But before many years pass, Ben-Hur, a prince of the Jews, and Messala, a Roman soldier, will also share a deep hatred for each other. An unforgettable account of betrayal, revenge, and redemption, *Ben-Hur* tells the tale of a nobleman who fell from Roman favor and was sentenced to live as a slave - all at the hands of his friend, Messala. Once nearly brothers, any hope of reconciliation is dashed after Messala is injured during a vicious chariot race won by the vindictive Ben-Hur. But what makes this story unforgettable is the changed man Ben-Hur becomes after seeing Christ on the cross, showing the power of God's love and true forgiveness are the only forces stronger than hatred and revenge.

Units 31-34: *Twice Freed* by Patricia St. John, 1999 CF4kids
Onesimus is a slave, and Eirene is a rich merchant's daughter. Onesimus longs to gain his freedom and Eirene's love. However, he doesn't realize where true freedom lies. He wants nothing to do with Jesus Christ. His master, Philemon, may follow the teachings of Christ and his apostle Paul, but Onesimus has other plans. This fictional story is based on Onesimus and his master Philemon - two people from the New Testament. While Philemon becomes a Christian, Onesimus resents his master and begins running from both his master and Christ's love. But, Onesimus keeps running into those who have been saved and caught up in this strange new religion: Christianity. Historical details and descriptive language make the story come alive, while the Biblical truth woven throughout the book is inspiring.

Bibliography: Self-Study Extension Package for Older Readers
(continued)

Note: History readings are broken down into manageable daily assignments that coordinate with the various time periods in *Hearts for Him Through Time: Creation to Christ*. The reading assignments are meant for your older students to read independently. Depending on your goals for your older students' independent readings, you may want to assess their reading comprehension. Some suggestions for assessment include:
- orally retell what they've read (suggested once during each unit; use the "Narration Tips" found in the Appendix for help as needed)
- write a two to three paragraph summary of the reading (suggested twice during each unit; use the "Written Narration Skills" found in the Appendix for help in editing)
- notebook by drawing a picture about the reading and write a one paragraph summary about what you read that goes along with your picture (suggested once during each unit)

These assessments are meant to relieve parents of the need to preread the extension books and take the pressure off the parent to be all knowing about the book. They let the students do the work of thinking about a book instead, causing it to be more firmly placed in their minds. For example, on the oral narration day, the student would hand the parent the extension package book open to the starting page of the reading. As the student narrates, the parent skims through the pages in order and listens to see how well the student is narrating (which is easy to do with the book in hand). At the end of the narration, the parent might mention a missed part by saying, "Could you tell me a bit more about what Alexander the Great did when..." Then, the parent would give a lead for the student to narrate the missed part. This puts the focus on the student interacting with the text, rather than on the parent coming up with great discussion questions (which is an area already thoroughly covered in *Drawn into the Heart of Reading*).

On the written narration days, the student would hand in the extension package book marked to the opening page of the reading, along with the written narration. When the parent has a free moment, the parent calls the student to read the narration out loud, which helps the student catch any mistakes and fix them. Meanwhile, the parent is looking through the pages as the student reads the written narration to see if the high points of the story are mentioned. In written narrations, the parent can always expect a less thorough narration and shouldn't make the student go back and add more. Instead, after complimenting the student on what was done well, the parent may mention one thing to work on, like, "On your next written narration, try to add a few more details... or cover more of the story... or mention the characters' names...". The parent would then watch for that skill, and if it isn't there, help the student add it. Again, the focus is on the student's interaction with the text, and not on the parent's ability to come up with questions. The "Written Narration Skills" section in the Appendix should also be used to help with editing.

On the notebooking day, students should draw something, or print and paste in a picture printed from the Internet that goes with what they read that day. The page should be given a heading, and the picture should be given a caption. Last, students should either copy a paragraph or so from the text that goes well with the picture they chose, or write something original that goes with their notebooking page. The students hand in both the bookmarked page of their book and their assignment. When the parent checks it, the parent should call the student to read and explain it (while the parent is looking over the reading). The parent makes a few guiding comments at the end for students to attempt for the next notebooking session. The notebooking time does not have to be an overview, but can focus in a more key way on one aspect the children found interesting. It moves into a more research type mode, as students get older. The parent should not usually have the student redo or add to the current entry. The focus is on students interacting with the text and showing the parent what they individually processed within the reading.

Self-Study History Extension Package Schedule

Unit 1:
     <u>Day 1</u>: *Dinosaurs by Design* p. 6-17
     <u>Day 2</u>: *Dinosaurs by Design* p. 18-27
     <u>Day 3</u>: *Dinosaurs by Design* p. 28-37
     <u>Day 4</u>: *Dinosaurs by Design* p. 38-49

Unit 2:
     <u>Day 1</u>: *Dinosaurs by Design* p. 50-59
     <u>Day 2</u>: *Dinosaurs by Design* p. 60-69
     <u>Day 3</u>: *Dinosaurs by Design* p. 70-79
     <u>Day 4</u>: *Dinosaurs by Design* p. 80-87

Unit 3:
     <u>Day 1</u>: *A Cry from Egypt* "Preface," p. xiii-xiv, and p. 1-7 (Note: p. 2-3 include violent beatings by Egyptian overseers.)
     <u>Day 2</u>: *A Cry from Egypt* p. 9-20 (Note: p. 14-15 describe a violent beating from the past.)
     <u>Day 3</u>: *A Cry from Egypt* p. 21 – middle of p. 27
     <u>Day 4</u>: *A Cry from Egypt* middle of p. 27-35 (Note: bottom of p. 31 – top of p. 32 briefly describe a beating.)

Unit 4:
     <u>Day 1</u>: *A Cry from Egypt* p. 37-46
     <u>Day 2</u>: *A Cry from Egypt* p. 47-57
     <u>Day 3</u>: *A Cry from Egypt* p. 58-63
     <u>Day 4</u>: *A Cry from Egypt* p. 65 – top of p. 71

Unit 5:
     <u>Day 1</u>: *A Cry from Egypt* top of p. 71-77 (Note: p. 72 – top of p. 75 describe a violent beating from an overseer and a struggle for life.)
     <u>Day 2</u>: *A Cry from Egypt* p. 79-88
     <u>Day 3</u>: *A Cry from Egypt* p. 89 – top of p. 98
     <u>Day 4</u>: *A Cry from Egypt* top of p. 98-108

Unit 6:
     <u>Day 1</u>: *A Cry from Egypt* p. 109-120
     <u>Day 2</u>: *A Cry from Egypt* p. 121-126 (Note: bottom of p. 125-126 include a vivid description of the death of an asp.)
     <u>Day 3</u>: *A Cry from Egypt* p. 127-133
     <u>Day 4</u>: *A Cry from Egypt* p. 135 – middle of p. 142

Unit 7:
     <u>Day 1</u>: *A Cry from Egypt* middle of p. 142 – top of p. 150
     <u>Day 2</u>: *A Cry from Egypt* top of p. 150-155
     <u>Day 3</u>: *A Cry from Egypt* p. 157-166 (Note: p. 158-159 include the death of a lamb for the Passover meal, and p. 162-165 include the deaths of Egyptian first-born sons.)
     <u>Day 4</u>: *A Cry from Egypt* p. 167-176

Unit 8:
     <u>Day 1</u>: *Hittite Warrior* p. 1-13
     <u>Day 2</u>: *Hittite Warrior* p. 14-22
     <u>Day 3</u>: *Hittite Warrior* p. 23-33
     <u>Day 4</u>: *Hittite Warrior* p. 34-43

Unit 9:
     <u>Day 1</u>: *Hittite Warrior* p. 44-57
     <u>Day 2</u>: *Hittite Warrior* p. 58-71
     <u>Day 3</u>: *Hittite Warrior* p. 72-83
     <u>Day 4</u>: *Hittite Warrior* p. 84-98

Unit 10:
> Day 1: *Hittite Warrior* p. 99-112
> Day 2: *Hittite Warrior* p. 113-124
> Day 3: *Hittite Warrior* p. 125-131
> Day 4: *Hittite Warrior* p. 132-141

Unit 11:
> Day 1: *Hittite Warrior* p. 142-152
> Day 2: *Hittite Warrior* p. 153-162
> Day 3: *Hittite Warrior* p. 163-176
> Day 4: *Hittite Warrior* p. 177-183

Unit 12:
> Day 1: *Hittite Warrior* p. 184-195
> Day 2: *Hittite Warrior* p. 196-209
> Day 3: *Hittite Warrior* p. 210-225
> Day 4: *Hittite Warrior* p. 226-237

Unit 13:
> Day 1: *Within the Palace Gates* p. 9-26
> Day 2: *Within the Palace Gates* p. 27-37
> Day 3: *Within the Palace Gates* p. 38-47
> Day 4: *Within the Palace Gates* p. 48-59

Unit 14:
> Day 1: *Within the Palace Gates* p. 60-75
> Day 2: *Within the Palace Gates* p. 76-85
> Day 3: *Within the Palace Gates* p. 86-99
> Day 4: *Within the Palace Gates* p. 100-112

Unit 15:
> Day 1: *Within the Palace Gates* p. 113-122
> Day 2: *Within the Palace Gates* p. 123-133
> Day 3: *Within the Palace Gates* p. 134-147
> Day 4: *Within the Palace Gates* p. 148-169

Unit 16:
> Day 1: *Within the Palace Gates* p. 170-184
> Day 2: *Within the Palace Gates* p. 185-192
> Day 3: *Within the Palace Gates* p. 193-205
> Day 4: *Within the Palace Gates* p. 206-220

Unit 17:
> Day 1: *Within the Palace Gates* p. 221-232
> Day 2: *Within the Palace Gates* p. 233-247
> Day 3: *Within the Palace Gates* p. 248-264
> Day 4: *Within the Palace Gates* p. 265-288

Unit 18:
> Day 1: *Within the Palace Gates* p. 289-308
> Day 2: *Peeps at Many Lands: Ancient Greece* Chapter I, p. 1-9
> Day 3: *Peeps at Many Lands: Ancient Greece* Chapter II, p. 10-19
> Day 4: *Peeps at Many Lands: Ancient Greece* Chapter III, p. 20-28

Unit 19:
  Day 1: *Peeps at Many Lands: Ancient Greece* Chapter IV, p. 29-36
  Day 2: *Peeps at Many Lands: Ancient Greece* Chapter V, p. 37-48
  Day 3: *Peeps at Many Lands: Ancient Greece* Chapter VI, p. 49-56
  Day 4: *Peeps at Many Lands: Ancient Greece* Chapter VII, p. 57-66

Unit 20:
  Day 1: *Peeps at Many Lands: Ancient Greece* Chapter VIII, p. 67-80
  Day 2: *Peeps at Many Lands: Ancient Greece* Chapter IX, p. 81-91
  Day 3: *Peeps at Many Lands: Ancient Greece* Chapter X, p. 92-100
  Day 4: *Peeps at Many Lands: Ancient Greece* Chapter XI, p. 101-115

Unit 21:
  Day 1: *Alexander the Great* p. 3-18
  Day 2: *Alexander the Great* p. 19-26
  Day 3: *Alexander the Great* p. 27-39
  Day 4: *Alexander the Great* p. 43-58

Unit 22:
  Day 1: *Alexander the Great* p. 59-70
  Day 2: *Alexander the Great* p. 71-82
  Day 3: *Alexander the Great* p. 83-96
  Day 4: *Alexander the Great* p. 97-107

Unit 23:
  Day 1: *Alexander the Great* p. 108-122
  Day 2: *Alexander the Great* p. 125-139
  Day 3: *Alexander the Great* p. 140-149
  Day 4: *Famous Men of Rome* p. 5-10

Unit 24:
  Day 1: *Famous Men of Rome* p. 11-17
  Day 2: *Famous Men of Rome* p. 19-23
  Day 3: *Famous Men of Rome* p. 25-31
  Day 4: *Famous Men of Rome* p. 33-38

Unit 25:
  Day 1: *Famous Men of Rome* p. 39-45
  Day 2: *Famous Men of Rome* p. 47-50 (half)
  Day 3: *Famous Men of Rome* p. 50-56
  Day 4: *Famous Men of Rome* p. 57-65

Unit 26:
  Day 1: *Famous Men of Rome* p. 67-70
  Day 2: *Famous Men of Rome* p. 71-76
  Day 3: *Famous Men of Rome* p. 77-84
  Day 4: *Famous Men of Rome* p. 85-91

Unit 27:
  Day 1: *Famous Men of Rome* p. 93-100
  Day 2: *Famous Men of Rome* p. 101-105
  Day 3: *Famous Men of Rome* p. 106-110
  Day 4: *Famous Men of Rome* p. 111-113

Unit 28:
  Day 1: *Famous Men of Rome* p. 115-120
  Day 2: *Ben Hur* Audio Disc 1 – Tracks 1-3
  Day 3: *Ben Hur* Audio Disc 1 – Tracks 4-6

    Day 4: *Ben Hur* Audio Disc 1 – Tracks 7-8

Unit 29:

    Day 1: *Ben Hur* Audio Disc 1 – Tracks 9-11

    Day 2: *Ben Hur* Audio Disc 1 – Tracks 12-16

    Day 3: *Ben Hur* Audio Disc 1 – Track 17 and Disc 2 – Tracks 1-2

    Day 4: *Ben Hur* Audio Disc 2 – Tracks 3-5

Unit 30:

    Day 1: *Ben Hur* Audio Disc 2 – Tracks 6-8

    Day 2: *Ben Hur* Audio Disc 2 – Tracks 9

    Day 3: *Ben Hur* Audio Disc 2 – Tracks 10-12

    Day 4: *Ben Hur* Audio Disc 2 – Tracks 13-17

Unit 31:

    Day 1: *Twice Freed* p. 9-27

    Day 2: *Twice Freed* p. 29-37

    Day 3: *Twice Freed* p. 39-57

    Day 4: *Twice Freed* p. 59-76

Unit 32:

    Day 1: *Twice Freed* p. 77-93

    Day 2: *Twice Freed* p. 95-113

    Day 3: *Twice Freed* p. 115-129

    Day 4: *Twice Freed* p. 131-151

Unit 33:

    Day 1: *Twice Freed* p. 153-162

    Day 2: *Twice Freed* p. 163-180

    Day 3: *Twice Freed* p. 181-195

    Day 4: *Twice Freed* p. 197-214

Unit 34:

    Day 1: *Twice Freed* p. 215-221

    Day 2: *Famous Men of Rome* p. 121-125

    Day 3: *Famous Men of Rome* p. 127-130

    Day 4: *Famous Men of Rome* p. 131-132

Unit 35:

    Day 1: *Famous Men of Rome* p. 133-137

    Day 2: *Famous Men of Rome* p. 139-141

    Day 3: *Famous Men of Rome* p. 143-146

    Day 4: *Famous Men of Rome* p. 147-150

Science Lab Sheet

Question:

_____

_____

_____

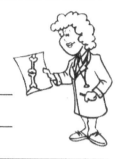

Guess:

_____

_____

_____

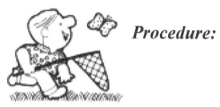

Procedure:

Conclusion:

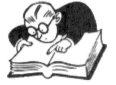

_____

_____

_____

NARRATION TIPS: TEACHER'S LIST

Notes: When children narrate, they tell back in their own words what they have just read or heard. It allows them to share their own version of the passage with accuracy, individual personality, spirit, and originality.

Narrating is an essential skill in life. To be able to give an opinion of a book, relay a telephone message, summarize a letter, give driving directions, write an article, or share a doctor's instructions – are all examples of practical applications of narration skills. Narrating is an important skill to learn. You can begin to teach your children to narrate by following the steps listed below. Just be patient, and have fun with it! Narration is a way of life.

BEFORE NARRATING:

1. **Choose a living book.** Living books are alive with ideas and have a story aspect to them. The books read in this curriculum are living books.

2. **Skim the section your child will use for narration.** Children's narrations usually show how well they understand the book, but sometimes a child gives a confident, articulate narration that is eloquently wrong.

3. **Introduce the section being read.** Review **briefly** what was read last time. Other **optional** ideas: Use Charlotte Mason's "informing idea" (i.e. *The Pilgrims weren't allowed to worship God. I wonder what they'll do? Let's read to find out.*). Or, write a list of difficult names or words and pronounce them. Children may use the list during narrating.

4. **Tell children they will narrate after the reading.** When children know they will narrate, they will attend the reading with sharper attention.

5. **Read the selected passage once.** The teacher or the child may read it. Move toward having children do their own reading by age 9. This will help improve narrations. Have only one child narrate at a time. Keep the readings short at first. You can even read a bit, ask for a narration, read some more, and narrate some more. Don't define words during the reading.

DURING NARRATING:

1. **Have children tell you all they remember about the reading.** Say, *Tell me all you can about what you just read.* They should not be looking at the book. Do not interrupt a narration. It distracts the train of thought. Do not correct children while they are narrating.

2. **The teacher is a listener; not a lecturer.** Let the child's mind do the sorting, rejecting, and classifying of what should be shared.

3. **Children may use exact phrasing from the book.** They may pick up phrasing and vocabulary that strikes them. This allows children to make the language of good living books their own.

4. **Children may share connections made.** Children may compare what was read to another book, situation, or memory of their own. However, the connection should not take over the narration.

5. **The length of the narration is not the point.** If children can retell the most pertinent information in a few sentences, that may be enough. The purpose of narration is the process of ordering and selecting what to tell. Every narration doesn't need to be in full detail.

6. **There is not one "right" narration.** A dozen children could read the same section and give a dozen different good narrations. A teacher should not listen for a long list of words to be shared from the text.

AFTER NARRATING:

1. **Share comments or details.** You can ask questions, correct misinformation, and ask for clarification at this point. However, avoid being overly critical. Limit what you say to a few important points.

2. **Do not grade narrations.** Grading a narration gives the impression that there is only one right way to do it. Children are left searching for the elusive "one right narration", rather than using their own originality.

OTHER HELPFUL NARRATING TIPS:

1. **Be patient with your child.** If your child is frustrated or seems to be missing the meaning of the reading, shorten the sections he narrates on or take a turn narrating yourself. Try to be as encouraging as possible; make sure not to be overly critical or to give too lengthy advice.

2. **Help your children develop the habits of listening and attention**. If your children have been used to "gobbling up" books instead of giving focused attention to reading, shorten the sections used for narration and focus on what they know – not on what they don't know.

3. **Children begin written narrations at age 10**. They need extensive practice in oral narrations first. Instructions for written narrations will be included in the next level of this curriculum.

HOW TO NARRATE: STUDENT'S LIST

1. Listen carefully to what your teacher tells you about the book.

2. If you are in the middle of a book, think about what was read last time.

3. During the reading, think carefully about what is being read. Pay attention to names, places, events, and things that grab your attention.

4. Be ready to tell all you can remember when the reading is done.

5. Retell what was read with as much detail as you can. There is not one right way to do this.

6. It's fine to repeat words or phrases that sound just like the book. It's fine to share connections you made with what was read.

7. Do not make things up or begin everything you say with, "And then…".

8. Listen to what your teacher says after you narrate. Try to do these things the next time you narrate.

WRITTEN NARRATION SKILLS: TEACHER'S LIST

Notes: When children do written narrations, they use their writing to tell back in their own words what they have just read or heard. Written narrations allow children to use their writing to share their own version of the passage they have just read or heard with accuracy, individual personality, spirit, and originality.

You can begin to help your children with their written narrations by following the steps listed below. If you are new to Heart of Dakota and have not yet worked through the copywork, oral narration, and dictation in the guides, then you should plan to spend longer moving through the list of skills below. This is quite normal, so don't be surprised if you do not get through all of the skills in the list this year.

The skills listed below range from beginning writing skills to more difficult writing skills that require knowing higher levels of grammar, usage, and punctuation. Skills are based on a continuum of increasing difficulty, so related skills may be spread out to be placed where they each fall best on the overall continuum. For example, the third skill on the list is beginning and ending sentences correctly, as well as correcting sentence fragments. But, fixing run-on sentences, which is a related skill, is not addressed until the seventh skill. For this reason, it is best to read the list over in its entirety, so you can see the overall flow of the continuum. Focusing on teaching <u>one</u> new numbered skill at time <u>in the order it is listed</u> will help you to avoid overwhelming your child with too many skills at once, and will give your child a manageable plan for successfully learning to do written narrations.

For new or struggling writers, you should start with the skill listed first on the list below. Once that skill is <u>mastered</u>, move on to the next skill. The skills should be cumulative, meaning <u>each time a new skill is added, the old skills are still required</u>. You may either make <u>gentle</u> comments as students are writing each sentence of their narration, or wait until the narration is complete to make your <u>gentle</u> comments then.

If your child already routinely does the beginning skills on the list, you should jump to the first skill on the list that your child has not mastered. Before editing, always have your children read the narration aloud to you so they can catch any of their own mistakes first.

The skills list below is for the teacher's use. There is also a list for students' use that can be used for their reference; however, it should not be used in place of the teacher's list since written narration is a new skill being taught.

WRITTEN NARRATION SKILLS LIST:

1.   **Indent each paragraph.** Leave a space about the size of one thumb tip at the beginning of the first sentence in each paragraph.

2.   **Make sure the first sentence is on the right topic.** Reword it if necessary.

3. **Begin each sentence with a capital letter, and end each sentence with the correct punctuation mark (. ! ?).** To do this you will also need to correct any sentence fragments to make complete sentences.

4. **Begin working on writing with correct spelling by using a combination of the following options.** Note: Option 1 is a better habit for students to acquire than Option 2, and Option 2 is a better habit for students to acquire than Option 3, and so on. Option 4 should only be used for very poor spellers, as it is not the same as having students write something in their own words.

   Option 1: Have students look back in the book to copy the correct spelling of key words.
   Option 2: Write words that students ask you to spell for them on a markerboard or paper while they are writing. Then, they can copy the word(s) as they write.
   Option 3: Spell orally any words the students ask you to spell for them while they are writing.
   Option 4: Allow students to dictate the narration to you for you to write, and have them copy it at the end.

   Spelling will also be addressed more fully later on in the skills list, so when students have become good at using these spelling options, move on to number 5.

5. **Make sure that sentences do not all start with the same word or words.** Vary the first word of the sentences within each paragraph as much as possible.

6. **Use correct capitalization within each sentence.** Check to be sure all proper nouns, titles, etc. are capitalized.

7. **Fix any sentences that are run-ons by providing a gentle reminder while students are writing.** For example, "That's the start of a new sentence now."

8. **Write a good closing sentence.** This sentence should wrap up the paragraph in an interesting way, and make the reader feel like your writing is coming to a close. Ideas for a strong closing sentence include the following:
   * restating the introduction using different words
   * using a quote
   * asking a question
   * stating the main theme or idea
   * giving your personal opinion

9. **Use correct spelling within your writing.** Edit the student's narration for spelling by underlining incorrect spelling in pencil and writing the correct spelling of the word in the margin of their paper or on a markerboard.

10. **Use correct punctuation within the sentences.** Check to be sure students have properly used commas in a series, commas between two sentences, apostrophes, etc.

WRITTEN NARRATION SKILLS: STUDENT'S LIST

1.   **Indent each paragraph by leaving a thumb tip space at the beginning.**

2.   **Make sure the first sentence is on the right topic.**

3.   **Begin each sentence with a capital letter, and end each sentence with the correct punctuation mark: .   ?   !**

4.   **Begin working on writing with correct spelling by using the different options your teacher suggests.**

5.   **Make sure that sentences do not all start with the same word or words.**

6.   **Use correct capitalization within each sentence, like for special names or places.**

7.   **Fix any sentences that are run-ons.**

8.   **Write a good closing sentence.**

9.   **Use correct spelling within your writing.**

10.   **Use correct punctuation within the sentences.**

Dictation Passages – Level 3

<u>Special instructions for the dictation passages</u>: Each student needs a notebook for dictation. A wide-lined notebook is best. On each dictation day, your student will study the dictation passage. It is helpful to write any difficult words on markerboard or paper for the students to focus on. New words are in bold. Also, call attention to any capital letters and punctuation marks in the passage. Discuss them briefly as needed.

When students feel ready, remove the dictation passage from the students' sight. Call out the passage one phrase at a time. Pause after each phrase for students to repeat it back to you and write it. Continue until the entire passage has been dictated.

Give students a moment to look over their passage for mistakes. Then, have them compare their sentences with the key. Students should circle any mistakes they made on the key and correct the mistakes in their own notebook. If the passage was correct, place a checkmark next to the passage in the key. All items in the sentence must be correct, including punctuation marks, before going on to the next passage. If students made any mistakes, they'll repeat the same passage as many days as it takes to get it right.

Always begin the next session where the student left off. If your child is repeatedly stuck on passages, he or she may need to move to an easier level of dictation passages. Three different levels of passages are provided in this guide.

*Dictation passages are taken from *Dictation Day by Day: Book One* by Kate Van Wagenen. (MacMillan Company 1916, 1923).

Level 3 – Dictation Passages Key

1

The **children** who did not study **their** lessons last year are **sorry** now. Are you one of these **lazy** children?

2

Do you want a **flower** in the **schoolroom**? If you have **none**, you must plant some seeds in a pot of **earth**.

3

All plants have a root, a **stem**, and leaves. **Most** plants **also** have flowers, fruit, and seeds. Can you find **each** part?

4

Please open the **door**. I want to take a peep at the snow. Here is the **key**.

5

In March, April, May and June the farmer is very busy. **There** are a **dozen things** to be **done** on a farm.

6

Next Saturday I shall go to the farm to see my **aunt**. I like to take **dinner** with her.

7

How much **salt** did you **put** in the **soup**? Come here and I shall show you.

8

I **always** help my mother before I come to school. As soon as I **reach** home, I help her **again**.

9

Every Monday **morning** we begin a new week. We must **learn** each lesson well.

10

In **September** and **October** the leaves of the **maple** turn red and yellow and brown. They look pretty in a glass.

11

September, October, and **November** are the three **autumn months**. Then the birds fly to their winter home.

12

The **eagle** feeds on **rabbits**, small birds, and fish. He makes his nest in some **high** spot.

13

We can see an eagle on every **quarter** and **fifty**-cent **piece**. On **what** other piece do we find the eagle?

14

The **ox** is useful to the farmer. It **moves** very slowly. **Its neck** is big and strong.

15

Please **bring** me the **orange, which** is on the **table**. I bought it for my dinner. It came from the **south**.

16

Dogs and sheep **carry** seeds around and drop them. Some seeds are **carried away** by **wind** and water.

17

The **butcher** and the **baker** call at our home every **Tuesday** and Saturday. **Julia** buys meat and bread for our dinner.

18

I like to play with Kate's doll very much. It can **lie** down and **shut** its **eyes**. Can you **guess** its name?

19

My mother and sister have **been** away from home **since** Friday, and we shall be **happy** to see them **once** more.

20

We feed Anna's **canary** every day at **twelve o'clock.** He likes all kinds of seeds, and he eats fruit **too**.

21

When my father was sick, we called a **doctor** who lives in **New York**. He **said** that father must have rest and **sleep**.

22

As Julia's home was a **mile** away, I took the **car** at **First Street**. I did not get the right one, so I was not on time.

23

Helen gave a **party** to **thirty** little boys and girls. They had cakes and ices and many nice things to eat.

24

When Jack hurt his **finger**, he could not help his father. He was such a good boy that his sister told him a **story almost** every day.

25

When I go into our **parlor**, I can hear the **clock** tick. My mother will not let me **touch** this clock.

26

My father gave my brother and me **silver** pencils. Fred's pencil was soon **broken**, but I **kept** mine a month.

27

How many **inches** are there in a **foot**, **George**? There are twelve inches in a foot, and three feet in a yard.

28

December, **January**, and **February** are the winter months. Then we have many storms, but we also have **skating**.

29

Does John go out **early** in the morning? Yes, he wants to **earn** money for his **mama**.

30

There are three classes of **bees**. They all live **together** in a hive and feed on honey, which they **collect** in the summer.

31

The **queen** bee lays the eggs. The **drones** do no work and have no **sting**.

32

The **workers** get food for the **entire** hive. They get this honey from the flowers. They like **clover** very much.

33

Friday noon I went to the store **myself** and bought a large **squash**, a quart of **pears**, and a pound of **tea**.

34

While mother was busy, I **read** to my little sister near the old **elm** tree. Did you ever try to keep a little sister **quiet**?

35

Do you read **word** by word? If you do, read a **page** a day for a month, and you will soon **improve**.

36

When we **raise** plants, we must give them sun and **air** and water. By the **middle** of March some of them may begin to bloom.

37

Last Saturday I saw **twenty merry children** on their way to the park. Can you tell me **why** they **smiled** and were so happy?

38

Frogs lay their eggs in a kind of **jelly**. It takes about a month for these eggs to hatch. Then we see the tadpole.

39

A tadpole is all **head** and tail. Did you ever watch the **gills disappear** and the legs grow?

40

As the **legs** of the tadpole grow, the tail disappears. Then the tadpole is **changed** to a **perfect** little frog. It feeds on **insects**.

41

Everything **else** one can turn and turn about, and make old look like new, but there's no **coaxing** boots and **shoes** to look better **than** they do.

42

I don't like the cold days of winter. Jack **Frost bites** my fingers and my **toes**. I like April and May better.

43

Nearly every day the rose's pretty **face** was **washed** by the dew. Was the dear little flower happy when it **felt** the drops of dew?

44

Said young **Dandelion**
With a sweet air,
I have my eye on
Miss **Daisy** fair.

        - Miss Mulock

45

Do you see those black clouds **coming** up in the west? I think it will rain in **fifteen** or twenty **minutes**.

46

I **tried** to drive my **uncle's** big black horse to the **barn**. I soon found I could not **whip** him.

47

Is it too early to light the **lamp**? No, I wish to **write** a letter, and it must be done by nine o'clock **tonight**.

48

Do not **forget** to **speak** to your uncle **today** about the fruit which I bought for him. I have grapes, peaches, and pears.

49

Mother took me to the **circus**. I was **afraid** when the **lion roared**.

50

We went for a sail, but the wind **drove** the ship **along** very fast. When the water **dashed** into our boat, we were in great **danger**.

51

The horse helps men in their work. He is also **useful** in **war**. Did you ever look at his **iron shoes**?

52

Alice is a **gentle loving** child. She has a kind **heart**, and always does her very best to please both father and mother.

53

We get silk from the **tiny** silkworm. It feeds upon the **leaf** of the **mulberry** tree. It eats every leaf it can find.

54

Then the silkworm **spins** a little ball of silk **around** its **body** and goes to sleep. Did you ever see **any** of these balls of silk?

55

May I go with you on **Thursday** to see the **beaver** dams? **Henry** and I were there last Monday and saw **eight**.

56

The beaver **builds** these dams so that the door of his **house** will be **under** water. Did you ever see any of these **queer** houses?

57

Mr. Beaver does not make his house **until** September. I am **sure** he wants the coat of mud to **freeze** so hard that it will be quite **safe.**

58

Can the beavers cut **down** trees? **Yes**, it is **true** that they do this with their teeth **unless** the wood is too hard.

59

The fox and the **wolf** are **about** as **large** as dogs. Their teeth are very sharp, as they are made to **tear** their food.

60

The **nose** of both the wolf and the fox is more **pointed** than a dog's nose. Their tails are much more **bushy**.

61

The **puppies** of the fox do not open their eyes till they are **between** ten and twelve days old. They are **twice** as fond of play as a dog's puppies.

62

Here are **eighteen lemons** to make a **cool** drink for the children. Are they coming on Tuesday or **Wednesday**?

63

Did Harry **break** his **arm** some time **ago**? His mother told me he cried with pain when he fell from his **pony**.

64

When I pull the **string**, the **kitten follows** it from place to place. She likes to jump up in the air for it too.

65

We live in **America**, and we love our home. Every day when we **behold** the flag, we say that it is good to be an **American**.

66

In the summer months, June, July, and August, we use very little **coal**. Sometimes we get a **bushel**, which the coal man sends in a **bag**.

67

How many eggs does your sister **Emma** get for a dollar? I bought **fourteen** last Wednesday at our **own grocer's**.

68

The **lily grew** under glass till we could put it with the other flowers. We want it as a gift for Aunt **Ellen**, who will soon be **seventy** years old.

69

At home I have my own **soap**, **brush**, and **comb**. I never go away in summer **without** them.

70

Have you ever seen an **ostrich**? Yes, my **cousin** and I saw some of these big birds **yesterday** in **Central** Park. They are very strong and can run fast.

71

Among the flowers sent to **church** were **nineteen** or twenty **lilies**. We've never before seen such pretty white ones.

72

Some of **grandma's friends** took a long ride to see her on her seventy-**ninth birthday**. Did Emma show you the fruit which the children gave to grandma?

73

The **butterfly** lives only for one summer. It does not fly at night. It goes to rest about five o'clock in the **afternoon**. I **caught** a live one today down **beside** the brook.

74

I learned to add and **subtract** very well, but I cannot **multiply** and **divide** so **easily**. I **spent** months trying to learn.

75

You've been out to **gather wild** flowers, I am sure. Did you **climb** the rocks for them, or did you find them near the **river**?

76

Frank's father, Dr. West, sent him one **hundred** dollars for **Christmas**. What do you think he will do with that **amount** of money?

77

My rabbit likes to run in the **field**. When I feed him **carrots** or **tender cabbage** leaves, he looks at me as if he would like to **thank** me.

78

The **earthworm** bores **through** the **soil** and **softens** it. Then the rain can reach the roots of plants, and also any seeds which **happen** to be in the ground.

79

What did you see in the country? I saw a number of things, but I liked the lovely flowers best of all. One day I picked an apron full before six o'clock in the morning.

80

Woodpeckers have strong bills so that they can bore for insects. The farmer does not like these birds, **because** they **sample** his best fruit and often **hammer** his trees full of holes.

81

Dr. White and his **wife** spent **Easter** week at the **seashore**. Their home is in **Boston**, but they do not live there **during** June, July, or August.

82

Does Ruth's **music teacher** let her play by **ear**? No, she doesn't, because she wishes Ruth to play every piece as it is **written**.

83

All **parents** like to have **people praise** their children. They like to feel that their children never forget to be **polite**.

84

Sarah studies her lessons at night. She has **breakfast** early and is always **ready** for school at eight o'clock.

85

One day in September my sister's **husband wrote** me a letter saying he **expected** to come to the city in October. He also said he hoped I would not leave until he came.

86

The teacher told her children, when they worked an **example** in **division**, to be sure that the **remainder** was smaller than the **divisor**.

87

James asked whose **candy** he had found **lying** on the **shelf**. As no one said a word, he ate it.

88

Any child who wants to **become** strong and **healthy** must have **plenty** of **sunshine**. How much time do you **spend** in the air each day?

89

A **hungry** fox saw some grapes on a vine. He **sprang** up and tried to get them. Finding them **beyond** his reach, he said that he **thought** those grapes were **sour**.

90

Our **family** is so very large that we eat a loaf of bread at each **meal**. Can you tell me how many **loaves** we shall use in **December**?

91

Every Saturday Henry did the **different errands** very **quickly**. Then he had **nothing** else to do the remainder of the day.

92

The robin and the **bluebird**
Soon after flew away,
But as they left the **treetop**,
I think I **heard** them say,
"If birds and flowers have work
    to do,
Why, so have the little children
    too."
              - Helen C. Bacon

93

The **poplar** tree is so tall and **straight** that it doesn't give much **shade**. When the wind blows, the leaves shake and shiver as **though** they would fall to the ground.

94

The **fir**, pine, **cedar**, and **spruce** trees **wear** their green leaves during the entire year. Their **twigs** are as green in February and March as they are in May.

95

The American **bison**, called by most people the **buffalo**, is a wild ox. Years ago it was found in our country from ocean to **ocean**, but now none is to be seen.

96

Buffaloes feed on grass and chew a cud like the cow. They always seek a **valley** near the **edge** of some **stream** so that the **herd** may get both food and drink.

97

When the white men came to this country, they **built** their homes on the **plains** near streams. Then they **began** to kill these **animals** for their fur and their flesh.

98

The buffaloes went West, where the **Indians** caught many of them by **throwing** a rope **over** their horns. Now we have no buffaloes **except** those found in our parks.

99

As I passed the grocer's, I saw **thirteen** or fourteen **melons** in the **window**. I did not see any **berries**.

100

Agnes has a small **place** in her garden where she is raising **tomatoes**. We all like them much better than those we buy in the **market**.

101

The **policeman** at our **corner** is quick to see people who do wrong. We **trust** him, because he is a friend of the children. He helps them to **avoid** all danger.

102

Firemen are **brave** and quick to **act**. They **rush** into **blazing** buildings and carry out helpless women and children.

103

All things **whatsoever** ye would that men should do to you, do ye **even** so to them, for this is the **law** and the **prophets**.
- The Bible

Dictation Passages – Level 4

Special instructions for the dictation passages: Each student needs a notebook for dictation. On each dictation day, your student will study the dictation passage. It is helpful to write any difficult words on markerboard or paper for the students to focus on. New words are in bold. Also, call attention to any capital letters and punctuation marks in the passage. Discuss them briefly as needed.

When students feel ready, remove the dictation passage from the students' sight. Call out the passage one phrase at a time. Pause after each phrase for students to repeat it back to you and write it. Continue until the entire passage has been dictated.

Give students a moment to look over their passage for mistakes. Then, have them compare their sentences with the key. Students should circle any mistakes they made on the key and correct the mistakes in their own notebook. If the passage was correct, place a checkmark next to the passage in the key. All items in the sentence must be correct, including punctuation marks, before going on to the next passage. If students made any mistakes, they'll repeat the same passage as many days as it takes to get it right.

Always begin the next session where the student left off. If your child is repeatedly stuck on passages, he or she may need to move to an easier level of dictation passages. Three different levels of passages are provided in this guide.

*Dictation passages are taken from *Dictation Day by Day: Book One* by Kate Van Wagenen. (MacMillan Company 1916, 1923).

Level 4 – Dictation Passages Key

1

Let us take **pride** in our school. Children who make it a **rule** not to **scatter** papers, and who pick up such things when they find them, are **forming** good **habits**.

2

Our room must be clean and **cheerful**. Then a glass **vase** filled with a few **sweet** flowers will **brighten** our entire day.

3

What a **blessing** to have a policeman on the **avenue**! He **warns drivers** to go slowly around corners. He takes lost children home or finds their parents.

4

A fireman's **life** is often in **great** danger. He dashes into the **flames** and never thinks of **himself**. He must be brave to do this.

5

William bent the **blade** of his **knife** so much that he broke it. He's very sorry now, because his grandma, who is dead gave it to him on his birthday.

6

Last Wednesday we went to **Coney Island** by boat. It's only a short sail from New York, but the **ship** was **loaded** with people, and we had a very **rough** trip.

7

On Sunday and every **holiday** we have **either turkey** or **chicken** for dinner. We all like these dinners very much.

8

When **Emily** is nineteen, her father has **promised** to let her **travel** for a year. Isn't it **strange** that he will let her stay away from home for such a long time?

9

In winter I get up at night
And dress by the yellow **candle** light.
In summer, quite the **other** way,
I have to go to bed by day.

          - Robert Louis Stevenson

10

There were **forty angry geese** flying here and there, trying to get away from the dog. He wanted to drive them into that **dirty** water.

11

Hear the **steam** cars **whistle** as they fly down the **track**! I am sure that **eighty** trains pass here each day. Sometimes the noise almost makes me **deaf**.

12

When I went to market on Saturday, I bought a **peck** of **potatoes**, some **onions**, and a few **peppers**. The grocer very politely said he would send them home.

13

"I cannot stay the **east** wind
Or **thaw** its **icy smart**;
But I can keep a corner warm
In mother's loving heart."

14

This is the sixth lace collar I have made since April. I hope to finish making it by Tuesday. Your friend, Miss Lamb, said she would give me seventy cents for it, but I think that is not enough.

15

I'm going to **Brooklyn** at four o'clock. It is a great **distance** from home, and I fear I **cannot** go to the party. I shall be too **tired**.

16

In June we sold **ninety** yards of red, white, and blue **ribbon**. It was useful both for Flag Day and for **Fourth** of July.

17

All the **front** rooms in our house are much **larger** than the rear rooms. I know that it takes an **hour** to **sweep** each one, and it is not **easy** work.

18

Alice and Helen were on the lake during the **heavy shower**. Whose **fault** was it that they were caught in the storm and nearly **drowned**?

19

Tomorrow I expect to go to a small town **sixty** miles from here. I hope it will be **pleasant**, so that Frank and I may go down to the beach and gather **shells**.

20

When I brushed my **clothing**, I found that my **sleeve** was **loose** and torn about an inch above the **elbow**. Please wait until I find some **thread** to mend it.

21

Some time during Sunday night a **thief** went into our garden and picked all the ripe **vegetables**. Monday morning it **seemed** as though he had also **destroyed** every leaf and flower.

22

Boughs are **daily rifled**
By the gusty thieves,
And the book of **Nature**
Getteth short of leaves.
- Thomas Hood

23

The **sparrow's** eggs have many colors. She lays five or six. They hatch in sixteen or seventeen days. Did you ever see one?

24

The mother bird feeds her young ones **only** for a week. Then they must pick up their own food from the **ground** or **wherever** they can find it.

25

Last Friday Uncle Henry left New York at 2:30 P.M. and reached Chicago at 9:30 A.M. on Saturday. As he had most **important business** to **attend** to, he was very glad to pay an **extra price** to travel on this fast train.

26

Did you ever see a bird picking up grains of **wheat** in the farmer's field? We eat the same food, but the **miller grinds** it into **flour** for us, and **finally** it is baked into bread.

27

Martha went to the **kitchen** to see what she could do. Her mother, who **stood** near the table, asked her to put the oranges and melons on the shelf near the **pineapple**.

28

"I love little **Pussy**,
Her coat is so warm;
And if I don't hurt her,
She'll do me no harm.

So I'll not pull her tail,
Nor drive her away,
But Pussy and I
Very **gently** will play."

29

When **Richard** I was king of **England**, Robin Hood and his merry men lived in the **beautiful** Sherwood **Forest**. They dearly loved its hills, its valleys, its flowers, and its **carpet** of bright green.

30

These men **searched** people passing through the woods, and killed four or five of the king's deer every day. Robin Hood never **robbed** a **woman**. He **shared everything** with his men.

31

Robin Hood was **captain** of the band.
Little John was **second** in **command**.
Friar Tuck was **another** one of Robin
Hood's men. Maid Marian also lived in
the forest and **cheered** them all with her
sweet music.

32

As the **ruler desired** to see Robin
Hood, whose men did so much
mischief, he went to their forest home.
The bold robber stopped the king's horses
with **ease**. Then he blew three times on
his horn.

33

When Robin blew his horn, all his men
appeared in **answer** to his call. The
king saw he was not **frightened**, and he
admired Robin's wit and **wisdom** so
much that he told him it was King
Richard who stood before him.

34

Then the king **invited** the entire band
to go home with him. Robin **ordered** his
men to **mount** and go **forward**, and as
they **departed**, Robin Hood rode beside
the king.

35

Alfred's manners are quite different
from those of **David**. When Alfred meets
me on the street, he raises his hat and
bows very politely. David passes as
though he were **ashamed** to see me.

36

Philip's mother, who saw him looking
down the **road, knew** he could not finish
his lessons that way; so she told him not
to sit there **idly dreaming**.

37

Captain Church has a **cargo** of
hickory logs which he is **obliged** to
deliver in England. If all goes well, he
may reach the other side before the first
of the year.

38

When I am **grown** to man's **estate**,
I shall be very **proud** and great,
And tell the other girls and boys
Not to **meddle** with my toys.
- Robert Louis Stevenson

39

Amy, if you saw a **greedy spider** on the **branch** of a tree, wouldn't you **believe** that you were looking at an insect? And yet the spider is not a true insect, because it has eight legs and its body is divided into two parts.

40

Doesn't that spider look queer, **running** to a place of **safety** with a big white **bundle**! This holds **several** eggs; and her young, when hatched, are **content** to ride on her back.

41

If you spend a few minutes looking **closely** at a spider, you will **certainly** see that there are six points on its back. From these points comes the **sticky fluid** which makes the spider's **dainty** web.

42

"If Mother Nature **patches**
The leaves of trees and vines,
I'm sure she does her **darning**
With the **needles** of the pines."

43

Robert Bruce, king of **Scotland**, was **defeated** in six battles. At last his men disappeared, and **escaping alone** he hid himself in a barn. He thought he would give up the fight.

44

One **forenoon** as Bruce lay on a **blanket** in the barn, he **noticed** a spider trying to **fasten** its threads from one beam to another. Six times the spider failed. The next time it caught the beam.

45

When Bruce saw what the spider did, he sprang to his feet and cried that he would not give up and be beaten by a spider. He gathered his **soldiers** together, met the **enemy**, and **won** back his **kingdom**.

46

Last Tuesday, as we neared the **shore**, the **gulls surrounded** our ship. I **threw** half of my orange into the sea, and several birds tried to **seize** it at once.

47

When Mr. and Mrs. Miller went to the country, **Thomas** remained with friends until their **return**. He **meant** to be good, but I'm afraid he was often very **naughty**.

48

When George **Washington** was a boy at school, he was fond of **sport**, but he also liked his lessons. He never **broke** his word and always took **care** to speak the **truth**.

49

One Thursday in September the farmer put a load of **celery** and **lettuce** in his **wagon** and went to the **village**. After he sold these vegetables, he bought some fresh meat and a few yards of **cloth**.

50

In October and November, before our **furnace** is lighted, we have a **grate** fire in our **sitting** room. Here we gather every evening for a pleasant hour, and each one **describes** the **pictures** he sees in the fire.

51

Bertha's mother **taught** her to mend her own **stockings**. It was not easy for her to learn to **sew**, because her needle always broke and her thread always **knotted**.

52

When I go to see my aunt, I always take an **express** train. Before I get on the train, I **check** in my **trunk**. The man who gives me my check stands **behind** a **counter**.

53

Washington **planned** our flag. It was **begun** in May, 1777, by Mrs. **Betsey** Ross, and her **task** was **completed** in June of the same year.

54

June 14, 1777, **Congress approved** the flag **submitted** by Mrs. Ross. **Everyone** admired the red, white, and blue then, as we love and admire our flag today.

55

Dr. White gave **Isabel** a **couple** of plants for her birthday. She knew that to **produce** flowers, one must give them **sunshine**, and as it was cold **outside** she put them in her window.

56

Children, sing to Him whose care
Makes the land so rich and fair;
Raise your tuneful voices high
To our Father in the sky.

      - Margaret Sangster

57

Isabel soon noticed the **effect** of the sun. The buds began to **swell**, and the entire plant bent toward the light. If you wish to know **whether** this is true, you can **prove** it at any time.

58

The peas became yellow, and the shell turned yellow. "All the world's turning yellow," said they. Suddenly the shell was torn off and put in to the pocket of a jacket.

      - Andersen

59

Columbus went to **Spain** because no one in his **native** land had **faith** in him. He believed that the earth was round. The people in those days **imagined** it was flat.

60

The people of Spain were looking for a short way to **Asia**, because they wanted to **trade** with that **distant** place. The queen **granted** Columbus three ships and made him **commander** of the fleet.

61

Columbus and his men spent days of **terror** on the sea, but finally, by means of the **compass**, they **succeeded** in reaching land. When they first saw land, they **exclaimed** that hey had reached **India**.

62

Last June I was the **guest** of Dr. Frank's **nephew**, whose **cottage** stands near the **margin** of a large lake. We had great fun playing in the water. Each little wave seemed to **murmur**, "Catch me if you can."

63

One day in April as **Joseph hurried toward** the garden, he called to his sister, "Please help me dig some **angleworms**. Father is going to take Dick and me fishing. We are sure to catch nine or ten **perch**."

64

Only a tender flower
Sent us to rear;
Only a life to love
While we are here.
Only a baby small,
Never at rest,
Small, but how dear to us,
God knoweth best.

    - Matthias Barr

65

Bright little **dandelion**,
Downy, yellow face,
Peeping up among the grass
With such gentle grace;
Minding not the April wind,
Blowing rude and cold,
Brave little dandelion,
With a heart of gold.

66

As Miss Roberts left the **classroom** to meet the Reverend George King, who called to see about his son **Albert**, she said, "I do not wish to leave a **monitor**. I am quite sure you will all **behave** well when I am **absent**."

67

Oysters are **protected** from high waves by living at the **bottom** of small bays. From the first of May to the last of August they lay their eggs. During that time we eat **clams instead** of oysters.

68

When I was down beside the sea,
A **wooden spade** they gave to me
To dig the **sandy** shore.
My holes were **empty** like a cup.
In every hole the sea came up
Till it could come no more.

    - Robert Louis Stevenson

69

Last Wednesday when **Jane** came home from the South and called, "**Prince**, come here!" The dog tried to give her both **paws** at once, and showed by his **joyful actions** that he was glad to see her.

70

The **wheels** of the farmer's wagon caught in the mud. In his **trouble** he called for help. He heard a voice say: "Put your **shoulder** to the wheel, and then I may **aid** you. Heaven helps those who help **themselves**."

71

There once lived in **Rome** a lady named **Cornelia**. She was a woman of great **intelligence** and spent all her time in **educating** her two sons, who grew up wise and strong.

72

One day a lady called upon Cornelia and asked to see her **jewels**. Cornelia, instead of showing **rubies** or **diamonds**, sent for her two sons and, when they **approached**, said, "These are my jewels."

73

Everybody who lived near the northern woods tells us that each **season** has its own **beauty**. Would you believe that the **dull** winter colors are as lovely as those of the spring and summer?

74

In July the **Atlantic** Ocean is often so **calm** that it looks like a **mirror**. If you cross in February or March, however, there is a **chance** that you may run into a **blinding** snowstorm.

75

Our teacher, Miss Wild, **refused** to call upon the **pupils** who always guessed the answers. She was most **careful** during the **grammar** and **arithmetic** lessons.

76

"Look! Here's a pretty pigeon house!
In every narrow cell
A **pigeon** with his little wife
And family may **dwell**."

77

The little flower **listened** to the **oriole's** song until she **understood** its **language**. She knew the bird was saying: "**Rejoice**! Rejoice!"

78

Switzerland is a small country in **Europe**. It is **famous** for its high mountains and its many lovely lakes. The Swiss are fond of **freedom**, and for that **reason** love the story of William Tell.

79

Switzerland was once ruled by the **cruel** Gessler. To show the Swiss that they must **obey** him, he placed his hat on a pole in the **public square**, and ordered everyone who passed to bow the **knee**.

80

Several men obeyed. At **length** Tell passed **beneath** the hat, and his friends were **dismayed** to see that he did not even bend his head. Tell said, "Does Gessler **suppose** he can make all the Swiss obey him?"

81

The soldiers near the pole at once **reported** Tell's **conduct** to Gessler, who **directed** Tell to be **brought** before him. Then Gessler said, "You're a very fine **archer**, and you shall have a chance to save your life by your skill."

82

Tell was **informed** that, if he could **shoot** an apple from his son's head, his life would be **spared**. However, if he failed or **injured** his son in any way, he should die **instantly**.

83

Tell **selected** two **arrows**, and after **putting** one in his belt, **aimed** at the apple and cut it in half. Gessler asked why he had selected two arrows. Tell replied, "The second arrow was for you **tyrant**, in case I missed my first shot."

84

My country, 'tis of **thee**,
Sweet land of **liberty**,
Of thee I sing;
Land where my fathers died,
Land of the **pilgrim's** pride,
From every mountain side,
Let freedom ring.
- Samuel F. Smith

85

Those who visited Mrs. Archer saw at once what an **excellent housekeeper** she was. The rooms were clean, the **furniture** was **polished**, and the flowers, books and pictures gave an air of **comfort** to her home.

86

In the fall when many of my **favorite** flowers are **dying**, I think that the woods are pleasanter than the **meadows**. If I find good **company**, I **enjoy** walking until the snow flies.

87

The first snowfall has **arrived**. The children have watched **eagerly** for it. Now they are **anxious** to leave their **cozy** room, and join some boys who are making a snowman on the **sidewalk**.

88

The wind blows a gale, but the boys are so **excited** that their mother has promised to allow them to go out in the **bitter** cold. The **largest** boy is twelve, and he will not find it very **difficult** to care for his brothers.

89

The snow had begun in the **gloaming**,
And **busily** all the night
Had been **heaping** field and **highway**
With a **silence** deep and white.
— James Russell Lowell

90

Did you ever read anything about **Florence Nightingale**? Both her parents were **English**, but as she was born in 1820 in Florence, **Italy**, she was named for the city of her **birth**.

91

When she was a child, she often **pretended** that her dolls had been injured, and she would **nurse** and **bandage** them. She was very fond of animals too, and her first living **patient** was a **shepherd's** dog.

92

From nursing animals, she passed to **human beings**, and her **chief pleasure** was caring for the sick and **suffering**. Her family had a great deal of money, but she did not care for the **enjoyments** of the rich.

93

In 1854 there appeared in the papers long **accounts** of the suffering of the **wounded** soldiers in **Eastern** Europe. These men lacked not only **medicines** but also the **commonest** things needed by the sick and dying.

94

Florence Nightingale collected a large amount of **hospital supplies**, and with thirty or forty nurses **prepared** to leave England at once. When she reached the Crimea, both **officers** and men gave her a hearty **welcome**.

95

She soon had ten **thousand invalids** under her care and had **general** charge of all the hospitals on the **peninsula**. Her **labors** finally **affected** her health, and she was obliged to return to England.

96

Here she lived for many years and wrote on the **subjects** of light, fresh air, **warmth**, and quiet in **dealing** with the sick. Longfellow has written a **poem** on her **relief** work in the East.

97

In our home we obey the **law** about fire escapes. We know that, if there is an **alarm** of fire and fire escapes are **blocked**, our lives and the lives of people on the **upper floors** may be in danger.

98

A good king of Atri once hung a bell in the market place. He **allowed** any **person** to ring the bell who had been harmed in a way he did not **deserve**. The king told his people to **remember** that he would always **answer** their call.

99

In Atri lived a man who loved his **wealth** more than anything else. He said he did not **intend** to **waste** it feeding useless animals, so his **faithful** old horse was turned out to die. This horse happened to go in the **direction** of the bell.

100

A passing **traveler** had once mended the rope of the bell with a vine growing **against** a neighboring wall. The horse seeing the vines **rapidly** ate them, with the **result** that the bell began to ring. A **group** of people gathered, and for the **honor** of the town forced the owner to care for his horse.

101

The soldiers marched up the avenue in regular **columns**, and were **reviewed** by the mayor. Our **nation** owes a **debt** of **gratitude** to these men who stand ready to give their lives for the **union**.

102

When we go to our country place everyone arrives in an ill **humor**, because the **journey** is a long one and can be made only by a **local** train. This year we **solved** our difficulties by making the trip in an **automobile**.

103

My brother's return home always gives us great **happiness**. This year he wanted to visit a **secret** place in the woods where he played as a boy, so we **borrowed** a big lunch basket and planned a **picnic**. Then the **steady** rain came and stopped our fun.

Dictation Passages – Level 5

Special instructions for the dictation passages: Each student needs a notebook for dictation. On each dictation day, your student will study the dictation passage. It is helpful to write any difficult words on a markerboard or have students trace over the word in the passage with a pencil. New words are in bold. Also, call attention to any capital letters and punctuation marks in the passage. Discuss them briefly as needed.

When students feel ready, remove the dictation passage from the students' sight. Call out the passage one phrase at a time. Pause after each phrase for students to repeat it back to you and write it. Continue until the entire passage has been dictated.

Give students a moment to look over their passage for mistakes. Then, have them compare their sentences with the key. Students should circle any mistakes they made on the key and correct the mistakes in their own notebook. If the passage was correct, place a checkmark next to the passage in the key. All items in the sentence must be correct, including punctuation marks, before going on to the next passage. If students made any mistakes, they'll repeat the same passage as many days as it takes to get it right.

Always begin the next session where the student left off. If your child is repeatedly stuck on passages, he or she may need to move to an easier level of dictation passages. Three different levels of passages are provided in this guide.

*Dictation passages are taken from *Dictation Day by Day: Book Two* by Kate Van Wagenen. (MacMillan Company 1916, 1923).

Level 5 – Dictation Passages Key

1

Let us do our **duty** in our **shop**, or our kitchen, the market, the street, the **office**, the home, just as well as if we stood in the front **rank** of some great battle.

- Theodore Parker

2

Whether our **stove** is fed by **oil**, coal, or gas, we must always use it with the greatest care. Fire **itself** is a good **servant** but a bad **master**.

3

Hear the rain **whisper**,
"Dear **Violet**, come!
How can you stay in your **underground**
home?
Up in the pine boughs
For you the winds sigh,
Homesick to see you
Are we – May and I."

- Lucy Larcom

4

Fire has been known to cause **awful damage**, because someone **forgot** what he had been told. It is **impossible** to be too careful in obeying the laws made for our **benefit**.

5

In City Hall Park, New York, there is a **statue** of the young **patriot**, Nathan Hale. Have you ever heard why this **monument** was **erected** to his **memory**?

6

During the **Revolution** Washington wished to **obtain** some **information** about General Howe's plans. As **somebody** of great bravery was needed, Captain Hale was **chosen** to go to the enemy's camp.

7

It **required** great **courage** to venture **inside** the enemy's lines, but Hale did not **hesitate**. He **probably** thought he would return in safety.

8

Captain Hale was **unable** to **accomplish** his **purpose**, for he was **arrested** by the English as a **spy**, tried, and sentenced to be **hanged**. He met his death with the same courage that had marked his life.

9

Though he was not **permitted** to write to his mother, he did not **complain**. When the moment for his **sacrifice** arrived, he said, "I **regret** that I have but one life to give for my country."

10

Is life so dear, or peace so sweet, as to be purchased at the price of chains and slavery? Forbid it, Almighty God! I know not what course others may take, but as for me, give me liberty or give me death!

- Patrick Henry

11

Between the dark and the **daylight**,
When the night is **beginning** to **lower**,
Comes a **pause** in the day's **occupation**,
That is known as the children's hour.

- Longfellow

12

The **flight** of the **Monkey** People through treeland is one of the things **nobody** can describe. They have their **regular** roads from fifty to seventy feet above ground, and by these they can travel at night if necessary.

- Kipling

13

One Saturday morning Lillian's mother asked her whether she'd like to go **shopping**. "Oh, mother, what a **question!**" laughed Lillian. Then she ran **upstairs** to dress and in her haste nearly **knocked** down her tiny brother Robert.

14

Joseph **begged** me to leave the **piazza** and go to see his fine vegetables. I was delighted to see that the **spinach** and **asparagus** were almost ripe and that there were quarts of **strawberries** on the vines.

15

When **Bessie** does not **recite** her lessons **promptly** to her brother, she always **copies** each **sentence** very carefully in her **composition** book. I am sure that if she does this very often she will soon surprise her teacher with perfect lessons.

16

How much time he gains, who does not look to see what his **neighbor** says or does or thinks, but only at what he does himself to make it **just** and holy.

- Marcus Aurelius

17

Sir **Walter** Raleigh was a famous Englishman who lived in the **reign** of Queen **Elizabeth**. He gained her goodwill by a very **simple** act of **courtesy**. Have you ever heard the story?

18

History tells us that Queen Elizabeth was about to cross a **muddy** road, when Raleigh noticed that she paused for a moment. He took from his shoulders a beautiful **velvet cloak** and **spread** it in her pathway.

19

When Raleigh spread his cloak in queen Elizabeth's path, she was so pleased with this **attention** that she **smiled** and ordered him to appear at **court**. There she gave him his **title** and **bestowed** rich lands upon him.

20

"Is that a man's cub? I have never seen one," said Mother Wolf. A wolf **accustomed** to **moving** his cubs can mouth an egg without breaking it, and though Father Wolf's **jaw closed** right on the child's back, not a **tooth scratched** the skin.

- Kipling

21

The same leaves over and over again!
They fall from giving shade above
To make one **texture** of faded brown
And fit the earth like a **leather** glove.

-Robert Frost

22

If we **separate** a **unit** into any number of **equal** parts, each part is a **fraction** of that unit. The word "fraction" comes from a Latin word which means "to break". We have many other words **derived** from the same root.

23

Last Wednesday my sister **Blanche** was six years old. She **received** a doll's **carriage** and a **scarlet** cloak. She laughed **merrily** when she saw her birthday cake with its six lighted candles on the table.

24

The earth is the Lord's and the **fullness thereof**; the **world**, and they that dwell therein. For He hath **founded** it upon the seas, and **established** it upon the **floods**.

- The Bible

25

There was once a **violent** sea fight off the **coast** of New England, and Captain Lawrence commanded the American **vessel**. He was noted for his **bravery**, and though wounded and dying, cried with his last **breath**, "Don't give up the ship!"

26

And out again I **curve** and flow
To **join** the **brimming** river;
For men may come, and men may go,
But I go on **forever**.

- Tennyson

27

Grace **Darling** was the **daughter** of a lighthouse **keeper**. It was her father's business to keep the light burning in all sorts of **weather**. They both knew that **failure** to do this might cause great loss of life.

28

One **cloudy** night Grace was **awakened** by loud screams. She knew that the **current** had driven some ship on the rocks. She cried, "Oh, father, there's a wreck in the **harbor**, and the people are calling for help!"

29

The wind **swept** across the water, and Grace's father said, "It won't be **possible** to go until morning." At dawn the ship was **discovered** in the distance, and though they feared the waves would **swallow** their small boat, **nevertheless** they started.

30

Grace took an oar and helped her father until they reached the wreck. Those who were on **board crowded** into the **frail** boat, and the **sailors** with their **precious freight** rowed back to the lighthouse.

31

Tired little baby clouds,
Dreaming of fears,
Turn in their air **cradles**
Dropping soft tears.
Great snowy mother clouds,
Brooding o'er all,
Let their warm mother tears
Tenderly fall.

— Mrs. L. L. Wilson

32

The **Puritans** who first **settled** in New England came to this country for **religious** freedom. As soon as they had **provided shelter** for themselves, they built a church.

33

These early Puritans also knew the **value** of a **thorough education**. In every **colony** schools were established as soon as churches. Sometimes the teaching and the **preaching** were done in the same building.

34

A crow had had no water to drink for a long time. Seeing a pitcher she flew to it with great **eagerness**, but she found the water so low that she could not reach it. She tried to break the pitcher with her beak and then to **overturn** it with her foot but her efforts were all in vain.

35

At last she thought of a plan: She picked up a number of little stones and dropped them one by one into the **pitcher**.

They fell to the bottom, and the water was soon raised so high that the thirsty crow was able to **quench** her thirst.

36

For **Thanksgiving** dinner we had a fine big turkey with **chestnut** dressing. We had onions, **turnips**, **cranberries**, and several other things. I thought the **pumpkin** pie was best of all. Do you **agree** with me?

37

For my vacation I went into the **mountains** of **western** Maryland, where I stayed until **harvest**. There were eighty head of **cattle** on the place, besides several turkeys, chicken, and geese. My **playmates** and I spent many pleasant days in the woods and fields.

38

My **geography** tells me that New York is the largest city on this **continent**. Its five **boroughs** contain **millions** of people, and it owes its **importance** to its excellent **position** on the Atlantic coast.

39

Hush, my dear, lie still and **slumber**,
Holy **angels guard** thy bed;
Heavenly blessings without number
Gently fall on thy head.

- Isaac Watts

40

In the **French capital** the people are **familiar** with every sort of dress. It would certainly be a very queer **style** that would **cause** these people to **stare.**

41

Our **handsome** ocean **steamers** are **wholly** different from those of thirty years ago. Instead of narrow **berths**, many of them have fine brass beds, and each steamer has a **library** where one may spend many pleasant hours.

42

I am sorry you had a **headache** and could not attend Andrew's party. The children played games awhile and then sang several songs. Louise played the **piano**. Before we went home, we had **currant** cake and **chocolate** ice cream.

43

From the **trolley** we saw some boys **teasing** an **odd** looking old man. We were very much pleased to see the **janitor** of our house **treat** these boys so roughly that they were glad to escape.

44

To be a **gentleman** one does not **depend** on the **tailor** or the grooming. Good **clothes** are not good habits. A gentleman is just a gentle-man, - no more, no less.

- Bishop Doane

45

Our country, which is called the **United States** of America, was **originally** a **dense** forest where cities and **railroads** were entirely **unknown**. Can you picture the deep woods and silent rivers of those early days?

46

When Columbus reached America, he found it **inhabited** by a **copper**-colored race whom he called Indians. Many of these **singular** people gathered round and **gazed** at Columbus in **astonishment**.

47

These men lived in huts or **wigwams** made of **birch** bark. From this bark they also made their **canoes**, which were light in **weight** and most beautiful in **appearance**.

48

They lived by hunting and fishing. They were **industrious**, raising some corn and **tobacco**. They enjoyed trading **valuable** furs for a handful of **brilliantly** colored beads.

49

These men at their **worst** could be cruel and unforgiving, but they had great pride, and **therefore** never showed by their **expression** that they felt pain, anger, or **sorrow**. What do you think of this side of their **character**?

50

Some day I hope you will have the **opportunity** of reading Helen Hunt Jackson's **charming** story of Indian life, called "Ramona". In **addition** to this piece of **prose**, many poems have been written about the Indians.

51

Oliver brought a note asking his teacher to **excuse** him for being **tardy**. On his way to the bakery for a loaf of bread, he lost his **nickel** and was obliged to return home for another.

52

Last Wednesday I went to the grocer's for some sweet **biscuit**, four bunches of **radishes**, a box of **raspberries**, and three ounces of **ginger**. As these things cost eighty-five cents, what change did I receive from two dollars?

53

Lost yesterday, **somewhere** between **sunrise** and **sunset**, two golden hours each set with sixty diamond minutes. No **reward** is **offered**, because they are gone forever.

- Horace Mann

54

The **fact** is that to do anything in the world **worth** doing, we must not stand back shivering and thinking of the cold and danger, but jump in and **scramble** through as well as we can.

55

If you've tried and have not won,
Never stop for crying;
All that's great and good is done
Just by **patient** trying.

Though young birds, in flying fall,
Still their wings grow stronger;
And the next time they can keep
Up a little longer.

56

Though the **sturdy** oak has known
Many a blast that bowed her,
She has risen again, and grown
Loftier and prouder.

If by easy work you beat,
Who the more will prize you?
Gaining victory from **defeat**,
That's the test that tries you!

- Phoebe Cary

57

One day, a crow who had found a piece of cheese started to take it home to her little ones. As she was resting in a tree, a fox passed by. He wished to have the cheese, so he began to talk to the crow. The crow did not **reply**.

The fox told her how **beautiful** she was, and how **glossy** her feathers were, but the crow made no **answer**.

58

At last he told her he had heard that her voice was very beautiful, but he could not be sure of it until he had heard her sing. He begged for one little song. The crow was so pleased with the words of the fox that she opened her mouth and gave a loud caw.

As she did so the cheese fell to the ground, and the fox quickly ate it up.

59

Four things a man must learn to do,
If he would make his record true:
To think without confusion clearly;
To love his fellow-man **sincerely**;
To act from honest **motives** purely;
To trust in God and heaven **securely**.

- Henry Van Dyke

60

Oh, say, can you see, by the dawn's early
      light,
What so proudly we hailed at the **twilight's**
      last **gleaming**?
Whose broad stripes and bright stars,
      through the **perilous** fight,
O'er the **ramparts** we watched, were so
      gallantly streaming?

61

And the rocket's red glare, **bombs bursting**
      in air,
Gave proof through the night that our flag
      was still there.

Oh, say, does that star-**spangled** banner yet
      wave,
O'er the land of the free and the home of the
      brave?

- Francis Scott Key

62

Not gold, but only men can make
      A people great and strong –
Men who, for truth and **honor's** sake,
      Stand fast and suffer long.

Brave men, who work while others sleep,
      Who dare while others fly –
They build a nation's **pillars** deep
      And lift them to the sky.

- Ralph Waldo Emerson

63

He thinks of you before himself;
He **serves** you if he can;
For in whatever company,
The manners make the man.
At ten or forty 'tis the same,
The manner tells the tale;
And I **discern** the gentleman
By **signs** that never fail.

- Margaret Sangster

64

Thomas Jefferson was the third
President of the United States. He was
born in **Virginia**, and like all **Southern**
gentleman **addressed** everyone in the most
agreeable manner.

65

One day as Jefferson was walking through his estate with his grandson, he **observed** that one of his **slaves** raised his cap and bowed politely as they passed. The **master** returned the **salute**.

66

The grandson **scarcely** seemed to have an **idea** that the **servant** was there. Noticing his **careless** conduct, Jefferson said, "Thomas, do you permit a slave to be more of a gentleman than you are?"

67

Oh, the doll's house! It was a stone-fronted **mansion** with real glass windows and a real **balcony**. There were three **distinct** rooms in it; a sitting room and a bedroom **elegantly furnished** and a little kitchen.

- Charles Dickens

68

Whenever I buy **bacon**, beef, **mutton**, or **veal**, I go to the store of J.B. Frank and Co., whose meat is both **cheap** and good. As they treat their **customers** well, I'm sure they do an excellent business.

69

When Mr. Bird goes to the city, he will find that **conductors** give **transfers** only at the time **passengers** pay their fare. I believe this rule was made because many **dishonest** people tried to **cheat** the company.

70

One morning about eleven o'clock **Edith decided** to make a cake as soon as the **oven** was hot. "This large **bowl**," said her aunt, "is the one to use when you put flour through the **sieve**."

71

A wind came up out of the sea,
And said, "O **mists**, make room for me."
It said unto the forest, "**Shout!**"
Hang all your **leafy banners** out!"
It touched the wood bird's folded wing,
And said, "O bird, **awake** and sing."

- Longfellow

72

Does your sister ever order **groceries** by **postal**? Thursday I sent for a pound of **cheese**, a box of **sardines**, and two quarts of **molasses**. Today the grocer said that he had not received my **message**.

73

I once heard a blind man say, "What do you think I'd give to know what my mother's face looks like?" When **impatient** or **inclined** to **grumble**, **compare** your lot with his and try to **imagine** how he felt.

74

Before you leave school, I hope you will read "The Life of **Laura** Bridgman." When she was two years old, scarlet **fever deprived** her of both sight and hearing. This book will **explain** to you how she was **instructed.**

75

It may **astonish** you to know that she received her education entirely through the **sense** of touch. On several **articles**, such as forks, knives, and spoons, were placed the names of the **objects** in raised letters.

76

Laura **examined** these **labels** until she knew the **difference** between them. Then she was given **similar** labels on separate pieces of paper, and she **usually** placed the word "fork" on the fork, and the word "spoon" on the spoon.

77

These **exercises** were **repeated**, until she finally saw that these signs gave her **power** to tell her thoughts to others. When she was **successful**, she became so **interested** that she studied constantly.

78

Her **brain** soon became very **active**, and she was taught grammar, and arithmetic through fractions. She gained a **knowledge** of geography from a raised map. She was fond of sewing and **knitting** and never spent an **idle** moment.

79

Her **judgment** of distances was very **accurate**. She had the **ability** to walk straight toward a door, put out her hand at the **proper** time, and **grasp** the handle.

80

Laura Bridgman received her education at Perkin's **Institute** in Boston. Her **peculiar** case **aroused** an **immense** amount of interest, because she was the first deaf, **dumb**, and blind person to be taught the use of language.

81

A good deed is never lost. He who **sows** courtesy **reaps friendship**; and he who plants kindness gathers love.

- Basil

82

"Come," cried the mouse, "let's play hide and seek!" Then all the **funny** little mice began to run through the **cellar**, till suddenly their play was **interrupted** by what seemed to be a **horrible giant.**

83

Did you ever notice the **glory** of the **heavens**? Be sure to look out of your **chamber** window this evening. See whether you can find the **Dipper** and the North Star.

84

Aunt Helen and her two **nieces** were obliged to wait an hour for a train at a small mountain village. "Oh, **Elsie**," cried Emma at last, "see that **smoke**! It surely must be the **engine** that has just come through the **tunnel**!"

85

As Virginia entered the **dining** room, she saw a butterfly on the **ceiling**. "Would you **really** believe," said she, "that this beautiful **shining** creature was ever a **horrid caterpillar**?"

86

As soon as my brother **graduates** from **college**, mother will take the children to Atlantic City for the **swimming**. She says that I must remain at home until after **promotion**, as I can't **afford** to lose so much time from school.

87

There are many forms of **amusement** at Atlantic City. My brother, who is a **fearless swimmer**, often goes to the end of the long **piers**. Margaret and I are fond of watching the **surf** from the boardwalk.

88

Have you ever seen one of those **huge old-fashioned bedsteads** that used to be found in every **household**? Mother often describes the one which she remembers, with its tall posts and snowy muslin curtains.

89

Balboa was a **Spanish** subject who came to America in search of gold. After a long stormy **voyage** he landed at the **Isthmus** of **Panama** and with several **companions** began to **explore** the country.

90

Some friendly Indians told Balboa of a **wonderful** country beyond the mountains. Although wild beasts often **threatened** to **devour** him and his men, nevertheless they **continued** their journey across the isthmus.

91

When they reached a great **height** and looked down upon the **glistening** waters of the **Pacific** Ocean, Balboa felt that no man had ever made a more **glorious discovery** than he.

92

In his youth Lincoln was a **clerk** for a small village **merchant**. He once gave a customer the wrong change, and when he found his mistake, he **hastily** closed the store and walked miles to **correct** his **error**.

93

Don't waste your life in **doubts** and fears. Spend yourself on the work before you, well **assured** that the right **performance** of this hour's duties will be the best **preparation** for the hours or ages that follow it.

- Ralph Waldo Emerson

94

It is only in some corner of the brain which we leave empty, that Vice can obtain a **lodging**. When he knocks at your door, be able to say, "No room for your **lordship**, pass on!"

- Bulwer Lytton

95

Ships from **foreign** ports enter the harbor of the City of New York through a **channel** at Sandy Hook. They are then in the Lower Bay, which has such a large **area** that an immense **fleet** can be **anchored** there.

96

From the Lower Bay ships pass to the Upper Bay through a **passage** or **strait** called the Narrows. This **magnificent** harbor contains **Governor's** Island, Ellis Island, and Bedloe's Island, which is crowned with an immense statue.

97

This **lofty figure** is called "Liberty **Enlightening** the World." It was **designed** by Bartholdi and was given to the United States by the French **Republic**.

98

France truly showed a **kindly spirit** when she gave us the Statue of Liberty to celebrate the first one hundred years of American **independence**. It was not placed in position, however, until 1885. Have you ever read Whittier's poem on this subject?

99

"**Marion**," said her sister as she **motioned** to her, "let's **steal** out toward the woods and gather some **daisies**. I'm sure I saw several down near the old **fountain**."

100

During **colonial** days the Liberty Bell was brought from England to **Philadelphia**, and **afterward** the **following** words were written upon it: "**Proclaim** liberty **throughout** all the land unto all the inhabitants thereof."

101

This bell first proclaimed the **adoption** of the **Declaration** of Independence, July 4, 1776. It was rung **annually** until the **metal** finally **cracked**. It was then placed in the State House, where its **echoes** are forever silent.

102

A large amount of **cotton** has always been raised in the South. In colonial days **African** slaves separated the seeds from the **raw** cotton by hand.

103

This handwork was slow and **costly** even for the **wealthy** planters of that day. In 1793, however, Eli Whitney **invented** the cotton gin, which is a **machine** used to separate the seeds from the cotton.

104

As the slaves gained **skill** in the **operation** of this "gin" or engine, cotton raising was **introduced** more largely in the South. The **fiber** was **spun** into threads, and the threads were **woven** into cloth.

Math Schedule: *Singapore Primary Mathematics 5A & 5B* (U.S. Edition)
(Times Media Private Limited, 2003)

NOTE: This schedule is written to coincide with the **four** day a week plan used in *Hearts for Him Through Time: Creation to Christ*. If you find you need to use the fifth day for math, you can easily do so by spreading out this schedule. When using this plan, remember that the "Textbook" pages should be used as a <u>teaching tool</u> with your child. We highly recommend that, as much as possible, the Textbook portion be done together with your child on a markerboard with markers. This will help your child understand that each math lesson has 2 parts; the Textbook portion completed with your teaching and assistance, and the Workbook portion completed independently. On days that there is only a Textbook portion assigned, part of it can be done on markerboard and part of it can be done on notebook paper. The end-of-the-year review lessons are all scheduled in Week 35. If you wish to spread out the reviews more, you may use the extra Week 36 to do so.

Unit 1:
<u>Day 1:</u> *Textbook 5A* p. 6-7; *Workbook 5A* p. 5
<u>Day 2:</u> *Workbook 5A* p. 6
<u>Day 3:</u> *Textbook 5A* p. 8-9; *Workbook 5A* p. 7-8
<u>Day 4:</u> *Textbook 5A* p. 10

Unit 2:
<u>Day 1:</u> *Textbook 5A* p. 11-12; *Workbook 5A* p. 9-10
<u>Day 2:</u> *Textbook 5A* numbers 7, 8, and 9 on p. 13; *Workbook 5A* p. 11
<u>Day 3:</u> *Textbook 5A* numbers 10, 11, and 12 on p. 13; *Workbook 5A* p. 12-13
<u>Day 4:</u> *Textbook 5A* p. 14

Unit 3:
<u>Day 1:</u> *Textbook 5A* p. 15-16; *Workbook 5A* p. 14-15
<u>Day 2:</u> *Textbook 5A* p. 17-18; *Workbook 5A* p. 16-17
<u>Day 3:</u> *Textbook 5A* p. 19 – number 3 on p. 20; *Workbook 5A* p. 18-20
<u>Day 4:</u> *Textbook 5A* numbers 4, 5, and 6 on p. 20; *Workbook 5A* p. 21-23

Unit 4:
<u>Day 1:</u> *Textbook 5A* p. 21
<u>Day 2:</u> *Textbook 5A* p. 22-23; *Workbook 5A* p. 24-25
<u>Day 3:</u> *Textbook 5A* p. 24; *Workbook 5A* p. 26-27
<u>Day 4:</u> *Textbook 5A* p. 25

Unit 5:
<u>Day 1:</u> *Textbook 5A* p. 26 – number 4 on p. 27; *Workbook 5A* p. 28
<u>Day 2:</u> *Textbook 5A* numbers 5 and 6 on p. 27; *Workbook 5A* p. 29
<u>Day 3:</u> *Textbook 5A* p. 28-29; *Workbook 5A* p. 30
<u>Day 4:</u> *Textbook 5A* p. 30; *Workbook 5A* p. 31

Unit 6:
<u>Day 1:</u> *Textbook 5A* numbers 12, 13, and 14 on p. 31; *Workbook 5A* p. 32
<u>Day 2:</u> *Textbook 5A* numbers 15 and 16 on p. 31; *Workbook 5A* p. 33
<u>Day 3:</u> *Textbook 5A* p. 32
<u>Day 4:</u> *Workbook 5A* p. 34-35, 38

Unit 7:
<u>Day 1:</u> *Workbook 5A* p. 36-37, 39
<u>Day 2:</u> *Textbook 5A* p. 33-35; *Workbook 5A* p. 40-41
<u>Day 3:</u> *Textbook 5A* p. 36
<u>Day 4:</u> *Textbook 5A* p. 37-38; *Workbook 5A* p. 42-43

Math Schedule: *Singapore Primary Mathematics 5A & 5B* (U.S. Edition)

Unit 8:
> <u>Day 1:</u> *Textbook 5A* p. 39; *Workbook 5A* p. 44-45
> <u>Day 2:</u> *Textbook 5A* p. 40
> <u>Day 3:</u> *Textbook 5A* p. 41 – number 1 on p. 42; *Workbook 5A* p. 46-47
> <u>Day 4:</u> *Textbook 5A* numbers 2 and 3 on p. 42; *Workbook 5A* p. 48-49

Unit 9:
> <u>Day 1:</u> *Textbook 5A* p. 43
> <u>Day 2:</u> *Textbook 5A* p. 44-46; *Workbook 5A* p. 50-51
> <u>Day 3:</u> *Textbook 5A* numbers 7, 8, and 9 on p. 47; *Workbook 5A* p. 52-53
> <u>Day 4:</u> *Textbook 5A* number 10 on p. 47; *Workbook 5A* p. 54-55

Unit 10:
> <u>Day 1:</u> *Textbook 5A* p. 48
> <u>Day 2:</u> *Textbook 5A* p. 49 – number 6 on p. 51; *Workbook 5A* p. 56-57
> <u>Day 3:</u> *Textbook 5A* number 7 on p. 51; *Workbook 5A* p. 58-59
> <u>Day 4:</u> *Textbook 5A* p. 52

Unit 11:
> <u>Day 1:</u> *Textbook 5A* p. 53 – number 2 on p. 54; *Workbook 5A* p. 60-61
> <u>Day 2:</u> *Textbook 5A* number 3 on p. 54; *Workbook 5A* p. 62-63
> <u>Day 3:</u> *Textbook 5A* p. 55
> <u>Day 4:</u> *Textbook 5A* p. 56; *Workbook 5A* p. 64

Unit 12:
> <u>Day 1:</u> *Textbook 5A* p. 57; *Workbook 5A* p. 65-67
> <u>Day 2:</u> *Textbook 5A* p. 58; *Workbook 5A* p. 68
> <u>Day 3:</u> *Textbook 5A* p. 59; *Workbook 5A* p. 69-71
> <u>Day 4:</u> *Textbook 5A* p. 60

Unit 13:
> <u>Day 1:</u> *Textbook 5A* p. 61-62
> <u>Day 2:</u> *Textbook 5A* p. 63-64
> <u>Day 3:</u> *Textbook 5A* p. 65-67; *Workbook 5A* p. 72-75
> <u>Day 4:</u> *Textbook 5A* number 2 on p. 68; *Workbook 5A* p. 76-78

Unit 14:
> <u>Day 1:</u> *Textbook 5A* number 3 on p. 68-69; *Workbook 5A* p. 79-81
> <u>Day 2:</u> *Textbook 5A* p. 70
> <u>Day 3:</u> *Textbook 5A* p. 71-74; *Workbook 5A* p. 82-83
> <u>Day 4:</u> *Textbook 5A* p. 75-76; *Workbook 5A* p. 84-85

Unit 15:
> <u>Day 1:</u> *Textbook 5A* p. 77-78; *Workbook 5A* p. 86-87
> <u>Day 2:</u> *Textbook 5A* p. 79
> <u>Day 3:</u> *Textbook 5A* p. 80-81; *Workbook 5A* p. 88-90
> <u>Day 4:</u> *Textbook 5A* p. 82

Unit 16:
> <u>Day 1:</u> *Textbook 5A* p. 83 – number 1 on p. 84; *Workbook 5A* p. 91-94
> <u>Day 2:</u> *Textbook 5A* number 2 on p. 84; *Workbook 5A* p. 95-96
> <u>Day 3:</u> *Textbook 5A* p. 85-88; *Workbook 5A* p. 97-98
> <u>Day 4:</u> *Textbook 5A* p. 89 – number 15 on p. 90

Unit 17:
> <u>Day 1:</u> *Textbook 5A* number 16 through 21 on p. 90 – p. 92
> <u>Day 2:</u> *Textbook 5A* p. 93-94
> <u>Day 3:</u> *Textbook 5A* p. 95-96
> <u>Day 4:</u> *Workbook 5A* p. 99-100, 103

Math Schedule: *Singapore Primary Mathematics 5A & 5B* (U.S. Edition)

Unit 18:
    <u>Day 1:</u> *Workbook 5A* p. 101-102, 104
    <u>Day 2:</u> *Textbook 5B* p. 6 – number 2 on p. 7; *Workbook 5B* p. 5
    <u>Day 3:</u> *Textbook 5B* numbers 3 and 4 on p. 7; *Workbook 5B* p. 6-7
    <u>Day 4:</u> *Textbook 5B* numbers 5 and 6 on p. 7; *Workbook 5B* p. 8

Unit 19:
    <u>Day 1:</u> *Textbook 5B* p. 8 – number 6 on p. 10; *Workbook 5B* p. 9
    <u>Day 2:</u> *Textbook 5B* number 7 on p. 10 – number 11 on p. 11; *Workbook 5B* p. 10
    <u>Day 3:</u> *Textbook 5B* numbers 12, 13, and 14 on p. 11; *Workbook 5B* p. 11
    <u>Day 4:</u> *Textbook 5B* p. 12 – number 6 on p. 14; *Workbook 5B* p. 12

Unit 20:
    <u>Day 1:</u> *Textbook 5B* number 7 on p. 14 through number 11 on p. 15; *Workbook 5B* p. 13
    <u>Day 2:</u> *Textbook 5B* numbers 12, 13, and 14 on p. 15; *Workbook 5B* p. 14
    <u>Day 3:</u> *Textbook 5B* p. 16 – number 1 on p. 17; *Workbook 5B* p. 15
    <u>Day 4:</u> *Textbook 5B* numbers 2 and 3 on p. 17; *Workbook 5B* p. 16-17

Unit 21:
    <u>Day 1:</u> *Textbook 5B* p. 18-19; *Workbook 5B* p. 18
    <u>Day 2:</u> *Textbook 5B* numbers 6 through 10 on p. 20; *Workbook 5B* p. 19
    <u>Day 3:</u> *Textbook 5B* numbers 11 and 12 on p. 20; *Workbook 5B* p. 20
    <u>Day 4:</u> *Textbook 5B* p. 21

Unit 22:
    <u>Day 1:</u> *Workbook 5B* p. 21 – number 15 on p. 23
    <u>Day 2:</u> *Workbook 5B* number 16 on p. 23 – p. 25
    <u>Day 3:</u> *Textbook 5B* p. 22 – number 13 on p. 23
    <u>Day 4:</u> *Textbook 5B* number 14 on p. 23 – p. 24

Unit 23:
    <u>Day 1:</u> *Textbook 5B* p. 25-26; *Workbook 5B* p. 26-27
    <u>Day 2:</u> *Textbook 5B* numbers 5 through 8 on p. 27; *Workbook 5B* p. 28-29
    <u>Day 3:</u> *Textbook 5B* numbers 9 and 10 on p. 27; *Workbook 5B* p. 30
    <u>Day 4:</u> *Textbook 5B* p. 28-29; *Workbook 5B* p. 31-32

Unit 24:
    <u>Day 1:</u> *Textbook 5B* p. 30; *Workbook 5B* p. 33-34
    <u>Day 2:</u> *Textbook 5B* p. 31; *Workbook 5B* p. 35-36
    <u>Day 3:</u> *Textbook 5B* p. 32
    <u>Day 4:</u> *Textbook 5B* p. 33 – number 3 on p. 34; *Workbook 5B* p. 37-38

Unit 25:
    <u>Day 1:</u> *Textbook 5B* number 4 on p. 34 – number 5 on p. 35, *Workbook 5B* p. 39-40
    <u>Day 2:</u> *Textbook 5B* number 6 on p. 35 – number 7 on p. 36; *Workbook 5B* p. 41-42
    <u>Day 3:</u> *Textbook 5B* numbers 8 and 9 on p. 36; *Workbook 5B* p. 43
    <u>Day 4:</u> *Textbook 5B* p. 37

Unit 26:
    <u>Day 1:</u> *Textbook 5B* p. 38 – number 3 on p. 40; *Workbook 5B* p. 44-45
    <u>Day 2:</u> *Textbook 5B* p. numbers 4 and 5 on p. 40; *Workbook 5B* p. 46-47
    <u>Day 3:</u> *Textbook 5B* number 6 on p. 40 – number 8 on p. 41; *Workbook 5B* p. 48
    <u>Day 4:</u> *Textbook 5B* number 9 on p. 41 – number 12 on p. 42; *Workbook 5B* p. 49-51

Unit 27:
    <u>Day 1:</u> *Textbook 5B* numbers 13 and 14 on p. 42; *Workbook 5B* p. 52
    <u>Day 2:</u> *Textbook 5B* p. 43
    <u>Day 3:</u> *Textbook 5B* p. 44 – number 2 on p. 45; *Workbook 5B* p. 53
    <u>Day 4:</u> *Textbook 5B* numbers 3 and 4 on p. 45; *Workbook 5B* p. 54

Math Schedule: *Singapore Primary Mathematics 5A & 5B* (U.S. Edition)

Unit 28:
Day 1: *Textbook 5B* p. 46; *Workbook 5B* p. 55-56
Day 2: *Textbook 5B* p. 47; *Workbook 5B* p. 57-58
Day 3: *Textbook 5B* p. 48-49; *Workbook 5B* p. 59-60
Day 4: *Textbook 5B* p. 50

Unit 29:
Day 1: *Textbook 5B* p. 51-52; *Workbook 5B* p. 61-64
Day 2: *Textbook 5B* p. 53; *Workbook 5B* p. 65-66
Day 3: *Textbook 5B* p. 54 – number 12 on p. 55
Day 4: *Textbook 5B* number 13 on p. 55 – p. 56

Unit 30:
Day 1: *Textbook 5B* p. 57-58; *Workbook 5B* p. 67
Day 2: *Textbook 5B* p. 59; *Workbook 5B* p. 68
Day 3: *Textbook 5B* p. 60; *Workbook 5B* p. 69
Day 4: *Textbook 5B* p. 61-62; *Workbook 5B* p. 70

Unit 31:
Day 1: *Textbook 5B* number 4 on p. 63; *Workbook 5B* p. 71
Day 2: *Textbook 5B* number 5 on p. 63 – p. 64; *Workbook 5B* p. 72-73
Day 3: *Textbook 5B* p. 65-67; *Workbook 5B* p. 74
Day 4: *Textbook 5B* p. 68-70; *Workbook 5B* p. 75-76

Unit 32:
Day 1: *Textbook 5B* number 4 on p. 71; *Workbook 5B* p. 77-78
Day 2: *Textbook 5B* numbers 5 and 6 on p. 71; *Workbook 5B* p. 79-80
Day 3: *Textbook 5B* p. 72-75; *Workbook 5B* p. 81-82
Day 4: *Textbook 5B* p. 76-77; *Workbook 5B* p. 83-85

Unit 33:
Day 1: *Textbook 5B* p. 78; *Workbook 5B* p. 86-87
Day 2: *Textbook 5B* p. 79; *Workbook 5B* p. 88-91
Day 3: *Workbook 5B* p. 92-93
Day 4: *Workbook 5B* p. 94-96

Unit 34:
Day 1: *Textbook 5B* p. 80 – number 5 on p. 82; *Workbook 5B* p. 97-98
Day 2: *Textbook 5B* number 6 on p. 82; *Workbook 5B* p. 99
Day 3: *Textbook 5B* p. 83-84; *Workbook 5B* p. 100
Day 4: *Textbook 5B* p. 85

Unit 35:
Day 1: *Workbook 5B* p. 101-104
Day 2: *Textbook 5B* p. 86-89
Day 3: *Textbook 5B* p. 90-93
Day 4: *Textbook 5B* p. 94-9

Books by This Author:

Little Hands to Heaven
A preschool program for ages 2-5

Little Hearts for His Glory
An early learning program for ages 5-7

Beyond Little Hearts for His Glory
An early learning program for ages 6-8

Bigger Hearts for His Glory
A learning program for ages 7-9, with extensions for ages 10-11

Preparing Hearts for His Glory
A learning program for ages 8-10, with extensions for ages 11-12

Hearts for Him Through Time: Creation to Christ
A learning program for ages 9-11, with extensions for ages 12-13

Hearts for Him Through Time: Resurrection to Reformation
A learning program for ages 10-12, with extensions for ages 13-14

Hearts for Him Through Time: Revival to Revolution
A learning program for ages 11-13, with extensions for ages 14-15

Hearts for Him Through Time: Missions to Modern Marvels
A learning program for ages 12-14, with extensions for ages 15-16

Drawn into the Heart of Reading
A literature program for ages 7-15 that
works with any books you choose

Hearts for Him Through High School: World Geography
A learning program for ages 13-15, extending to grades 10-11
with adjustments in the 3R's and science

Hearts for Him Through High School: World History
A learning program for ages 14-16, extending to grades 11-12
with adjustments in the 3R's and science

Hearts for Him Through High School: U.S. History I
A learning program for ages 15-17, extending to grade 12
with adjustments in the 3R's and science

Hearts for Him Through High School: U.S. History II
A learning program for ages 16-18

See the website: www.heartofdakota.com
For placement information, product details, or to order a catalog
For ordering questions, email: orders@heartofdakota.com
Or, call: 605-428-4068